Doctors, dissection and resurrection men: excavations in the 19th-century burial ground of the London Hospital, 2006

MOLA Monograph Series

For more information about these titles and other MOLA publications visit the publications page at www.mola.org.uk

1 Excavations at the priory and hospital of St Mary Spital, London

2 The National Roman Fabric Reference Collection: a handbook

3 The Cross Bones burial ground, Redcross Way, Southwark, London: archaeological excavations (1991–8) for the London Underground Limited Jubilee Line Extension Project

4 The eastern cemetery of Roman London: excavations 1983–90

5 The Holocene evolution of the London Thames: archaeological excavations (1991–8) for the London Underground Limited Jubilee Line Extension Project

6 The Limehouse porcelain manufactory: excavations at 108–116 Narrow Street, London, 1990

7 Roman defences and medieval industry: excavations at Baltic House, City of London

8 London bridge: 2000 years of a river crossing

9 Roman and medieval townhouses on the London waterfront: excavations at Governor's House, City of London

10 The London Charterhouse

11 Medieval 'Westminster' floor tiles

12 Settlement in Roman Southwark: archaeological excavations (1991–8) for the London Underground Limited Jubilee Line Extension Project

13 Aspects of medieval and later Southwark: archaeological excavations (1991–8) for the London Underground Limited Jubilee Line Extension Project

14 The prehistory and topography of Southwark and Lambeth

15 Middle Saxon London: excavations at the Royal Opera House 1989–99

16 Urban development in north-west Roman Southwark: excavations 1974–90

17 Industry in north-west Roman Southwark: excavations 1984–8

18 The Cistercian abbey of St Mary Stratford Langthorne, Essex: archaeological excavations for the London Underground Limited Jubilee Line Extension Project

19 Material culture in London in an age of transition: Tudor and Stuart period finds c 1450–c 1700 from excavations at riverside sites in Southwark

20 Excavations at the priory of the Order of the Hospital of St John of Jerusalem, Clerkenwell, London

21 Roman and medieval Cripplegate, City of London: archaeological excavations 1992–8

22 The royal palace, abbey and town of Westminster on Thorney Island: archaeological excavations (1991–8) for the London Underground Limited Jubilee Line Extension Project

23 A prestigious Roman building complex on the Southwark waterfront: excavations at Winchester Palace, London, 1983–90

24 Holy Trinity Priory, Aldgate, City of London: an archaeological reconstruction and history

25 Roman pottery production in the Walbrook valley: excavations at 20–28 Moorgate, City of London, 1998–2000

26 Prehistoric landscape to Roman villa: excavations at Beddington, Surrey, 1981–7

27 Saxon, medieval and post-medieval settlement at Sol Central, Marefair, Northampton: archaeological excavations, 1998–2002

28 John Baker's late 17th-century glasshouse at Vauxhall

29 The medieval postern gate by the Tower of London

30 Roman and later development east of the forum and Cornhill: excavations at Lloyd's Register, 71 Fenchurch Street, City of London

31 Winchester Palace: excavations at the Southwark residence of the bishops of Winchester

32 Development on Roman London's western hill: excavations at Paternoster Square, City of London

33 Within these walls: Roman and medieval defences north of Newgate at the Merrill Lynch Financial Centre, City of London

34 The Augustinian priory of St Mary Merton, Surrey: excavations 1976–90

35 London's Roman amphitheatre: excavations at the Guildhall

36 The London Guildhall: an archaeological history of a neighbourhood from early medieval to modern times

37 Roman London and the Walbrook stream crossing: excavations at 1 Poultry and vicinity, City of London

38 The development of early medieval and later Poultry and Cheapside: excavations at 1 Poultry and vicinity, City of London

39 Burial at the site of the parish church of St Benet Sherehog before and after the Great Fire: excavations at 1 Poultry, City of London

40 London's delftware industry: the tin-glazed pottery industries of Southwark and Lambeth

41 Early and Middle Saxon rural settlement in the London region

42 Roman Southwark settlement and economy: excavations in Southwark 1973–91

43 The Black Death cemetery, East Smithfield, London

44 The Cistercian abbey of St Mary Graces, East Smithfield, London

45 The Royal Navy victualling yard, East Smithfield, London

46 St Marylebone church and burial ground in the 18th to 19th centuries: excavations at St Marylebone school, 1992 and 2004–6

47 Great houses, moats and mills on the south bank of the Thames: medieval and Tudor Southwark and Rotherhithe

48 The Rose and the Globe – playhouses of Shakespeare's Bankside, Southwark: excavations 1988–91

49 A dated type series of London medieval pottery: Part 5, Shelly-sandy ware and the greyware industries

50 The Cluniac priory and abbey of St Saviour Bermondsey, Surrey: excavations 1984–95

51 Three Ways Wharf, Uxbridge: a Lateglacial and Early Holocene hunter-gatherer site in the Colne valley

52 The impact of the railways in the East End 1830–2010: historical archaeology from the London Overground East London line

53 Holywell Priory and the development of Shoreditch up to 1600: archaeology from the London Overground East London line

54 Archaeological landscapes of east London: six multi-period sites excavated in advance of gravel quarrying in the London Borough of Havering

55 Mapping past landscapes in the lower Lea valley: a geoarchaeological study of the Quaternary sequence

56 Disease in London, 1st–19th centuries: an illustrated guide to diagnosis

57 The Augustinian nunnery of St Mary Clerkenwell, London: excavations 1974–96

58 The northern cemetery of Roman London: excavations at Spitalfields Market, London E1, 1991–2007

59 The medieval priory and hospital of St Mary Spital and the Bishopsgate suburb: excavations at Spitalfields Market, London E1, 1991–2007

60 A bioarchaeological study of medieval burials on the site of St Mary Spital: excavations at Spitalfields Market, London E1, 1991–2007

61 The Spitalfields suburb 1539–1860: excavations at Spitalfields Market, London E1, 1991–2007

62 Doctors, dissection and resurrection men: excavations in the 19th-century burial ground of the London Hospital, 2006

Doctors, dissection and resurrection men: excavations in the 19th-century burial ground of the London Hospital, 2006

Louise Fowler and Natasha Powers

MOLA MONOGRAPH 62

MUSEUM OF LONDON ARCHAEOLOGY

Published by Museum of London Archaeology

Copyright © Museum of London Archaeology 2012

A CIP catalogue record for this book is available from the British Library

Production and series design by Tracy Wellman
Typesetting and design by Sue Cawood
Reprographics by Andy Chopping
Copy editing by Anne Marriott
Series editing by Sue Hirst/Susan M Wright

Printed in the United Kingdom by Henry Ling Ltd
at the Dorset Press, an ISO 14001 certified printer

MIX
Paper from
responsible sources
FSC
www.fsc.org FSC® C013985

Front cover: students in the dissecting room at the London Hospital in 1916 (Fig 160) (Royal London Hospital Archives, RLHMC/P/1)

CONTRIBUTORS

Principal author (stratigraphy)	Louise Fowler
Principal authors (human bone)	Natasha Powers, Don Walker
Documentary research	Louise Fowler, Natasha Powers
Ceramic building material	Ian Betts
Clay tobacco pipes	Jacqui Pearce
Pottery and glass	Nigel Jeffries
Accessioned finds	Beth Richardson
Plant remains	Anne Davis
Faunal remains	James Morris
Scanning electron microscopy (SEM) analysis	Jenna Dittmar-Blado, Andrew S Wilson
Chemical analysis	Andrew S Wilson, Eline Schotsmans
Graphics	Hannah Faux, Carlos Lemos
Photography	Andy Chopping, Margaret Cox
Project managers	Nick Bateman, Nicola Powell
Editor	Susan M Wright

CONTENTS

FIGURES

TABLES

FOREWORD

This volume not only contains the results of an important archaeological investigation but provides, too, the fruits of a vast amount of documentary research, much of it new. The authors have evidently worked tremendously hard to do justice to an arduous and difficult excavation in two old burial grounds belonging to the Royal London Hospital: soil full of the remains of buried Londoners. By putting together materials gleaned from the dig, and from an intense search of the historical record, their report offers an exemplary attempt to marry buried and documentary materials.

Reading through the report, I am struck by the manner in which the archaeology and the documentary record together allow revelatory glimpses of insight about the regime in operation at the London Hospital during the era straddling the enactment and early operation of the 1832 Anatomy Act. This applies not just to the administration governing the burial of the dead and their subsequent 'resurrection' for dissection, and later redisposal, but also to the manner in which the secondary burials were made: in coffins that contained parts from multiple bodies and, on some occasions, from animals, but whose contents suggest that efforts were sometimes made to keep together body parts belonging to one person.

Especially interesting is the way in which one man – the London Hospital's chaplain, William Valentine (1787–1873) – emerges as an influential figure. Valentine did his best to impose his conviction that there must be respectful treatment of the dead, and he seems to have effected at least a form of lip-service to the decencies of burial, including the secondary coffining-up of mixed batches of remains: effects now visible from the archaeological record.

The dig at the Royal London Hospital reveals a completely different regime to that in operation at University College, on the other side of London. A recent exhibition (spring 2012) at the Grant Museum showed finds from a trial excavation in the great front quadrangle of University College on Gower Street, where adventitiously – during the digging of a trench for maintenance plant – human remains were discovered buried hugger-mugger. Remains from the dissecting room of the medical school seem to have been treated simply as refuse, to be hidden from view as swiftly as possible. One wonders what patients and staff might have thought had they known of this manner of disposal, and cannot help considering what such a manner of disposal reveals about the institution: the very same that honours the dissected remains of Jeremy Bentham, drafter of the Anatomy Act.

The poor patients at the 'godless institution on Gower Street' would perhaps have appreciated a William Valentine, whose efforts at the London Hospital ensured at least a burial service, the provision of coffins and some circumspection in the treatment of the dead. Bedstead Square at the London Hospital was, moreover, known to be a burial ground, whereas at University College the fact that the great quadrangle was packed with human remains appears to have been forgotten.

At the London Hospital, as this report also memorably records, the graveyard in which dead hospital patients were buried was overlooked by wards, so that when bodysnatchers unrelated to the hospital tried to get in there to steal bodies, the living patients swiftly raised the alarm and in no time the hospital was in uproar. Such insights cast new light on the lived experience of hospital patients at the London, as well as allowing inferences about that of the hospital's servants, who behind the scenes were constantly arranging much of this in secrecy to keep the dissecting rooms supplied and, presumably, to line their own pockets. Such findings are very salutary for modern observers of the medical history of London.

This book is an extraordinary piece of work: a remarkable document that reveals how paper and earth can speak to one another across time. I feel privileged to have been able to study it.

Ruth Richardson, DPhil, FRHistS
Historian of medicine
King's College London; University of Cambridge; Hong Kong University

SUMMARY

The early 19th century was a pivotal time in the medical history of this country. This monograph tells the story of that period through the results of archaeological excavations carried out by Museum of London Archaeology (MOLA, formerly MoLAS) on the site of the Royal London Hospital, Whitechapel, London, in 2006. The London Hospital was founded in 1740; it has been known as the 'Royal London Hospital' since its 250th anniversary in 1990. Before the Anatomy Act of 1832, the only legal method for obtaining a body for dissection was to acquire that of an executed criminal, yet the human and animal remains that were recovered from the London Hospital date to *c* 1825–41, spanning the decades leading up to, and immediately following, the introduction of the Act.

The nature of the archaeological and historical evidence and the methods used to analyse these are outlined, with a brief introduction to the hospital movement, the rise of the voluntary hospital and the place of the London Hospital within the metropolis. Historical and archaeological data are combined to provide a chronological narrative of the site before the establishment of the excavated burial ground, from which the remains of a minimum of 259 people were recovered. Many of these unclaimed patients – mostly adult and male – had been the subject of anatomisation or autopsy, human dissection taking place alongside the vivisection and dissection of dogs, domestic rabbits, horse and cattle as well as exotic species such as the mona monkey.

Aspects of the osteological data are integrated throughout the text, with individual chapters focusing on particular themes. Health and disease are examined, using both osteological information and the written evidence for the response of the hospital to times of crisis. Healed infectious lesions were more prevalent than active ones, suggesting that these were a reflection of the general health of the population from which patients were drawn, rather than a consequence of the hospital-related nature of the assemblage. Just three primary inhumations displayed evidence of tuberculosis and eight had suffered from venereal syphilis. Traumatic conditions were common and included an unusual dislocation in the left hand of an adult male. Most of the fractures seen had healed and so represent trauma acquired earlier in life, but within the assemblage were a number of fracture types rarely observed in archaeological studies, together with peri-mortem injuries reflecting the hospital's function as an accident and emergency centre. The diagnosis of a probable aortic aneurysm was of particular interest as one of the surgeons specialised in this field, whilst pressure necrosis from bedsores, the result of long-term incapacity, was observed in the remains of one female. Other unusual conditions seen include secondary hypertrophic osteoarthropathy, Erlenmeyer flask deformity related to an undiagnosed condition and probable disuse atrophy.

The osteological indicators of health and the unusually short male stature seem to reflect a local population living in overcrowded and harsh conditions and in perilous employment. In contrast, the presence of adults who were sufficiently 'healthy' to survive a period of vitamin D deficiency during childhood suggests that the contributing population may not have been as compromised as might otherwise be assumed.

The daily life of the hospital can be characterised from the artefacts and faunal remains, which include the remains of cheap cuts of mutton and beef and ceramics used for serving and possibly storing food. Syringes and enema pipes, bottles that originally contained medicines, medical case studies from the governor's minute books and the remains of those who died after accidents or surgery help to paint a picture of the working life of the hospital, the staff who made this institution function and the treatment and care provided to the patients.

The background to human dissection in the early 19th century is discussed, and the resurrectionists and the Anatomy Act are introduced. The specifics of the London Hospital are described. It was purported to be the only London institution that could supply its needs from within its own walls, and the archaeological excavation provided evidence of teaching, coroner's inquests, the supply and use of cadavers, and the osteological and microscopic evidence for who was dissected, how and by whom. Patterns in the use of cadavers show the systematic sharing of bodies and indicate that dissection and surgical practice followed methods described by the contemporary textbooks and the surgeons of the London. Teaching specimens found included prosections and articulated osteological preparations of both humans and animals, stained specimens and unusual lead casts of the aorta and adjacent vessels. Perhaps most disturbing was a group of human bones that had been worked on a lathe.

The archaeological evidence for burial practices shows formal, if somewhat communal, burials. The reuniting of the human remains and placement of the animal bone in the lowest of the coffins suggests that there was a degree of sensitivity in the way in which the dissected cadavers were interred.

The personal views of those at the London Hospital regarding illegal activity also feature, such as diaries showing the frustrations of the house governor, the Revd William Valentine, first-hand accounts of the opinions of influential surgeons such as Richard Headington and the tragic story of the ex-superintendent of St Thomas's dissecting room and sometime resurrectionist, William Millard, which forms a case study in the relationship between the surgeon and his supplier, as told by his formidable widow, Ann. Such was Ann's determination to clear her husband's name that she acquired a printing press that was installed at her home in Southwark and found herself in legal dispute with the editor of *The Lancet*, Thomas Wakley.

ACKNOWLEDGEMENTS

The archaeological excavation was funded by SKANSKA Barts & The London, a joint venture between Skanska and Barts and the London NHS Trust. MOLA would like to extend particular thanks to Graeme Kirk of Skanska and Steve Eames of Barts and the London NHS Trust. David Divers advised the project on behalf of English Heritage's Greater London Archaeological Advisory Service.

The authors would like to thank Barts and the London NHS Trust archivist, Jonathan Evans, for his continued support and for sharing with us his great knowledge of the Royal London Hospital archives and museum. We are indebted to our MOLA colleagues: the site osteologists – Brian Connell, Rebecca Redfern, Don Walker and, from the Museum of London Centre for Human Bioarchaeology, Jelena Bekvalac and Tania Kausmally; the archaeologists – particularly Johanna Vuolteenaho, who supervised the original excavation work, and Stella Bickelmann, Pete Cardiff, Lindy Casson, Neville Constantine, Valerie Griggs, Daniel Jones, Victoria Markham, Adrian Miles, Adele Pimley, Rik Sayer, David Sorapure, Gemma Stevenson and Paul Wordsworth; and Graham Kenlin and Gabby Rapson, who processed the finds from the site. Alan Pipe and Damian Goodburn provided advice on the human worked bone.

We are grateful to Paul Bland, Carrie Jones and Carol O'Sullivan for carrying out the radiography at City University London and providing their professional opinion on diagnosis and to Keith Manchester for his opinion of the 'lime' tubes. The following people kindly provided copies of forthcoming work: Andrew Chamberlain (Newcastle Infirmary), Annia Cherryson, Claire Murphy (Dublin Anatomy School) and Gaynor Western (Worcester Royal Infirmary). We would also like to thank Niall Boyce of *The Lancet* for his interest in the project, Wendy Thompson for the enlightening discussion of her great-great-great-great-grandfather William Millard and Kirsty Chilton for information on the illicit dealings of the London resurrection men. At the Natural History Museum, London, Colin McCarthy and Louise Tomsett assisted with the identification of the tortoise and monkey bones. We are grateful to Brooklynne Fothergill for information on turkeys, to Sheila Hamilton-Dyer for information on rabbits and guinea pigs and to Richard Thomas for advice on exotic fauna in the United Kingdom. Finally, thanks go to Piers Mitchell and Ruth Richardson for their valuable comments on the publication draft.

1

Introduction

A hospital is, of all social institutions, the one in which perhaps the greatest mixture of motives, the most incompatible ambitions and the most vexatious vested interests are thrown together. (Langdon-Davies 1952, 2)

1.1 The hospital movement of the 18th and 19th centuries: introduction and historical background

Medieval hospitals were religious institutions, run by the church for the care of the sick and the elderly, and places of refuge where not only the acutely ill but also those with chronic illnesses or mental illnesses, or who simply could not look after themselves could apply for help. By the beginning of the 16th century, however, many hospitals had a bad reputation. In London the master and brethren of St Thomas's, for example, were accused of corruption and irregularities, including 'insomuch that a poor woman great with child was denied a lodging and died at the church door, while rich men's servants and lemans were readily taken in' (Barron and Davies 2007, 173). During the dissolution of the monasteries many hospitals were forced to close, creating a crisis in the care of the sick and the poor, who no longer had anywhere to seek asylum. Many were left to fend for themselves on the streets, and the situation in London – where most hospitals were dissolved in the 1530s and 1540s – became so bad that the Lord Mayor and citizens of London petitioned the king to re-establish the hospitals 'so that with Godd's grace fewe or no personnes shalbe seene abrode to begge or ask almesse' (Clark-Kennedy 1962, 4). To this end, five hospitals were eventually re-established or founded anew during the mid 16th century in order to cater for different groups of people who were unable, through poverty and circumstance, to provide for themselves: Christ's Hospital for the care of orphaned children; St Mary Bethlehem (Bedlam) for the insane; Bridewell, where homeless children were housed and vagrants, prostitutes and petty criminals were imprisoned and set to work; and two hospitals for the care of the sick – St Bartholomew's to the north and St Thomas's to the south of the River Thames (Clark-Kennedy 1962, 4–5; Barron and Davies 2007).

For those who could not afford to pay for their own treatment, the 1601 Elizabethan Poor Law (the 'Old' Poor Law) did not specify the level of medical care to be provided to paupers who were maintained by the parish. Although parishes were obliged to maintain the poor who were incapacitated by age or by illness they did not have to attempt to treat or cure the sick. However, surviving overseers' accounts suggest that many parishes paid a local surgeon or apothecary to provide basic medical treatment to paupers, often in their own homes. Some parishes also maintained poorhouses or workhouses to which incapacitated paupers might be admitted if they had no family or friends able to care for them (Lane 2001, 44–57). A small number of larger workhouses contained sick wards, particularly in London, such as the workhouse of St George's at Hanover Square, built in 1725–6 (Morrison 1999, 155).

Voluntary hospitals

The 18th century saw a boom in the establishment of new voluntary hospitals, which were started and maintained by charitable gifts and subscriptions. Unlike the endowed hospitals of St Bartholomew's, St Thomas's and Guy's, all of which had been established though single large donations sufficient to provide for their running in the longer term, the voluntary hospitals were constantly appealing for funds to enable them to continue to function and to grow. The first of these voluntary hospitals was the Westminster Infirmary in London, which opened in a rented house on Petty France in 1720. In the following 25 years, a further four voluntary hospitals were founded in London, including the London Hospital in 1740 (known since 1990 as the Royal London Hospital) (Table 1; Clark-Kennedy 1962, 19–20). Beyond the capital many counties also opened hospitals during the 18th century, such as the Newcastle Infirmary (founded in 1751 thanks to subscriptions from a number of prominent citizens) and the Worcester Royal Infirmary (Nolan 1998, 23; Western 2010).

Until later in the 19th century there were few treatments available that could not be administered in private homes. The wealthy and the moderately well-off would have paid a physician and surgeon to treat them at home or possibly, as treatments improved later in the 19th century, in a specialist hospital; charitable hospitals were founded in order to treat the working poor who could not afford to pay for their own treatment (Higgs 2009, 7). These hospitals were generally not intended for paupers, who were the responsibility of the parish, or for the incurable chronically sick, but for the labouring poor, who might be incapacitated through illness or injury but who could return to a useful working life once cured by the hospital (Rivett 1986).

The 'New' Poor Law passed in 1834 severely curtailed or entirely abolished the relief available to the poor outside the institution of the workhouse. After this date a greater number of workhouses were built with infirmaries, which in some cases were separate, large buildings with more in common with contemporary voluntary hospitals. They were not able to treat more complicated cases, which might still be sent to a hospital. Some parishes chose to subscribe to the new hospitals, enabling them to send a number of paupers there for treatment. However,

many of the elected guardians charged with implementing the 'New' Poor Law entertained the view that paupers were not entitled to the same level of care in sickness as the independent working poor (Morrison 1999, 159–60).

Charitable donations of all sizes were made to the voluntary hospitals, and in exchange for a donation of a certain size one could become a governor or life governor of the charity (ie, the hospital). Becoming a governor led to privileges, such as the right to vote in members of staff and the right to recommend patients for treatment. It was not always the extremely wealthy who donated money to become governors. Whilst the voluntary hospitals operated within the social structure of the period, the way in which one could subscribe opened them to a wide range of people, all of whom enjoyed the same rights to vote and to inspect the hospital accounts. This attracted the 'middling sort', who were then able to wield power and influence in a manner not available to them in other areas (Lawrence 1996, 49). Those with small businesses could, by becoming governors, secure treatment for their staff, associate with other governors of higher social standing and perhaps secure contracts to supply the hospital with services and provisions. Lawrence (1996, 50) found that at all the voluntary hospitals those governors who played the most active role were predominantly from the middling class, although a smaller number of titled gentlemen were also involved.

Patients

In contrast with the earlier medieval hospitals, which functioned as places of refuge for those with a wide range of both curable and incurable ailments, 18th- and 19th-century hospitals had strict rules about whom they would admit. With limited funds, many of the voluntary hospitals were especially careful to restrict admittance to the cases considered to be the most deserving, and it was important too that the cases admitted to the hospital should be curable. For many governors their most important privilege was the right to recommend patients for treatment. They did not want the hospital beds clogged up with

Table 1 Hospitals caring for the sick in 18th-century London (not including Bridewell, St Mary Bethlehem, or Christ's Hospital)

Hospital	Established	Method of funding	Payment, 1788 (Howard 1791)	No. of patients, 1788 (Howard 1791)
St Bartholomew's	re-established 1544 (Barron and Davies 2007, 153)	endowed by Henry VIII	2s (clean) £1 5s 8d (foul) 17s 6d (burial fee)	428
St Thomas's	re-established 1551	endowed by Edward VI	3s 6d (clean) 10s 6d + 4d per day (foul)	440
Westminster	1720	voluntary subscription (Rivett 1986, 24–5)	none	71
Guy's	1721 (Clark-Kennedy 1962, 19; Rivett 1986, 24–5)	legacy of John Guy	2s 9d (nurse) 6d (steward) 7s (foul) 20s (burial fee)	304
St George's	1733	voluntary subscription (Rivett 1986, 24–5)	none	150
London	1740	voluntary subscription (Rivett 1986, 24–5)	none	120
Middlesex	1745	voluntary subscription (Rivett 1986, 24–5)	none	70

chronic cases leaving no room for their recommended patients. Moral judgements could also play a part in deciding who was and was not entitled to hospital care. All the London hospitals had rules designed to ensure the moral well-being of the patients and emphasising the spiritual responsibilities of the staff (Lawrence 1996, 45). Many hospitals refused to treat patients suffering from venereal disease or mental illness, chronic cases, pregnant women and young children. Guy's Hospital was opened in 1724 as an annexe to St Thomas's for the incurable patients who were not admitted to that hospital, but subsequently it was also opened to curable patients (Clark-Kennedy 1962, 19).

At the voluntary hospitals, there was usually one occasion each week when patients were admitted. Prospective patients had to present themselves in front of a committee with their governor's letter. The committee decided which were to be admitted and might refuse admission, especially if the hospital was overcrowded. Patients could be admitted as inpatients within the hospital or treated as outpatients. For particularly deserving cases, the rules on admission might be relaxed (Rivett 1986).

Although it was not until the Metropolitan Free Hospital (later the Royal Free Hospital) opened in 1837 that there was a hospital in London that did not require either fees or governor's letters from prospective patients, urgent cases could in practice be admitted. Details of the admissions procedures at the London Hospital are discussed in Chapter 5.3.

In 1788, John Howard, a well-known campaigner for the reform of prisons and hospitals, reported on the conditions within the hospitals of London. At the endowed hospitals patients usually had to pay for treatment, or provide a deposit to cover the cost of their burial if they died whilst in the hospital. 'Foul' or venereal cases were accepted but had to pay higher fees. At the voluntary hospitals, in contrast, patients did not usually have to pay for treatment but they had to be given a letter of recommendation by one of the governors of the charity (Howard 1791).

Within the rapidly growing metropolis of early 19th-century London it was possible for many cases to fall between the gaps in the provision of medical care provided by the Poor Law and the charitable hospitals. In November 1822 the minutes of a meeting of the house committee of the London Hospital recorded the case of a man who had been treated by the hospital, most likely as an extra case 'necessary for the preservation of life' as no governor is recorded as having recommended him. As the hospital could do no more for him he was discharged, but his 'miserable and wretched' appearance meant that he was unable to secure a place of lodging. Without proven residence within the parish the Whitechapel parish officers refused to admit him to their workhouse, or even to remove him to his original parish of settlement, which was a long way away. Although he was clearly still very sick, and is described as being in 'a most abject state of distress and weakness' there was no institution willing to house or care for the man. His eventual fate is not recorded (RLH, LH/A/5/17, 174–6).

1.2 Hospitals and healthcare: the archaeological background

Considering the number of hospitals operating in the metropolis, and the propensity for redevelopment of these sites, it is perhaps surprising that little archaeological evidence of 19th-century healthcare has yet been recovered from London. There is scant evidence from parish churchyards of the remains of those used for the study of anatomy, or of the activities of the bodysnatcher (Chapter 6), leading some to suggest that such individuals did not receive a burial conforming to the normal funerary rituals of the time (Crossland 2009, 107).

The limited osteological evidence from St Bartholomew's includes three pieces of sawn adult femora and a female mandible that was cut through the right horizontal ramus behind the third molar. These bones were recovered from a rubbish pit underlying the old, clinical surgeons' theatre and were dated to c 1726–94 (West 1980). In addition, there is a larger collection of disarticulated bone representing at least 316 individuals that was found during excavations nearly 20 years later. These were located within a charnel pit thought to have resulted from the disturbance of medieval burials during the construction of the hospital basement. In this deposit, a right femur and left tibia bore signs of amputation without subsequent healing. In the case of the tibia, the bone found would have formed the discarded (distal) portion of the limb (Walker 2008).

During excavations on the site of New London Bridge House, Southwark, in 1991, at least three trenches forming mass graves associated with St Thomas's Hospital were discovered. The graves are thought to have dated to the 17th century and may have been used for the victims of epidemic (Jones 1991). Of the 227 individuals recovered, 193 were analysed as part of the WORD project funded by the Wellcome Trust. No evidence of surgical or post-mortem intervention was reported (http://www.museumoflondon.org.uk/Collections-Research/LAARC/Centre-for-Human-Bioarchaeology/Database/Post-medieval+cemeteries/StThomasHospital.htm).

Between 1999 and 2000, Oxford Archaeology exhumed 107 post-medieval individuals from the burial ground of the Royal Naval Hospital, Greenwich, finding evidence of both amputation and autopsy. With its peculiar patient base, almost exclusively adult and male, the hospital burial ground, opened in the mid 18th century, was full and closed by 1857 (Boston et al 2008, 8). A large collection of anatomised 19th-century individuals has also been recovered from the Medical College of Georgia in Augusta, USA (Blakely and Harrington 1997).

This volume is strongly focused on the London Hospital in the first half of the 19th century but comparative material excavated from a small number of non-hospital London sites — most significantly the assemblage of dissected human and animal remains found at Benjamin Franklin House, Craven Street, and associated with the 18th-century anatomist William Hewson (Kausmally 2010) – is also discussed.

When discussing the buried population we draw also on the

evidence of health, autopsy and amputation provided by the analysis of individuals from parish cemeteries across the metropolis. Although coroner's autopsies and those carried out at the request of families will be discussed in Chapter 7, the numerous sites with formal burials of individuals from the late 18th and early 19th centuries who had undergone such procedures are not referred to in detail. A summary of the current evidence for dissection, including those sites to which this volume refers, is given in Table 2. Much work is currently ongoing and the publication of analyses of material from Bristol, Dublin and London will provide further comparison in the future.

Throughout this volume, comparison will be made with the results of the excavation of Newcastle Infirmary and Worcester Royal Infirmary. Excavations at the former recovered a large sample of articulated burials and disarticulated material; a watching brief on the site of the latter uncovered two pits containing disarticulated human bone and a further layer of disarticulated bone (Nolan 1998; Western 2010).

1.3 Documentary sources for the London Hospital

Barts and The London NHS Trust maintains an archive of primary records from the London Hospital, which has been extensively consulted during analysis. The records include the

Table 2 *Archaeological excavations producing evidence of dissection*

Site type	Site/location	Date	Nature of assemblage	MNI with surgical intervention	Type of intervention	Dissected animal bone present?	Reference
Hospital	St Bartholomew's Hospital, London	medieval	disarticulated bone from charnel pit (MNI = 316)	2 adults	surgical waste/practice	no	Walker 2008
		1726–94	disarticulated bone from rubbish pit	2 adults (1 female)	dissection/surgical practice	no	West 1980
Hospital	St Thomas's Hospital, London	late medieval	227 burials (193 analysed)	none	none	no	Centre for Human Bioarchaeology (http://www.museumoflondon.org.uk/Collections-Research/LAARC/Centre-for-Human-Bioarchaeology/Home.htm)
Hospital	Worcester Royal Infirmary	18th–19th century	disarticulated bone from pits & disturbed ground	18	dissection/surgery	no	Western 2010
Hospital	Bristol Royal Infirmary	18th–19th century	disturbed burials & disarticulated bone	?	autopsy/dissection/surgery	?	A Witkin, pers comm
Hospital	Newcastle Infirmary	1753–1845	210 articulated burials & disarticulated bone from pits	14%	autopsy/dissection/surgery	no	Boulter et al 1998
Hospital	13 Infirmary Street, Edinburgh	1749–1821	MNI = 14 inhumations & disarticulated bone	2 autopsy & a selection of dissected bone	autopsy & dissection	no	Henderson et al 1996
Hospital	Surgeon's Square, Edinburgh	18th & 19th centuries	55 disarticulated bones	13	dissection	no	Henderson et al 1996
College	Medical College of Georgia, Augusta, USA	19th century	c 9800 bones	?62	dissection/surgical practice/waste	yes	Blakely and Harrington 1997
College	Old Anatomy School, Trinity College Dublin	1711–1825	MNI = 233 disarticulated individuals	?	dissection	yes	Murphy 2011
Museum	the first Ashmolean Museum (the Old Ashmolean Museum, now The Museum of the History of Science), Broad Street, Oxford	18th century	2050 bones	?15	?dissection	yes	Hull 2003
Parish cemetery	St Pancras, London	18th–19th century	715 burials	9 dissected, 16 autopsied	dissection & autopsy	yes	Emery and Wooldridge 2011
Prison	Oxford Castle	16th–19th century	62 burials	5	dissection	?	Boston and Webb 2012, 55
Private house	Benjamin Franklin House, Craven Street, London	18th century	disarticulated bone	?	dissection	yes	Hillson et al 1999; Kausmally 2010

MNI = minimum no. of individuals

minutes of the weekly meetings of the house committee of governors charged with the day-to-day running of the hospital, the reports of the house governor, the Revd William Valentine, annual reports, inventories, diet books, lists and various letters and communications. It is unfortunate that registers of patients and of deaths or burials in the hospital ground for the date range of the burials recorded during the excavation have not survived. In their absence the 1841 census return from the hospital was consulted, and provides a 'snapshot' of the patients in the hospital on the night of 6 June 1841 (TNA: PRO, 1841 England census, parish St Mary Whitechapel).

Notes of cases treated at the hospital were sometimes reported in medical publications, including *The Lancet* and the *London Medical Gazette*. Reports of some cases and of other occurrences at the London Hospital also appeared in papers such as *The Times*, the *Morning Post* and the *Morning Chronicle*. These newspapers, accessed via the Times Digital Archive (http://gale. cengage.co.uk/times.aspx) and the 19th-century British Library Newspapers database (http://gale.cengage.co.uk/product-highlights/history/19th-century-british-library-newspapers.aspx), have provided us with much anecdotal evidence. The online *Old Bailey proceedings* (http://www.oldbaileyonline.org) furnished details of a number of relevant inquests.

The London Hospital Medical College was founded in 1785. It was initially run independently of the hospital and few records that relate to it directly have survived for the period under investigation. The first-hand accounts of observers such as Ann Millard (wife of the resurrection man William Millard) and Bransby Cooper (nephew and biographer of Sir Astley Cooper) have provided information beyond that available in the hospital's own records about the more surreptitious practices associated with the medical college and the hospital burial ground.

1.4 Excavation and recovery at the Royal London Hospital

The Royal London Hospital is located on Whitechapel Road, about 1.6km to the east of the City of London (Fig 1). The excavation and watching brief carried out by MOLA (site code RLP05; NGR 534700 181705) took place within the area covered by the phase 1 works for the redevelopment of the hospital site, an area to the south-east of the original hospital building (Figs 1–2). This area was divided into several excavation, exhumation and watching brief areas, which were labelled A–J (Fig 3). A controlled archaeological excavation took place within the northern part of area A. In other areas, an archaeological watching brief during the ground reduction was conducted. The archaeological investigations revealed 262 burials in the north of area A, within the area formerly known as Bedstead Square, although factors such as the decay of coffins and the presence of non-standard burials and of multiple burials within graves make an exact count difficult. A second area of burials was located within area B, to the west of area A, within the hospital burial ground in use from *c* 1841. These burials were cleared by BGS Exhumation Specialists, monitored by MOLA, and reinterred without further study. Evidence for the construction and expansion of the hospital was also recorded, together with a small number of earlier features, including two ditches of medieval date.

All bone found within deposits removed by machine (Chapter 3.6) was screened on site by a team of human osteologists. Elements showing evidence of dissection or pathological changes were retained to provide examples of the location and type of cuts and specimens. Material from these contexts ([100], [650] and [660]) is, therefore, inherently biased

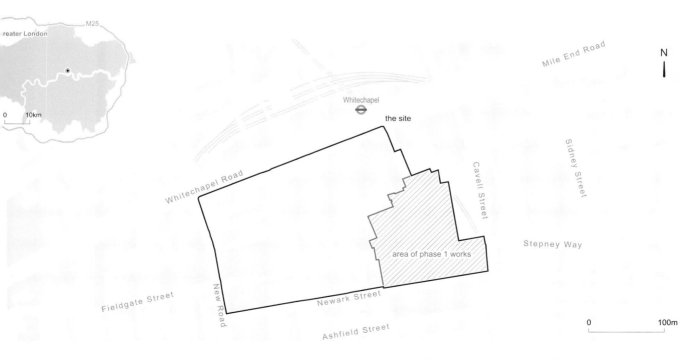

Fig 1 Location of the site superimposed on the modern Ordnance Survey street plan, showing the area of the phase 1 works (scale 1:5000)

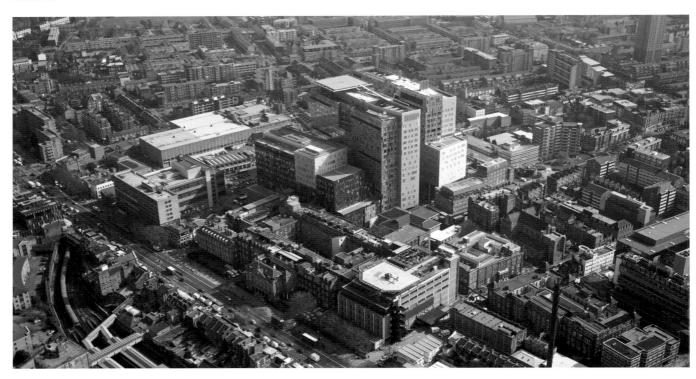

Fig 2 The new development at the Royal London Hospital, behind (south-east of) the original hospital buildings on Whitechapel Road; view looking south-east (courtesy of Skanska UK Plc)

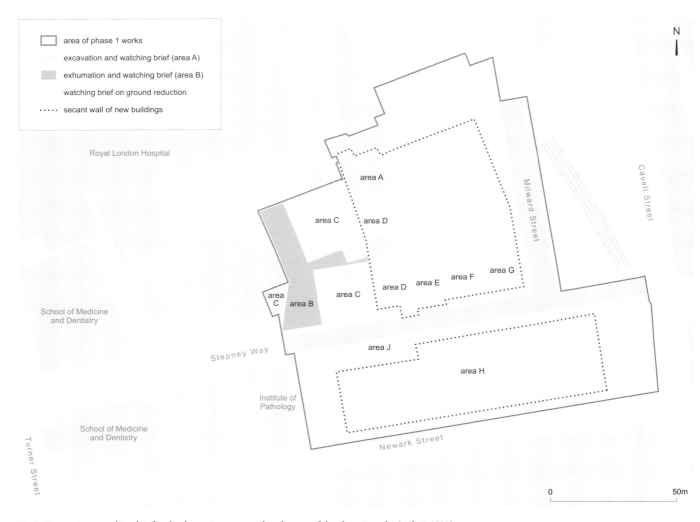

Fig 3 Excavation, watching brief and exhumation areas within the area of the phase 1 works (scale 1:1500)

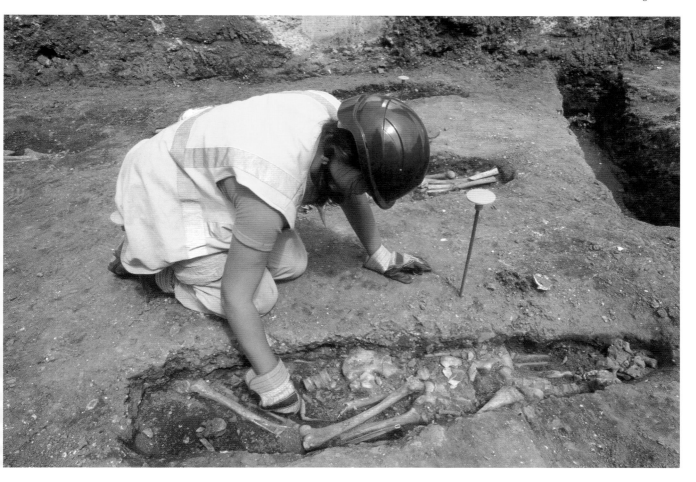

Fig 4 Excavation of a coffin containing partial remains in area A

towards anatomical specimens.

Stacked coffins containing a jumble of disarticulated bone and dissected portions of individuals posed a unique excavation challenge (Fig 4). The contents of each coffin were recorded under a single context number and articulated portions identified by the excavators were bagged separately and kept as such throughout the post-excavation process. Where substantial parts of more than one individual had been identified during excavation or could be reassociated at assessment or analysis, each was recorded as a separate 'individual'.

1.5   Outline of the historical and osteological aims

The history of medicine is a vast and complex subject and so this volume, in line with the date of the remains that were recovered (*c* 1825–41/2), focuses on the early years of the 19th century, that is, the decades leading up to and immediately following the introduction of the Anatomy Act in 1832. In London in 1882, 557 corpses were dissected, of which only 27 came from hospitals – the rest being from poorhouses – but in the early 19th century the picture was very different (Williams

and Price 2005, 139).

The aim of the project was to establish the origin and nature of this apparently forgotten cemetery, to determine whether those buried in the hospital grounds had been used for anatomical teaching and to place the buried population in context, both by comparison with other contemporary burial grounds and through an interrogation of the documentary evidence for the day-to-day working life of the London Hospital.

The excavated evidence was assessed (Vuolteenaho et al 2008) in accordance with the guidelines set out in *Management of archaeological projects* (MAP2; English Heritage 1991). After this, a series of detailed research questions was compiled. The aim was to chronicle the construction, expansion and redevelopment of the hospital, particularly in relation to the provision for burial, and to establish how the archaeological evidence could contribute to our understanding of the life of the patients and staff. The discovery of human and faunal remains showing marks consistent with sawing and cutting presented the opportunity both to examine the relationship the hospital had with medical teaching and to investigate attitudes to the living and the dead. Osteological analyses were carried out to characterise the health of the living population from which the buried remains were drawn through the examination of rates of disease and injury, to establish any significant differences from other contemporary groups and to examine the evidence of post-mortem intervention. A significant aim, given the date of the archaeological remains, was to examine any changes in behaviour before and after the introduction of the Anatomy Act.

A pamphlet published by Ann Millard in 1825 presented a further goal: to interrogate the evidence in support of (or refuting) her claims of illegal activity during the 1820s and the widespread tacit support of this within the medical establishment, with particular regard to the attitudes and opinions of those at the London (Millard 1825; Chapter 8).

Archaeology seeks 'the re-creation of Man – sentient, rational or even irrational Man – in the vicissitudes of his long life-history' (Wheeler 1956, 91). Once in a while, an excavation allows tantalising glimpses into the stories behind the objects and buildings. Yet more infrequently these glimpses can be connected with documented events, but to connect directly, using a combination of historical and archaeological evidence, with the thoughts and feelings of those who preceded us is an opportunity rarely afforded. The story of the London Hospital is just such an opportunity.

1.6 Textual and graphical conventions used in this report

During excavation a unique context number was assigned to each archaeological feature or deposit. These three-digit numbers are referred to throughout this volume and are presented in square brackets, thus: [100]. The unusual nature of the human remains from the site necessitated the generation of additional numbers during post-excavation analysis through the addition of a numerical suffix, where portions of different individuals were found within the same deposit. Thus the primary inhumation from within a grave would be numbered [100] and additional portions from within that same grave would become [10001], [10002], [10003] and so forth.

Following analysis of the site stratigraphic record, land-use numbers were assigned to Open Areas (OA) and Structures (S). Group numbers have been used where necessary to refer to a collection of context numbers within a land-use entity, such as a group of graves and burials within the cemetery.

Finds illustrated in the report are referred to by their catalogue number. This is preceded by the relevant category

code and shown in angled brackets, thus:

    <CP1>   clay pipe object no. 1;

    <G1>   glass object no. 1;

    <P1>   pottery object no. 1;

    <S1>   'small' or accessioned find no. 1;

    <T1>   tile object no. 1.

Summary catalogues of individual finds (tin-glazed wall tiles, clay pipes, post-medieval pottery, glass bottles) illustrated and discussed in this report are given in Tables 3–6; a catalogue of selected accessioned finds detailed in this report (some of which are illustrated) appears in Table 7; full details of finds may be found in Vuolteenaho et al 2008. Sample numbers are referred to in curly brackets, thus: {100}.

The following abbreviations are used within the text and in catalogue entries: D (depth); Diam (diameter); L (length); Th (thickness); W (width); Wt (weight). Pre-decimalisation sums of money given in the text are cited in £, s and d, where 12 pence (d) made one shilling (s) and 20 shillings (or 240d) one pound (£). One guinea represented one pound and one shilling (£1 1s). County names in the text refer to historic counties. Regarding the osteological data, all measurements and statistical calculations are expressed to one decimal place, with the exception of stature calculations; calculations resulting in rates of less than 0.1% have been expressed as such (ie, <0.1%). Tests of statistical significance were carried out on some of the osteological data; the results of the chi-square test (χ^2) for one degree of freedom (df) are quoted in Chapter 4.2 in the standard abbreviated form: χ^2, df, p[robability].

The graphical conventions used on the site plans are shown in Fig 5.

The full records are publicly accessible in the archive of the Museum of London under site code RLP05 and may be consulted by prior arrangement at the Museum's London Archaeological Archive and Research Centre (LAARC), Mortimer Wheeler House, 46 Eagle Wharf Road, London N1.

Table 3 Catalogue of the illustrated tin-glazed wall tiles <T1>–<T6>

Catalogue no.	Accession no.	Context no.	Land use	Period	Fig no.
<T1>	<79>	[653]	OA5	4	101
<T2>	<5>	[580]	OA6	4	101
<T3>	<76>	[650]	OA8	5	101
<T4>	<77>	[650]	OA8	5	101
<T5>	<157>	[850]	OA8	5	101
<T6>	<78>	[650]	OA8	5	101

Table 4 Catalogue of the illustrated clay pipes <CP1>–<CP2>

Catalogue no.	Accession no.	Context no.	Land use	Period	Description	Fig no.
<CP1>	<94>	[650]	OA8	5	form AO5, c 1610–40, marked	107
<CP2>	<150>	[865]	S1, OA5	4	form AO27, c 1780–1820, marked	107

Table 5 Catalogue of the illustrated post–medieval pottery <P1>–<P16>

Catalogue no.	Context no.	Land use	Period	Description	Fig no.
<P1>	[279]	OA6	4	sputum mug in refined whiteware with underglaze blue transfer-printed stipple and line decoration (TPW2)	98
<P2>	[279]	OA6	4	funnel in refined whiteware with underglaze blue transfer-printed stipple and line decoration	98
<P3>	[279]	OA6	4	bedpan in refined white earthenware (REFW)	99
<P4>	[300]	OA6	4	jug in refined white earthenware	103
<P5>	[279]	OA6	4	pot lid in refined whiteware with underglaze three-colour transfer-printed decoration (TPW5)	104
<P6>	[279]	OA6	4	bowl in refined whiteware with underglaze blue transfer-printed stipple and line decoration	122
<P7>	[279]	OA6	4	plate in refined whiteware with underglaze blue transfer-printed stipple and line decoration	122
<P8>	[279]	OA6	4	saucer in refined whiteware with underglaze blue transfer-printed stipple and line decoration	122
<P9>	[279]	OA6	4	mug in refined whiteware with underglaze blue transfer-printed stipple and line decoration	122
<P10>	[279]	OA6	4	jar in refined whiteware with underglaze blue transfer-printed stipple and line decoration	122
<P11>	[279]	OA6	4	feeding cup in refined white earthenware	123
<P12>	[279]	OA6	4	monogram of Staffordshire potter Thomas Dimmock junior	124
<P13>–<P16>	[279]	OA6	4	refined whiteware with underglaze blue transfer-printed stipple and line decoration: <P13> with the number 1; <P14> no. 2; <P15> no. 3; <P16> no. 4	125

Table 6 Catalogue of the illustrated glass bottles <G1>–<G4>

Catalogue no.	Context no.	Land use	Period	Description	Fig no.
<G1>	[100]	OA8	5	green-coloured champagne bottle	105
<G2>	[100]	OA8	5	aqua-coloured oval-shaped pharmaceutical or medicine bottle	134
<G3>	[100]	OA8	5	green-coloured cylindrical-shaped prescription bottle	134
<G4>	[100]	OA8	5	aqua-coloured cylindrical-shaped prescription bottle	134

Table 7 Catalogue of selected accessioned finds <S1>–<S36>

Catalogue no.	Accession no.	Context no.	Land use	Period	Description	Fig no.
<S1>	<56>	[615]	OA5	4	bone syringe: incomplete; surviving L 74mm; syringe applicator or 'pipe' with screw-fitting collar at top end, broken at lower end	14
<S2>	<17>	[256]	OA6	4	bone button: Diam 12mm; concentric groove around outer edge; central well has 3 attachment holes in a row	-
<S3>	<18>	[309]	OA6	4	bone button: Diam 16mm; concentric groove around outer edge; central well has 5 attachment holes	-
<S4>	<19>	[309]	OA6	4	bone button: Diam 16mm; concentric groove around outer edge; central well has 4 attachment holes	-
<S5>	<22>	[421]	OA6	4	button: Diam 14mm; bone disc with small central hole, probably originally textile-covered	-
<S6>	<90>	[444]	OA6	4	bone button: Diam 17mm; concentric groove around outer edge; central well has 4 attachment holes	-
<S7>	<91>	[137]	OA6	4	shell button: Diam 8mm; traces of petal-shaped decoration on upper surface, 4 attachment holes	-
<S8>	<12>	[443]	OA6	4	copper-alloy pin: L 25mm; globular wound-wire head	-
<S9>	<14>	[486]	OA6	4	copper-alloy pin: L 23mm; globular wound-wire head; slightly bent shaft	-
<S10>	<4>	[546]	OA6	4	lead strip: L 100mm, W (tapering) 11–15mm; folded at top, cut to near-horizontal hook shape at lower end	-
<S11>	<82>	[650]	OA8	5	iron pulley: L 85mm; hourglass-shaped	102
<S12>	<59>	[650]	OA8	5	bone brush: overall L 153mm; rectangular head has 5 rows of 14 holes, stained green by copper wire originally used to secure the bristles; leaf-shaped handle	106
<S13>	<60>	[650]	OA8	5	bone brush: rectangular (64 × 27mm) with rounded ends and corners; 8 rows of 12 holes with an additional row of 6 holes at each curved end; stained green by copper wire; probably nail brush or small scrubbing brush	106
<S14>	<85>	[282]	OA6	4	bone fan: incomplete; L 31mm; lower section of fan-stick of simple serpentine form; base has rivet hole	-
<S15>	<162>	[850]	OA8	5	bone toothbrush handle: L (incomplete) 100mm; oval section, rounded at end; stamped SEATON DALSTON	106
<S16>	<49>	[650]	OA8	5	bone cutlery handle: L c 95mm; 'pistol-grip' style with intact corroded iron scale-tang held with 3 or 4 attachment rivets	-
<S17>	<46>	[650]	OA8	5	ivory cutlery handle: L 90mm; 'pistol-grip' style with intact corroded iron whittle-tang; 2 circular impressions either side of the grip contain traces of inlay	-
<S18>	<51>	[650]	OA8	5	bone cutlery handle: surviving L 53mm; max W 13mm; circular section, slight bulge at top end	-
<S19>	<55>	[650]	OA8	5	ivory cutlery handle: surviving L 83mm; max W 15mm; circular section, slight bulge at top end	-
<S20>	<47>	[650]	OA8	5	ivory handle: incomplete, surviving L 50mm; rectangular section	-
<S21>	<52>	[650]	OA8	5	bone brush: incomplete ?toothbrush handle, L 96mm; rectangular section	-
<S22>	<57>	[650]	OA8	5	bone cutlery (probably knife) handle: incomplete, L 80mm, W 20mm tapering to 16mm; rectangular, flattened on underside, slightly rounded on top side	-

Table 7 (cont)

Catalogue no.	Accession no.	Context no.	Land use	Period	Description	Fig no.
<S23>	<48>	[650]	OA8	5	bone handle: L approx 95mm; oval section, whittle-tang; part of corroded curving blade survives	-
<S24>	<165>	[850]	OA8	5	ivory handle: incomplete, surviving L 64mm; 'pistol-grip' style whittle-tang handle	-
<S25>	<164>	[850]	OA8	5	ivory handle: incomplete, L 90mm; whittle-tang, cylindrical, with flat end	-
<S26>	<166>	[850]	OA8	5	bone handle: L 75mm; cylindrical handle, faceted from carving	-
<S27>	<43>	[650]	OA8	5	bone syringe: incomplete, L 86mm; syringe applicator or 'pipe' with screw-fitting collar at top end; broken at lower end	135
<S28>	<44>	[650]	OA8	5	bone syringe: incomplete, L 85mm; syringe applicator or 'pipe' with screw-fitting collar at top end	135
<S29>	<53>	[650]	OA8	5	bone syringe: incomplete; syringe applicator or 'pipe' with screw-fitting collar at top end	135
<S30>	<83>	[660]	OA8	5	copper-alloy tube: incomplete; L 90mm, Diam 8mm tapering to 6mm; ? from a syringe	139
<S31>	<45>	[660]	OA8	5	bone handle: L 120mm; 2-piece scale-tang knife handle with 3, possibly 4, central iron attachment rivets holding intact but corroded iron tang and 4 paired additional rivets securing rounded end; incised cross-hatched decoration on both sides	139
<S32>	<158>	[850]	OA8	5	bone brush: L 175mm, W 13mm; narrow and slightly curved with perforated handle; 3 rows of bristle holes and green copper-alloy wire staining	139
<S33>	<50>	[650]	OA8	5	bone cutlery (knife) handle and blade: surviving L 145mm; scale-tang construction, oval section, 3 surviving iron attachment rivets; iron tang and most of blade survive	-
<S34>	<54>	[650]	OA8	5	ivory handle: incomplete, L 96mm, Diam 20mm; tapering round section	-
<S35>	<86>	[234]	OA6	4	copper-alloy wires: 1 fragment of untwisted wire, surviving L 49mm; 2 fragments of twisted wire – 1 strand, doubled and twisted around itself with small loop at top, surviving L c 30mm, and 2 strands (unravelled at both ends so possibly originally 1 strand), surviving L c 45mm	190
<S36>	<20>	[341]	OA6	4	bone label: rectangular, 20 × 25mm, Th 2mm, with neat circular hole at top centre; inscribed with number '23'	193

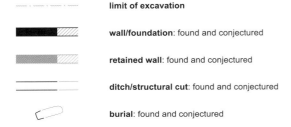

limit of excavation

wall/foundation: found and conjectured

retained wall: found and conjectured

ditch/structural cut: found and conjectured

burial: found and conjectured

Fig 5 Graphical conventions used in this report

1.7   Osteological methods

Human remains

Data for both articulated individuals and body portions from the cemetery (OA6; Chapter 3.4) were recorded directly on to an Oracle relational database system, by Don Walker, following standard criteria (Connell and Rauxloh 2007). As complete separation of the commingled remains proved impossible during excavation, remains were further separated and portions identified at analysis (above, 1.4, 1.6). Apparently associated elements (eg, paired long bones) were not added to the portions count unless there was evidence that they had been in articulation, and instead were added to a catalogue of disarticulated remains. The human remains were therefore placed in one of three categories: primary inhumation; portion; disarticulated bone. Data are presented using these classifications throughout.

An assessment was made of the state of preservation of each

skeleton as good, moderate or poor, and skeletal elements were catalogued as present where ≥50% complete. Subadult age estimation was carried out using epiphyseal fusion, diaphyseal length and dental development data (Moorees et al 1963a; 1963b; Maresh 1970; Gustafson and Koch 1974; Scheuer et al 1980; Scheuer and Black 2000). Adult age was estimated from observations of the pubic symphysis, auricular surface, ribs and dentition (Brothwell 1981; Iscan et al 1984; 1985; Lovejoy et al 1985; Brooks and Suchey 1990). Estimation of the sex of adult remains referred to observation of the morphological characteristics of the pelvis and skull, following the criteria of Buikstra and Ubelaker (1994, 16–20). Individuals were categorised as male, probable male, intermediate, probable female, female or (where the necessary elements were incomplete or otherwise unobservable) undetermined (eg, Tables 8–12). The calculation of stature was based on measurement of the right femur (Trotter 1970), whilst other metric observations and the calculation of indices followed Brothwell (1981, 82–3), Bass (1987, 69–70, 78) and Buikstra and Ubelaker (1994, 45–6, 74–84). The adult assemblage was scrutinised for the presence of non-metric or epigenetic traits (Berry and Berry 1967; Finnegan 1978; Brothwell 1981).

Pathological changes were recorded using standard guidelines and with reference to the clinical literature (Roberts and Connell 2004, 34). All significant or complex pathological conditions and surgical and post-mortem interventions were comprehensively documented and descriptions supported by digital photographs and electronic line drawings, employing colour coding for each type of tool mark (sawn cuts, knife/ scalpel cuts, false starts/skip marks/hesitation marks, residual spurs, burr holes and scrape marks). The direction of each saw cut was established, and where possible the position of the limb during the procedure was recorded (eg, supinated or pronated forearm).

Disarticulated bone was catalogued by element (loose teeth were omitted), with each row of data representing a set of articulated elements. Notes on the body portion present, pathology and demographic data, and digital record photographs supported this catalogue. The cataloguing of such bone raised a methodological problem. When using a cataloguing system that requires 50% or more of a bone segment to be present in an assemblage where a number of bones are sawn at the exact midpoint, and proximal and distal parts of the midshaft may subsequently have become separated, it would be theoretically possible to count the same element twice. With this in mind, the minimum number of individuals excluded counts of the midshaft. Vertebrae in the disarticulated sample were catalogued as present or absent, whereas in the articulated sample, the level of completeness (centrum, neural arch, complete) was also noted. When calculating prevalence rates by bone, a bone was counted as present where two or more segments (proximal, mid or distal) remained. Further details can be found in the Museum of London osteological method statement (Powers 2008), whilst full catalogue details are available in the project archive (above, 1.6).

The methodology of the analysis of the osteological data was to some extent driven by the need for clarity of result, in light of the mixed nature of the articulated skeletal assemblage. In addition to primary inhumations there were graves containing a number of portions of skeletons, often originating from several different individuals. Whilst it was sometimes possible to match portions from a single grave belonging to a single individual, there were many occasions when portions that possibly originated from a single individual could not be reassociated. For example, a shoulder joint portion could not be matched to an ankle joint without evidence from intervening parts of the skeleton. Therefore, whilst it was reasonable to establish a minimum number of individuals within the sample of portions, it would not be viable to attempt a detailed demographic analysis for comparison with the primary inhumations. Neither would it be productive to attempt the calculation of crude prevalence rates of disease (per individual) on the portions sample. These rates are presented for the primary inhumation sample only. However, the portions were suitable for true prevalence rate analysis (by bone element), and where appropriate these data were utilised together with, or in comparison with, those from the primary inhumations.

When combined, the primary inhumations and portions are referred to as the articulated sample. In addition to articulated skeletal remains, a large number of disarticulated elements were recovered from the graves. Many of these contained evidence of saw and cut marks. Except where noted in the text, the disarticulated remains are presented separately from the articulated skeletal assemblage. The disarticulated assemblage was also included in true prevalence rate analysis where appropriate.

A further level of analysis involved grouping by land use (Chapter 3.4). Any significant differences identified between these groups were investigated. Human remains from the post-1841 cemetery (OA7) and machined deposits (OA8) were recorded to assessment level only (Chapter 3.5, 3.6).

Faunal remains

The material was recorded on to the MOLA Osteology section Oracle animal bone post-assessment database. This includes species, skeletal element, completeness, zones present (using the MOLA zonal system), body side, epiphyseal fusion, dental characteristics and modification. Identifications of species and skeletal element referred to the MOLA Osteology section reference collection. Remains from the non-native animals were taken to the Natural History Museum for identification. When identification to species was not possible, the categories 'cattle-size' and 'sheep-size' were used, as were 'unidentified mammal', 'bird' and 'fish'.

Remains were aged using evidence from dental eruption, dental wear and epiphyseal fusion. Dental wear for cattle, sheep/goat, pig and horse was recorded following Grant (1982) and Levine (1982). Epiphyseal fusion was recorded as one of four categories: 'unfused', 'fused-open', 'fused-closed' and 'fully fused'. Measurements of complete and fully fused bones were taken using the methods recommended in von den Driesch (1976).

Alterations to the bones by either butchery or vivisection/dissection were recorded using the MOLA zonal system to indicate the location of the marks on the recorded element. The type of mark — cleaver, saw, knife, fine knife — was noted, along with its angle and direction; when necessary further textual description and diagrammatic drawings were utilised. If the marks appeared to relate to dissection or vivisection, the remains were discussed with the human osteologists and notes added to the textual description. Evidence of pathological change was also recorded using the MOLA zonal system along with descriptive text. The full records will be available from the London Archaeological Archive and Research Centre (LAARC).

The majority of the faunal remains results are displayed as the number of individual specimens present (NISP); this includes all the remains identified to species, including loose teeth, vertebrae and ribs. When necessary, the minimum number of individuals (MNI) was calculated for archaeological subgroups. This was done using zonal information for the most common elements present, taking into account side, epiphyseal fusion and metrical information.

Of the 2600 fragments of animal bone recovered during the excavation, 85% (2193) were found in association with the human burials. It appears that the vast majority of the animal remains had been deliberately placed within the coffins and graves. Of the 2193 elements from grave contexts, 84% (1705) were recovered in close association with the human skeletal material. Many of the animal remains from these contexts consisted of associated bone groups (ABGs), where the elements from the same individual animal are found in association. (The term 'associated bone group' is used rather than 'animal burial' to avoid any associated connotations (Morris 2011).)

One of the most challenging aspects of this assemblage was to identify remains that originated from the hospital's anatomy school. For remains such as the exotic species and dog ABGs with dissection marks it was relatively easy to surmise they originated from the anatomy school. The elements may not have stayed in articulation, owing to post-depositional movement, but it was still possible to identify many remains as originating from ABGs during the post-excavation process. This was achieved using the excavation records, the number and type of elements present, the completeness of the remains and metrical information. For the more commonly consumed domestic mammals (cattle, sheep/goat and pig) separation was much more challenging. The presence of individual specimens, such as the dissected cow first phalanx (see Fig 151) and the sheep mandible (see Fig 157), shows that domestic species were also utilised in anatomical teaching. It is not possible simply to assume that the remains of commonly consumed mammals originated from the hospital's kitchens. In identifying which parts of the assemblage might consist of 'kitchen waste', the nature of the elements present and taphonomic markers were therefore considered. This included evidence of butchery consistent with known practices from the period, burning and biostratonomic effects such as weathering and gnawing.

2

The growth of Whitechapel and the building of the London Hospital

In point of Air, Situation and Structure, there has not hitherto, it is apprehended, been erected in the Kingdom, any Asylum, for the relief of the distressed and sick Poor, better calculated to answer that important end than the LONDON HOSPITAL, the WARDS of which are large, and their Ceilings lofty. The Elevation of the Ground on which it stands appears to be no less than Thirty Feet above the level of the River at High Water.

Its proximity to the River, and the new West-India and East-India, and London-Docks, together with its Situation on one of the most public Roads, renders it liable to more applications, for the reception of Accidents, than any other Hospital in the Cities of London and Westminster. (RLH, LH/A/15/7; annual report of the London Hospital 1828, 36)

2.1 Before the London Hospital (periods 1–2)

Very few remains pre-dating the construction of the hospital were recorded during the archaeological investigations. The natural brickearth (period 1), exploited in the 18th century, and the overlying medieval subsoil (period 2) were exposed in various parts of the site (below, 2.2). A substantial boundary ditch was recorded in the northern part of area A, running parallel to Whitechapel Road (which was, from *c* 1110, the main London–Colchester road); it may have defined the southern edge of the strip of common land adjacent to the road (Fig 6). The ditch was cut by a small pit containing pottery dated *c* 1080–*c* 1200.

The Rocque map of 1746 shows the hamlet of Mile End, which had grown up around the new road to Colchester during the medieval period (Fig 7c). To the south of the road is a field, known during the 18th century as 'Mount Field', after the 'White Chappel Mount'. The origins of the mount are unclear, but it formed a substantial local landmark located immediately to the west of the field. Lysons (1811, 714) noted that the mount was '329 feet in length at the base, and 182 feet in breadth. The height above the level of the ground [was] about 25 feet'; the top of the mount was flat, 'except for where it [had] been dug away'. Joel Gascoyne's map of the area from 1703 labels the approximate location of the mount 'The Dunghill' (Fig 7b). A hornwork (a free-standing quadrilateral fortification in front of the main defence line) is shown occupying a similar position to the mount on Vertue's retrospective (*c* 1738) map of the defences constructed in 1642–3 to protect the City from Royalist attack during the Civil War (1642–6) (Fig 7a). It is possible that the

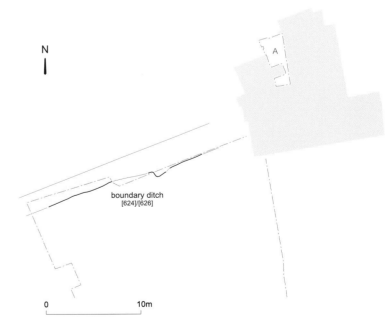

Fig 6 The medieval (period 2) boundary ditch recorded on the north edge of area A (scale 1:400); inset (top right) locates area A in relation to the overall area of phase 1 works (see Fig 3)

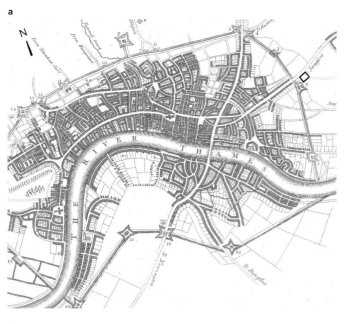

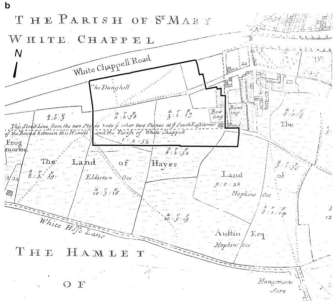

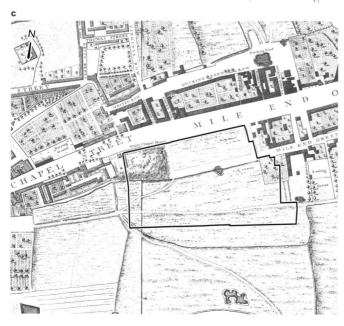

17th-century hornwork at Mile End encompassed an existing landscape feature. There may have been earlier, 15th-century, fortifications of some kind beyond Aldgate, along the Whitechapel Road to Mile End. Stow records (1603) that during Fauconberg's rebellion in 1471, when the rebels were denied passage over London bridge, some of them crossed the Thames, successfully attacked the London militia manning Aldgate, winning the 'Bulwarkes', and then entered the walled city where the fighting continued. Earl Rivers led a counter-attack that drove the rebels back to Mile End initially and then further east to Poplar, killing some and taking many prisoner (Kingsford 1971, vol 1, 30). Stow also notes that, previously, during Jack Cade's rebellion of 1450 'the commons of Essex in great number pight them a field upon the plaine of Miles end' (Stow 1592, 635).

Prior to the construction of the hospital, then, the majority of the site lay to the south of Mount Field, in an area of agricultural land crossed by numerous trackways. Rocque's map shows a pond immediately to the south of the field, although this feature does not appear on Gascoyne's map of 1703 (Fig 7b). No archaeological features were found that dated to this period, although residual pottery of medieval and early post-medieval date was found in later deposits associated with 18th- and 19th-century quarrying for brickearth, indicating activity in the area at this time.

2.2 Construction of the London Hospital from 1752 (period 3)

Historical background

The London Hospital was founded in 1740 and originally occupied cramped rented accommodation in the City, first at Moorfields and then on Prescott Street, near Aldgate. It was not long before the governors of the charity began to look for a more convenient location. As early as 1744 the Bishop of Worcester urged the governors to start a special fund for the purchase of a site and the construction of a new purpose-built hospital, inspired by the recent construction of Mr Guy's hospital in Southwark (opened 1725) (Clark-Kennedy 1962, 19, 111). The fund succeeded in raising over £5000, and the hospital surveyor Boulton Mainwaring was engaged in the search for a suitable location. In June 1748 he reported back to the

Fig 7 Historical maps showing the Whitechapel area in the mid 17th century and first half of the 18th century, with the outline of the Royal London Hospital site superimposed: a – Vertue's c 1738 map of London's Civil War defences in 1642–3 (LMA, main print collection, cat no. k1268650); b – Gascoyne's map of 1703 (LMA, main print collection, cat no. p5414427); c – Rocque's map of 1746 (Rocque 1746)

governors that 'The only Piece of Ground apprehended suitable for this occasion is situate near the River and commonly known as White Chapel Mount and the Mount Field' (ibid, 112–13) (Fig 7c). It was not until 1749 that the governors decided that Mount Field was indeed the most suitable location for the new hospital. The land had been let by the City of London to a builder on a lease of 60 years; he agreed to sell his interest in the property to the governors, and the City of London agreed to a ground rent of £15 per annum for the Mount and Mount Field (ibid, 114–15).

Construction work on the new hospital, designed by Boulton Mainwaring, started in 1752 (Clark-Kennedy 1962, 124). The original plan for the hospital consisted of a U-plan block of three storeys, with wings to the rear and the front facing on to what is now Whitechapel Road (Fig 8). Initially only the front block was built, opening in 1757 (ibid, 135). The east and west wings were added in 1775 and 1778 respectively (ibid, 159–60). The hospital's medical college opened in 1785, and was located within an eastwards extension of the front block of the hospital (ibid, 167). All the hospital buildings built during the 18th century occupied Mount Field (see, eg, Fig 10). An area of the Mount was levelled and used for the burial of patients who died at the hospital but whose bodies were not taken away by relatives or friends (ibid, 143).

During the 1750s, when the hospital was being constructed, most of the surrounding land consisted of fields and footpaths, with a small pond directly to the south of the hospital (Figs 7c, 9). To the east of the hospital and extending to the north of the main road was the village of Mile End Old Town, which was connected to the City by a string of development along the

roadside via Whitechapel and Aldgate. The governors also purchased – in two parts – around 20 acres (8ha) of land, known as Red Lyon Farm, to the south of the Mount and Mount Field, the first part in 1755 and the second in 1785 (RLH, LH/D/1). Eventually, these purchases provided a substantial part of the income of the hospital. From the 1780s onwards the governors actively developed the estate, constructing roads and letting plots on building leases. By the end of the 18th century, the Mount had been completely levelled, and the area to the south-west of the hospital had been developed (Fig 10).

The 18th-century landscape and brickearth quarrying: the archaeological evidence (OA4)

All the areas that subsequently underwent archaeological investigation (Fig 3) lay to the south of the later 18th-century hospital buildings, which were contained within Mount Field. Areas A, B, C and D lay within the area directly to the south of the hospital that was kept free from buildings and later enclosed. Area E was directly to the south of East Mount Street (marked on Horwood's 1799 map (Fig 10) as Mount Street), which at that time only extended along the eastern boundary of Mount Field. Areas F and G lay in undeveloped land to the east of the hospital and south of Mile End Green, and area H lay to the south of Oxford Street, this portion of which is marked on Horwood's map as the 'Foot Way from Whitechapel to Stepney, Limehouse, East India and West India Docks'. Area J comprised areas of undeveloped land and part of this footway. By 1799 the pond to the south of Mount Field shown on

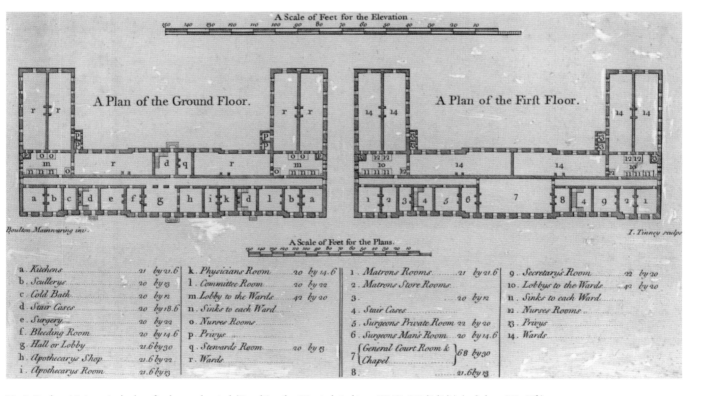

Fig 8 Boulton Mainwaring's plans for the new hospital (Royal London Hospital Archives, RLH, LH/S/2/1) (scale bars 150+10ft)

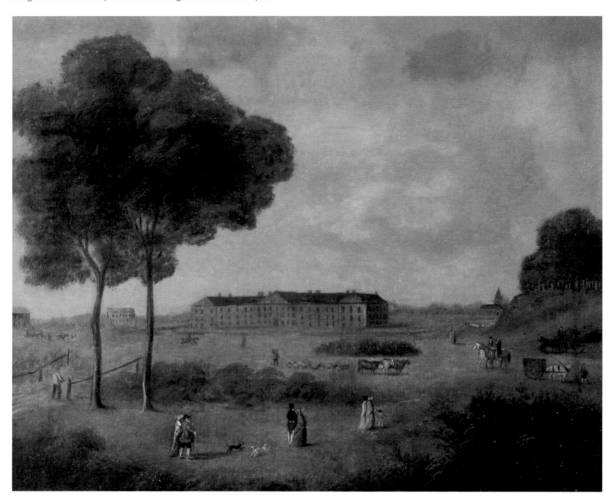

Fig 9 View of the London Hospital c 1760, in an open landscape with (right) Whitechapel Mount (18th-century British School) (Royal London Hospital Archives, RLHINV/18)

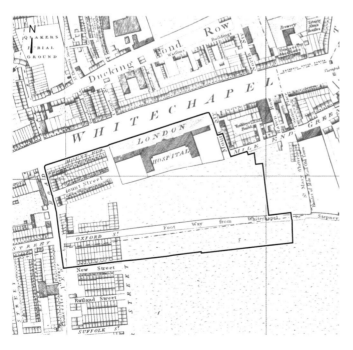

Fig 10 Horwood's map of 1799 showing the development of the area to the south-west of the hospital (Horwood 1813); outline of the Royal London Hospital site superimposed

Rocque's map of 1746 (Fig 7c) had disappeared.

By the end of the 18th century the land, although it had not been developed, lay within an increasingly urban landscape. Streets, houses, factories and institutions – including the hospital itself – were springing up in the vicinity at a furious pace, and the area was rapidly losing its former rural character. Many of the fields were quarried for brickearth in advance of development taking place (Fig 11). These brickearth quarries could cover large areas and be very lucrative: in *c* 1801 the land directly behind the hospital was said to be worth £100 per acre 'in respect of brick earth' (Clark-Kennedy 1962, 193).

Evidence for brickearth quarrying during the late 18th and early 19th centuries was recorded at the site in the form of extensive peaty deposits, comprising organic material that had been dumped into quarried areas. These deposits were recorded during the excavation and watching brief in areas A, B, E, F and G (OA4). They may also originally have extended across areas C and D, but these areas had been truncated to a greater extent by modern basements. At the northern limit of area G, the peaty deposits lay within a cut into the natural brickearth.

The quarrying activity had truncated the medieval subsoil in the northern part of area A, and the natural brickearth elsewhere.

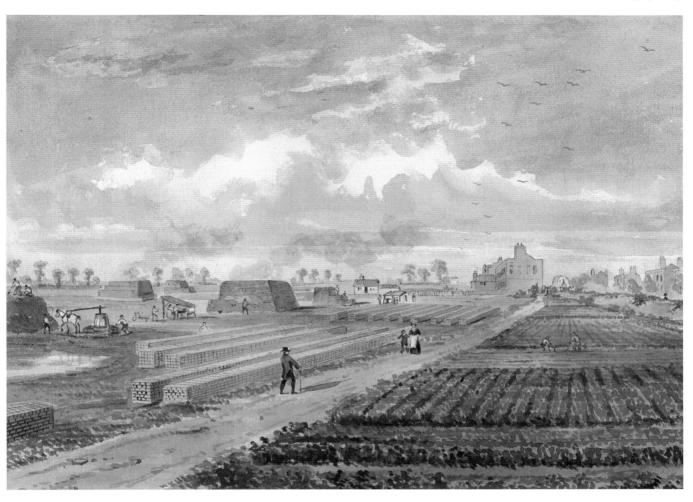

Fig 11 Fox going home to his dinner, of Haarlem's dyke the faithful image *by C H Matthews, c 1830, showing the complete process of brick production in Dalston, east London, with quarrying, drying out of the green bricks and the construction and firing of the brick clamps (LMA, SC/PZ/HK/01/019)*

The peaty deposits associated with the quarrying varied between *c* 0.30m and *c* 0.75m in thickness, up to a maximum of *c* 1.0m in area B. Pottery from both the medieval and the post-medieval periods was retrieved from the dumped deposits, although the majority was residual. Post-medieval pottery from the deposits in area A and area B is dated to *c* 1680–1700 and *c* 1480–1610 respectively. One clay pipe bowl, <74>, dated to *c* 1780–1829 (London type AO27), was retrieved from the deposit in area A, marked with the pipemaker's initials IC in relief on the sides of the heel.

A diverse assemblage of seeds and fruits was recovered from a sample taken from the deposit in area A ([654], {2}). Although a small number of the remains could be associated with plants growing on marshy ground, most were more representative of wasteland plants growing in and around the backfilled quarries, and perhaps also indicative of cultivated ground nearby. Several taxa, such as nettle-leaved goosefoot (*Chenopodium murale*), black nightshade (*Solanum nigrum*) and stinging nettle (*Urtica dioica*) are particularly characteristic of nitrogen-rich soils, such as those associated with manuring or dumped organic material.

The peaty nature of the deposit may indicate that the land here was fairly wet prior to the quarrying activity, and this is supported by the presence of a pond in this area as shown on

the 1746 Rocque map (Fig 7c).

A number of features were associated with the quarrying or with the dumping of the organic material that filled the quarries (Fig 12). Two narrow linear features, [669] and [675], aligned north–south and approximately parallel to each other, represent rough paths through the soft organic deposits, which may be contemporary with the quarrying activity. Both the tracks were *c* 0.30m wide, and the western path, [669], was recorded over a distance of at least 12.60m. The bases of both features had been consolidated: the fill of the eastern path contained red bricks laid in an almost wall-like fashion. To the west of the western path a shallow kidney-shaped pit associated with the quarrying activity was observed. The eastern side had a vertical edge, respecting the alignment of the path immediately to the east. A second trackway associated with the backfilling of the quarries was observed in the southern part of area A; it had been created by sinking brick rubble into the soft deposits below in two parallel tracks, [711] and [712] (not illustrated). The tracks were 0.30–0.40m wide, and *c* 1.60m apart, possibly for a cart. Although they had been truncated to the south-west (by machine), they were observed over a distance of 3.50m.

By 1799 (Fig 10) the pond shown on the Rocque map (Fig

N

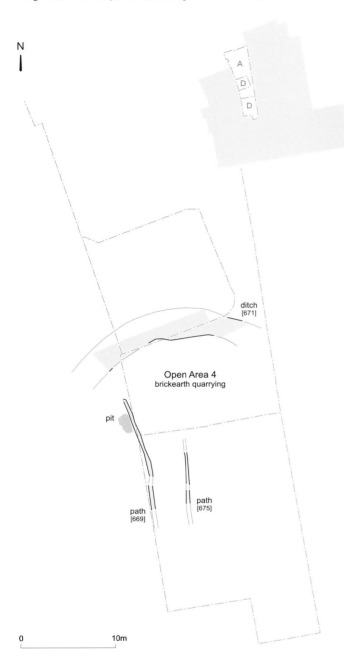

ditch
[671]

Open Area 4
brickearth quarrying

pit

path
[675]

path
[669]

0   10m

Fig 12 Features associated with brickearth quarrying (OA4, period 3) (scale 1:400); inset (top right) locates areas A and D within the overall area of phase 1 works (see Fig 3)

7c) had been drained. In the southern half of area A, a curved drainage ditch, [671], that may have been associated with this work was recorded. It was over 2.30m wide and 1.20m deep, and was recorded extending over *c* 19m east–west. The fill of the ditch contained dumps of brick rubble and fire debris together with lenses of a cess-like deposit similar to the organic deposits that filled the brickearth quarries.

Further to the east in area G a timber-lined rectangular pit, probably a soakaway, was recorded.

3

The early 19th-century enclosed ground and hospital cemetery

'We late-lamented, resting here,
Are mixed to human jam,
And each to each exclaims in fear,
"I know not which I am!"'
(Thomas Hardy, 'The levelled churchyard', 5–8 (Hardy 1994))

3.1 Hospital expansion and the development of the estate (period 4)

Historical background

Development of the hospital estate during the early 19th century

By 1800 the area to the south-west of the hospital had been laid out in streets and building plots had been let (Fig 10; Clark-Kennedy 1962, 192). To the south of the hospital work was in progress to construct Commercial Road, linking Whitechapel with the docks further to the east. This road greatly increased the value of the land that the hospital had purchased during the preceding decades, and plans were made for further streets to be laid out to the south of the hospital. The governors were concerned that any plans should take into account the necessity of maintaining 'the purity of the air round the Hospital', which was considered essential for the patients' well-being, and it was eventually decided therefore to keep a piece of ground directly behind the hospital free from buildings, and to develop the area to the south of Oxford Street (later known as Stepney Way). St Vincent Street (soon renamed Philpot Street) was laid out parallel to Turner Street, and New Street, Rutland Street, Suffolk Street and Norfolk Street were all extended to the east (ibid, 193). To the south of Oxford Street a large plot between Turner Street and Philpot Street was bought in 1816 for the construction of Stepney chapel, which was consecrated in January 1823 (RLH, LH/A/5/17, 183) (Fig 13).

In 1823 the house committee received estimates for 'filling up forming draining and gravelling … the whole of East Mount Terrace and the East end of Oxford Street from Raven Street to the South east Gate of the Enclosure behind the Hospital and likewise for draining that part of Oxford Street extending along the whole of the south side of the Enclosure behind the Hospital' (RLH, LH/A/5/17, 278). East Mount Terrace was the name given to the extension of Mount Street to the south (eg, on Fig 13), although subsequently both Mount Street and East Mount Terrace were known as East Mount Street. The eventual costs for East Mount Terrace were as follows (ibid):

> Scraping + cleaning the road preparatory to laying Rubbish: £5:14:-
> 236 cubic Yards of hard dry rubbish preparatory to gravelling: £11:16:-
> 95 cubic Yards of screened Gravel + levelling same: £20:10:-
> No. 4 cast Iron Gratings cesspools + drains into Services with Moor Stone kirbs + round gratings: £44:-:-
> Total: £90

The ground rents for the new plots were to be £2 10s per annum for houses in St Vincent Street, and £2 for those in the 'bye-streets' (RLH, LH/A/5/17, 35). The governors were keen to see the land developed and to this end they loaned money to builders taking plots, which they got back through increased ground rents (ibid, 107).

Maintaining the hospital estate was becoming increasingly time-consuming and costly, and fly-tipping appears to have been a problem in the immediate vicinity of the hospital. In 1821 the house committee appointed a subcommittee to inspect the roads on their estate, after receiving complaints from tenants about the state of the road near the Stepney chapel (RLH, LH/A/5/17, 51–2). In September 1831, they received a complaint from a tenant 'that rubbish was continually brought from the Hospital in a cart and shot on a piece of waste ground belonging to the Estate near east Mount Terrace' (RLH, LH/A/5/19, 309), and in November the trustees of St Mary's parish, Whitechapel, wrote 'requesting that the Committee would give orders to have a piece of waste ground behind East Mount Terrace, enclosed to prevent it being in future made a deposit for filth and rubbish' (ibid, 138). In 1833 the governors were forced to address the state of a piece of ground at the north end of Philpot Street, between Stepney chapel and the Brewers Almshouses. The ground was evidently becoming quite wet and drainage appears to have been an issue. A proposal to enclose the ground was rejected by the Building Committee in March 1834 as being too expensive, and they instead suggested 'enclosing the space in question with a Curb-stone + iron posts, + at the same time paving a channel on the outside thereof, + raising the ground enclosed, so as to give it such a declivity as will ensure the perfect dryness of the surface on all occasions' (RLH, LH/A/5/20, 237). This proposal was not approved by the house committee, perhaps because it was also considered too great an expense.

As well as maintaining their own estate, the governors attempted to act as a force for the improvement of the surrounding neighbourhood. In 1823 the house committee asked the secretary to write to the governors of Whitechapel

parish about the 'nuisances from Horse boiling Houses and shoots of night soil upon certain premises near Ticklebelly Common' (RLH, LH/A/5/17, 241).

The enclosed ground behind the hospital

By c 1815 the ground directly behind the hospital to the north of Oxford Street was in a pretty poor state as a result of the earlier brickearth quarrying (Chapter 2.2), and there were reports made to the house committee of horses trespassing on to the ground. In May 1816 the house committee, having decided that the ground needed to be enclosed, appointed a subcommittee to consider the best mode of doing this and the costs involved. Later they resolved 'that it is very desirable immediately to enclose the Ground adjoining the south wall of the Hospital with a view to render the Lots for Building more valuable and the ground itself in some way useful to the Hospital and prevent the inconvenience of its present state' (RLH, LH/A/5/16, 68–9). They settled on enclosing the ground with a dwarf wall and an iron palisade 5ft 6in (1.68m) high, to allow for the circulation of air. After this decision had been made it was still another year before the wall was constructed. Eventually Mr Bird, the contractor engaged to build the wall, was paid a total of £1093 4s 8d for the work, with the final balance paid to him in December 1817 (ibid, 153).

As a consequence of the earlier quarrying the enclosed ground lay at a considerably lower level than the surrounding streets, and the hospital made efforts to raise it. Money was paid for rubbish to be dumped in the enclosure, but hardcore was also needed to consolidate it. In December 1817 the house committee asked one of the governors, a Mr Tyler, 'to accept 1000 loads of good Mould at 6d per load to fill up the vacant Ground behind the Hospital' (below, 'Archaeological evidence

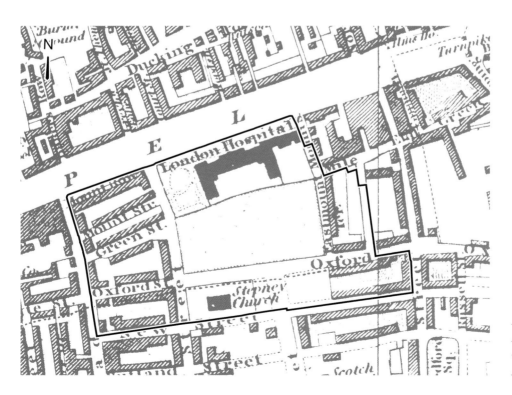

Fig 13 The Greenwoods' map of London, 1827 (Greenwood and Greenwood 1827), with the outline of the Royal London Hospital site superimposed

for the enclosed ground (OA5)'). The following week, with his eye on the costs, he managed to obtain the mould for 4d a load (RLH, LH/A/5/16, 150).

After the ground had been backfilled and enclosed it was utilised to provide the hospital with additional income. A succession of tenants occupied it, but the hospital placed fairly strict conditions upon what could be done with the land. In November 1821 the house committee received a letter from a Mr Gardiner of Bromley, who wished to take the ground for a market garden, but they thought that 'it would not be expedient to have the Ground cultivated in the mode' (RLH, LH/A/5/17, 56). There were concerns from some quarters that the ground would eventually be let on building leases as all the land around it was developed. In May 1822 the house committee received a letter from one of the governors regarding the matter (ibid, 111):

Gentlemen,
Having been very instrumental in procuring the long enclosure behind the Hospital to be railed in and preserved as an open space for keeping a good circulation of Air about the Hospital I take the liberty of giving my Opinion respecting a Question which has arisen of how far the Committee can bind their Successors in giving a Guarantee to the Builders who have recently taken Land that such Ground shall not be built upon during the continuance of their Leases. I think it a most fortunate circumstance that the committee are so called upon and I see no reason whatever why they may not with propriety commit the Governors for an object not merely beneficial to the present lettings but of the utmost importance to the health of thousands of Patients in succession. I regret that I cannot from other engagements stay here this morning and I hope I shall be pardoned for this intrusion.
I am … Mr Davis.

The following week the house committee resolved not to allow the enclosed ground to be built upon 'except for the use of the purposes of this Institution only' (RLH, LH/A/5/17, 113). However, it became increasingly difficult for the hospital to find suitable tenants. In March 1823 the house committee placed advertisements in the papers for tenders for occupying the enclosed ground behind the hospital 'either in whole or in part to be used as grazing Ground for sheep only'. They received a number of tenders for taking the ground, but none were considered to have come up to the expectations of the committee and so none were accepted (ibid, 202–3). In April the committee decided that the enclosed ground should be laid down in grass (ibid, 212), and in August of the same year a Mr Irwin Cooper of Redman's Row paid £25 for the grass that he mowed and carried away. The following year the ground was let for the sum of £35 to be used for the depasturing of sheep (ibid, 279), although it is possible that horses were kept there instead. In September 1824 William Sparks was convicted of stealing a black pony with a wall eye belonging to Daniel Hewitt from an open field at the back of the London Hospital where several other ponies were kept (*Old Bailey Proc*, September 1824, Willam Sparks (t18240916-137)). He was seen by a watchman in

Green Street, 300 yards from this field, leading it towards New Road (Fig 13).

By 1826, the ground was in a poor state again. In July that year, a tender was accepted from Mr E Boutle, who wished to rent the land 'and to fill up the same with good Mould from 1 foot to 1 ft 6 inches' (RLH, LH/A/5/18, 97). The lease was agreed on the condition that Mr Boutle maintained the fences (ibid, 98), but by the summer of 1828 the 'iron gates and fences [were] … in a dilapidated state' (ibid, 219), and in September the hospital repossessed the land, though they permitted Boutle to return to collect his crop of potatoes and 'scarlet beans' (ibid, 228).

A proposal to take the ground on a 21-year-lease in 1830 again noted the poor condition of the ground (RLH, LH/A/5/18, 342):

17th June 1830

Gentlemen
I beg leave to postpone taking the ground railed in at the back of the London Hospital on a lease of 21 years at the yearly rent of twenty five pounds per annum, the rent to be paid quarterly, but as the ground is in a dilapidated state at present I propose that the first year should be at a Peppercorn rent. Trusting gentlemen you will consider my present offer liberal, as I must depend on the produce of the ground for my family's livelihood – Your answer will oblige your most obedient humble servant James Workman.

The house committee refused the offer 'in consequence of the new buildings' (ibid, 342–3).

In June 1833 the house committee made an offer to the officers of Whitechapel parish to use the ground gratuitously for two years, 'on the condition that they clear + cultivate it with such crops as shall not be objectionable to the House Com^ee + keep it in order during the term' (RLH, LH/A/5/20, 87). They took over the ground in May 1834 and it was used by the parish officers to provide employment for the paupers under their care. In April 1837 the guardians of the newly formed Whitechapel Union wrote to the house committee and requested the continued use of the ground, which was granted on the same terms as it had been given to the parish (RLH, LH/A/5/21, 439).

Archaeological evidence for the enclosed ground (OA5)

During the archaeological excavation and watching brief, deposits relating to the improvement of the enclosed ground were recorded (Vuolteenaho et al 2008). Hardcore comprising rubble and fire debris had been dumped on the area, together with a substantial deposit of locally made redware pottery used in the sugar-refining process. Such were the quantities found that only a sample was taken, with up to seven sugar-collecting jars and six sugarloaf moulds retrieved conforming to the range of vessels identified by Brooks (1983) in her typology of sugar-equipment pottery vessels. The use of broken pottery from the sugar industry as make-up and hardcore has been observed on other archaeological sites in London's East End, particularly before the construction of Bishopsgate goods station in the 1840s (Pearce et al in prep). These deposits were probably dumped in 1817, when the hospital paid for rubbish and mould to be dumped to raise the ground at the same time as it was enclosed. In the southern half of area A these deposits were sealed by a layer of lime, which may have been deposited to prevent odours emanating from the wet organic deposits backfilling the brickearth quarries (Chapter 4.1). Unfortunately, the minutes of the house committee do not record when the lime was deposited and for what purpose, although as it was important to the committee to keep a good circulation of air around the hospital, it is likely that the stench of decaying organic matter would have been undesirable.

A small number of accessioned finds was retrieved from the deposits dumped to consolidate and raise the ground. A bone syringe applicator (<S1>, Fig 14) – one of four found on the site (Chapter 5.11) – is obviously associated with the hospital. Two other accessioned finds cannot be directly associated with the hospital but may well have been used within it. A fragment of bone comb (<61>) is a standard double-sided form, rectangular and made from ivory, with fine and coarse teeth. The type was in use throughout the 17th, 18th and early 19th centuries and the fragment cannot be closely dated. An unmarked flat cylindrical 2oz (57g) weight (<42>) is a standard 18th- or early 19th-century type (cf Thompson et al 1984, fig 58, no. 96, dated *c* 1750–70), perhaps used by one of the apothecaries. The deposits also contained two fragments of tin-glazed wall tile, which may have been installed in the original hospital building (Chapter 5.8; <T1>, Fig 101).

Three parallel linear features interpreted as bedding trenches were recorded in area B (Fig 15). These were undated but may have related to the use of the enclosed ground.

Also in area B and cut from the level of the raised ground was a large pit or soakaway (S1, Fig 15) backfilled with organic dumps containing a large number of cattle horncores and leather shoes, together with sherds of pottery and unidentifiable pieces of iron (Vuolteenaho et al 2008). This feature was partially exposed within a new manhole and drain run and was recorded during the watching brief. The base of the feature was not exposed during the excavation, but extended below 1.0m deep. The shoes and shoe parts are dated to the late 18th and early 19th century; the pottery is dated *c* 1807–40. The feature

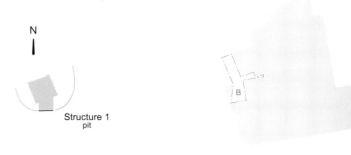

Structure 1
pit

Open Area 5
enclosed ground

? bedding trenches

0   10m

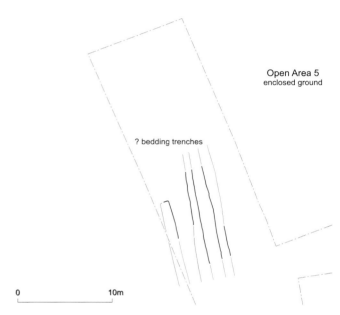

Fig 15 Archaeological features in the enclosed ground of the early 19th century (OA5, period 4) (scale 1:400); inset (top right) locates area B within the overall area of phase 1 works (see Fig 3)

also produced three clay pipe bowls, one of them in a fragmentary condition and decorated with moulded leaf seams. A type AO27 bowl (1780–1820) is marked BB in relief on the heel and has the name BADDELEY stamped incuse on the back of the bowl, facing the smoker (<CP2>, Fig 107). This may be Robert Baddeley, who was recorded in 1805 (Oswald 1975, 132).

A sample taken from the organic fill of the feature contained many plant stem fragments and other vegetation. Most were highly fragmented, but some resembled cereal straw. A number of cereal caryopses were seen, as was chaff, in the form of rye (*Secale cereale*) rachis nodes and internodes and, more unusually, several floret fragments from rice (*Oryza sativa*). Although food remains were rare in the sample, the rice florets are of particular interest as they have been found in only a few London sites to date, and represent an imported product. The most numerous seeds in the sample came from wild grasses (Poaceae) and buttercups (*Ranunculus acris/repens/bulbosus*), which, along with smaller numbers of remains from other grassland plants such as daisy (*Bellis perennis*), dandelion (*Taraxacum officinale*), self-heal (*Prunella vulgaris*) and field

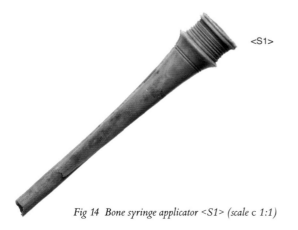

<S1>

Fig 14 Bone syringe applicator <S1> (scale c 1:1)

scabious (*Knautia arvensis*), suggest the presence of meadow or pasture in the vicinity. They may indicate that the soakaway was contemporary with the period when the enclosed ground was laid out in grass that was cut for hay (after 1823). Seeds from weeds of disturbed ground were also common. Several leafy shoots from heather (*Calluna vulgaris*) are more characteristic of heathland and may have been brought from further away, perhaps intended for fuel, animal bedding or in a besom broom. Occasional seeds of sheep's sorrel (*Rumex acetosella*) may have come from the same source.

Fifty-nine fragments of animal bone were hand recovered from the feature, of which 44 were cattle horncores from medium- and long-horn cattle, using the definitions of Sykes and Symmons (2007). Plotting of the minimum and maximum basal diameters against post-medieval examples of known sex suggests that the majority of the horncores came from bulls or oxen. Further details are available in the site archive (Chapter 1.6). The presence of large collections of cattle horncores is often viewed as evidence of tanning and leather working taking place on the site (Serjeantson 1989; Rielly 2011), but as the city horn works were clustered close to the hospital in Whitechapel (Yeomans 2006, 234), horncores would have been easy to come by. Perhaps they had originally been used as part of the pit's lining, or a useful filling material. The rest of the faunal remains from Structure 1 probably represent background rubbish gradually incorporated into the pit. A horse femur with indications of butchery from the feature may have come from one of the 'Horse boiling Houses' complained of by the house committee in July 1823 (RLH, LH/A/5/17, 241).

A brick culvert (S2; not illustrated) aligned north–south was also recorded in the area during the watching brief.

3.2 Provision for burial at the London Hospital

All hospitals operating during the 18th and 19th centuries had to make provision for the burial of those who died in the hospital with no friends or relatives to claim the body or pay for a burial. In 1788 St Bartholomew's charged a fee of 17s 6d, payable on admission, to cover the costs of burial in case of death during treatment and to be returned if the patient was subsequently discharged. At the same time Guy's charged a similar fee of 20s. In contrast to other hospitals in London, excepting the Westminster, the London Hospital did not charge a burial fee and thus the charity was liable to pay for the burial of unclaimed patients (Howard 1791, 131–42).

At the turn of the century Sir William Blizard, surgeon at the London Hospital, made efforts to ensure that greater respect was paid to those buried at the expense of the charity. He protested to the house committee, who resolved that 'the coffins or Shells provided for the Dead be painted or coloured black, and that a Bier be provided for carrying bodies, and also a black cloth to be thrown over the Coffin, and that the grass be

mounded up in a proper and usual way'. Patients who were well enough were expected to attend the funerals of those who died. The funeral service was to be read over each body by the chaplain's clerk 'separately and individually' (Clark-Kennedy 1962, 188). In November 1825 the governors resolved to provide '2 mourning cloaks for men and 2 hoods for women to attend the funerals of Patients' (RLH, LH/A/5/18, 53).

For those families who did claim the bodies of their friends and relations from the hospital, the cost of providing what was considered to be a decent burial for their loved ones could be crippling. A guide to the burial fees charged by the parish and private grounds in and around London in 1840 suggests that the cheapest burial fees in the area around the hospital could be as little as 5s, but most of the parish churches charged considerably more, often double the amount, to non-parishioners (Cauch 1840). Extra charges were made for funeral services held within the church, and for the bell. In 1843, the 'respectable' burial and funeral of a working-class adult could cost in the region of 4 guineas, to include a strong elm coffin, bearers to carry the corpse to the grave, pall and fittings for the mourners, but not the ground or burial fee (Chadwick 1843, 48). These figures can be compared with, for example, daily wage rates in the London building trades between 1820 and 1853 of 5s a day for carpenters and bricklayers and 3s for labourers (Schwarz 1985, 26, 38).

Many of the hospital's patients and their families could ill afford the costs of a private funeral, but the majority would do anything to avoid the fate of being buried at the expense of the charity. The house governor, William Valentine, was sympathetic to their fears, and in December 1822 he gave a contribution on behalf of the Samaritan Society (Chapter 5.6) towards the funeral costs of a woman who had died in the hospital (RLH, LH/A/17/3, 40–1):

The sister said she had promised, at the dying request of the deceased, that she would not allow the Body to be touched, + the husband declared he would not leave the door of the Receiving Room till he had the body of his wife – they represented themselves to be very poor, but that they would sell all they had rather than allow the Body to be buried at the expense, + consequently <u>in</u> the Hospital Ground – I said by way off inducement to their allowing the Body to remain till morning, but when I found it of no avail, I granted them that, which agreeable to the laws of humanity + of the Hospital, I thought they had a right to demand + permitted them to take the Body – I in my heart, could not but applaud the feelings from which their earnest entreaties proceeded, + I gave them 5s, as almoner of the Samaritan Society, to assist them.

Figures including the number of patients admitted and the number who died in the hospital each year were published in the annual reports of the hospital, together with the amount that was spent on burials for patients (RLH, LH/A/15). The number of burials in the hospital ground each year would have been considerably less than the number dying in the hospital, as only those with no friends or relatives to claim them would have been buried within the ground. Although factors such as changes in the cost of the coffins may have affected the costs incurred by the hospital, when the costs are compared with the numbers of deaths there is a clear relationship, indicating that more patients were buried in the hospital ground in years when there was an increase in the number of deaths in the hospital (Fig 16).

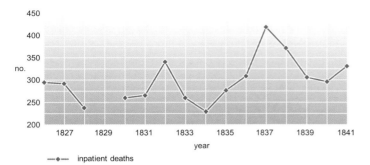

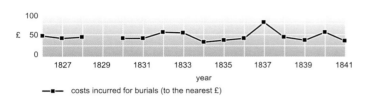

Fig 16 Number of deaths in the hospital and the costs incurred for burials, 1825–41 (data for 1829 not available), compiled from figures published in the annual reports (RLH, LH/A/15, 1–21)

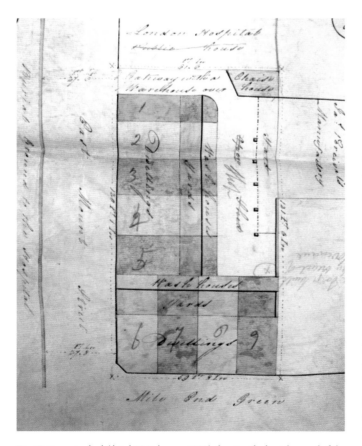

Fig 17 Property deed (dated 20 February 1822) showing the burial ground of the hospital to the west (left) of East Mount Street (north is to the top) (Royal London Hospital Archives, RLH, LH/ D/3/35)

3.3 The location of the London Hospital burial ground

During the 18th century, an area of the Mount was levelled and used for the burial of unclaimed patients. The City Corporation, however, in order to develop the land for its own benefit, decided not to renew its lease when it expired (Clark-Kennedy 1962, 194). The hospital burial ground was subsequently relocated to the east of the east wing of the hospital and south of the medical college. No contemporary plans showing the hospital burial ground in this location have survived, but a deed dated 20 February 1822 for a property on the east side of East Mount Street indicates the hospital burial ground on the opposite side of the street (Fig 17).

Initially the burial ground was located within the confines of Mount Field, to the north of the enclosed ground behind the hospital, but as the ground became increasingly full the house committee began to consider extending the cemetery southwards. In November 1825 the house governor suggested to the house committee that part of the enclosed ground be appropriated for burials: 'the committee attended on the ground and Resolved that Mr Mason Surveyor be requested to make a sketch of the present burial ground to enable the committee to judge whether it will be expedient or necessary to take any part of the enclosed Ground' (RLH, LH/A/5/18, 53–5). The following week the house committee resolved that Mason be asked (ibid, 56):

> to take measures to have the burial ground enclosed by low ramparts and chain agreeably to a plan now produced in order that it may be preserved from trespass by Waggons or by having any rubbish laid upon it and that when done the Committee to take into consideration the propriety of requesting the Bishop of London to consecrate the same.

The railing in of the ground was subsequently postponed because of the cost, 'the committee finding that the amount far exceeds their expectation' (ibid, 59).

Further discussion of the need to extend the burial ground took place in January 1826, but no decision was reached (RLH, LH/A/5/18, 64). It appears that at this time the hospital began to use a portion of the enclosed ground directly to the south of the existing burial ground for more burials. Further west, the hospital garden was also extended to the south.

In the early 20th century (probably 1907) J G Oatley, a surveyor of the hospital, created a set of historical plans of the hospital based on plans that he had traced, some then held by the Office of Works at the Guildhall. Oatley's plan of the hospital buildings as they existed in *c* 1830 indicates the extended burial ground, enclosed by a wall with a rounded corner and not reaching quite as far to the east as East Mount Terrace (Fig 18). It may be that this was a measure intended to minimise the possibility of trespassers entering the ground, although if so it was not entirely successful (Chapter 8.1)

The burial ground established on the north-east corner of

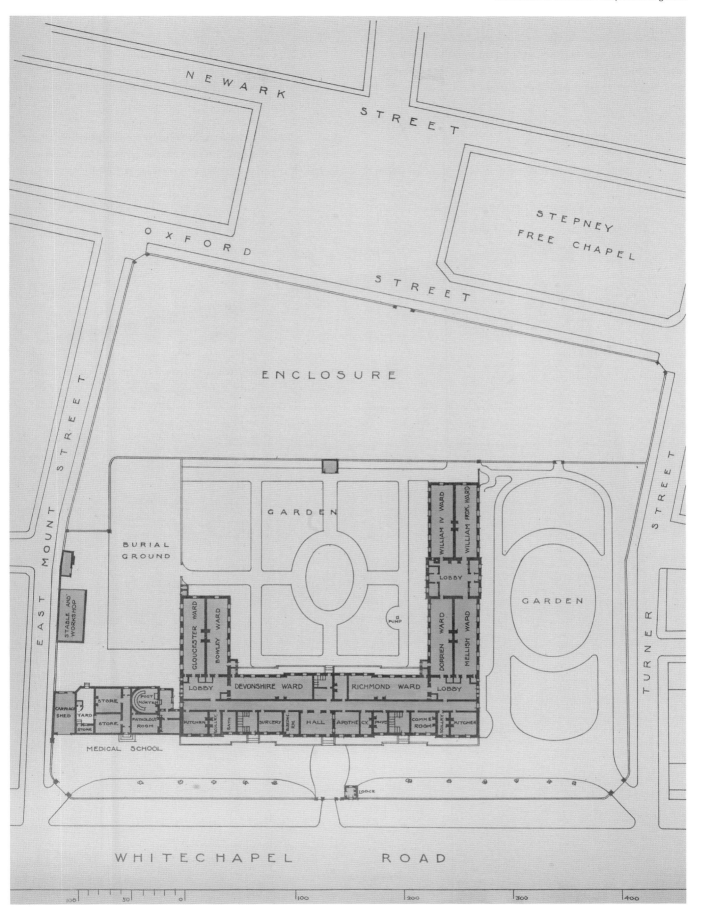

Fig 18 J G Oatley's (?1907) reconstructed plan of the hospital buildings in c 1830 (Royal London Hospital Archives, RLH, LH/S/1/21) (north is to the bottom of the page; scale is in feet)

the enclosed ground remained in use until a new area was laid out on the remainder of the enclosed ground to the south. The appropriation of the enclosed ground for burials had been suggested in 1832, when it was shown on plans of proposed improvements to the hospital drawn up by the surveyor, Mason (Fig 19). However, the existing ground was evidently still in use in October 1841, when the house committee resolved (RLH, LH/A/5/23, 142):

that the Walls at the South East Corner of the Burial Ground

be removed, that the South Garden Wall be continued to East Mount Terrace, and returned to the Wall at the back of the Workshops, in line of the present railing, and that so many of the Coffins, as may be required to be removed for the arrangements consequent on the new Building be deposited in the new enclosure.

The new burial ground to the south most probably came into use not long after this, after which the cemetery in area A was no longer used for burials. The cemetery officially remained in

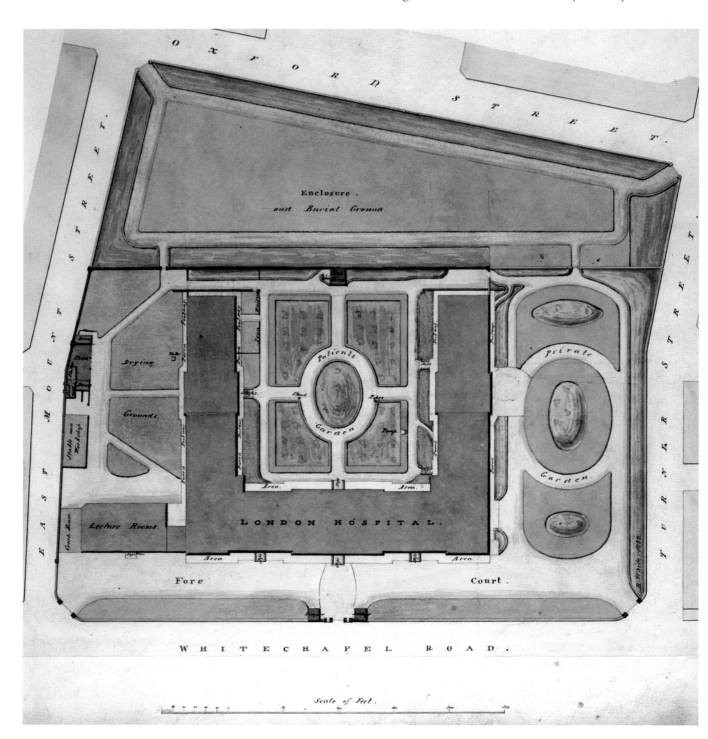

Fig 19 Alfred Richmond Mason's overall plan for the proposed development of the hospital, 1832 (north is to the bottom of the page; scale bar 60+250ft) (Royal London Hospital Archives, RLH, LH/S/2/4)

use until 1854, although burials may have continued until about 1860 (Holmes 1896, 174–5).

After the burial ground was relocated, the area that had been used as the cemetery previously became a drying ground (Fig 19), and was later known as Bedstead Square. Later in the

19th century the southern end of the new Grocers' Company Wing (opened by Queen Victoria in 1876: RLH, LH/A/26/43) was constructed to the north of the eastern half of the area, with workshops constructed over most of the southern part (Fig 20).

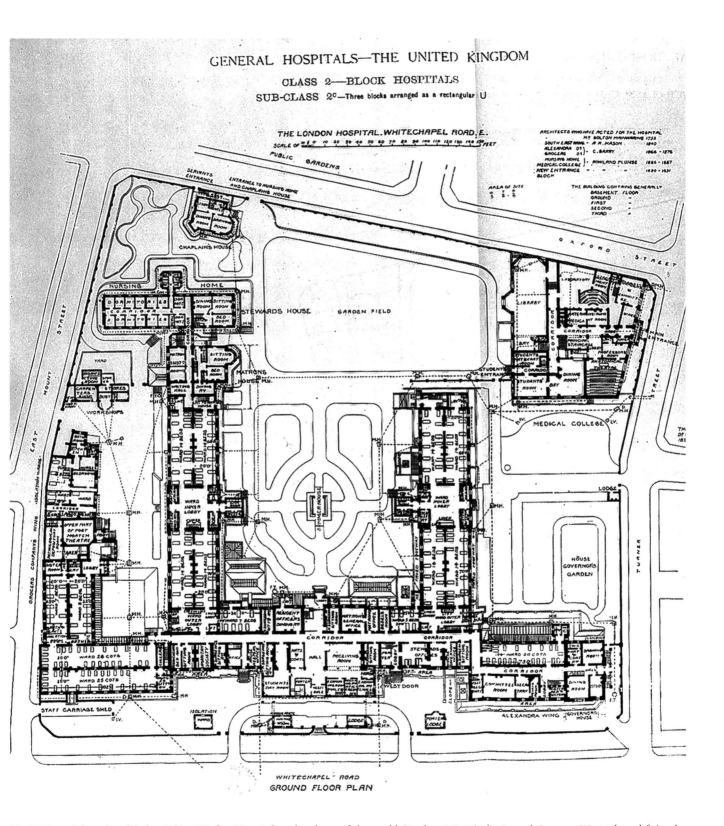

Fig 20 Ground-floor plan of the hospital in 1893, from Hospitals and asylums of the world *(Burdett 1893, 36); the Grocers' Company Wing is lower left (north is to the bottom of the page) (Wellcome Library, London, L0011804)*

3.4 Archaeological and osteological evidence for the cemetery of *c* 1825 to 1841/2 (OA6) (period 4)

The controlled archaeological excavation in area A comprised the entirety of the area used for burials between the point at which the burial ground was extended to the south in *c* 1825 and the time when the larger burial ground was established further to the south in 1841–2. This area (OA6) was bounded to the north by the earlier burial ground, to the east by East Mount Terrace (above, 3.1), to the south by the remainder of the enclosed ground, and to the west by the hospital garden (Fig 18). Parts of the area had been truncated by later drains and the foundations of hospital buildings, resulting in the disturbance of some of the graves (Fig 21). A large deposit of disarticulated bone, [457], containing remains from a minimum of 36 individuals, may be derived from such disturbance. As no burial registers survive, it is not possible to estimate the size of the excavated sample as a proportion of the total buried population.

In addition to standard individual (primary) inhumations, there were burials comprising body parts from more than one individual interred together within one coffin or box. In five of these burials the excavator noted seemingly empty areas within the coffin – these may have been filled with remains of soft tissue that have not survived, although it is also possible that

partial remains could have moved within the coffin if it was tilted as it was lowered into the ground. Seventy-five graves contained the remains of animals in addition to human remains.

All the primary inhumations were extended and supine, aligned east–west with, in all but two cases, the head to the west. The burials of partially articulated remains followed a similar pattern, so that where the remains could be seen to be within a standard kite-shaped coffin the 'head' was to the west.

Three distinct groups of burials were identified within the cemetery, defined on the basis of location and variation in burial rite.

Group 20

A portion of the curved wall built to enclose the extended cemetery shown on Oatley's plan of the *c* 1830 hospital (Fig 18) was recorded during the excavation, including the base of an archway that formed a gateway between the cemetery and the area between the cemetery and East Mount Terrace (S3, Fig 22). Fifty-two graves containing 118 burials lay within this extension and were excavated archaeologically. The graves were ordered and evenly spaced, arranged in up to six rows. Each grave generally contained between one and three burials; one grave contained four burials and another contained five. The tops of the graves lay at an average height of *c* 11.17–11.43m OD, and the bases of the graves lay at 10.63–11.37m OD.

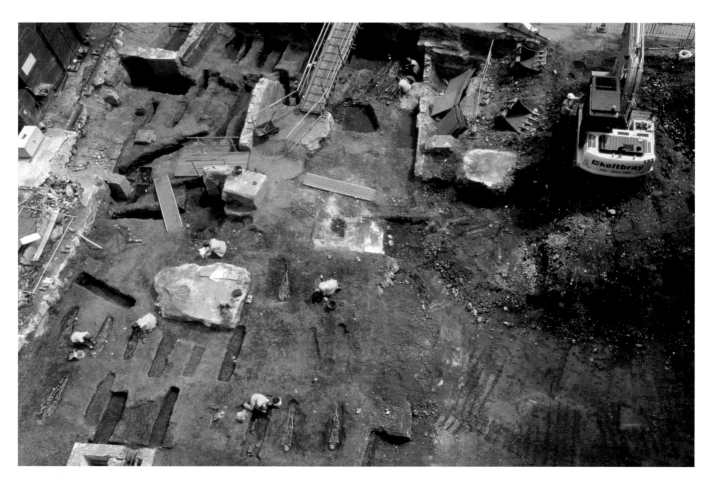

Fig 21   The cemetery (OA6) under excavation, looking east

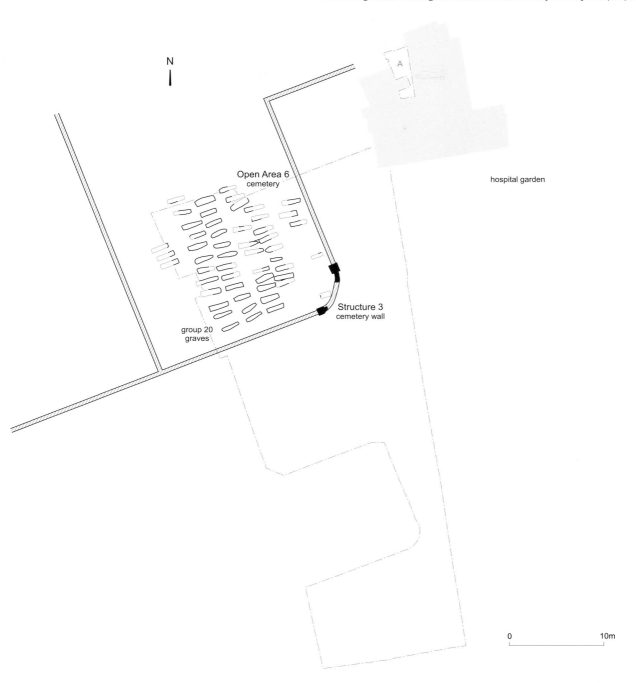

Fig 22 Plan of the initial phase of the cemetery (OA6, period 4): group 20 burials (scale 1:400); inset (top right) locates area A within the overall area of phase 1 works (see Fig 3)

The practice of stacking a number of burials within individual graves is well known from other 19th-century burial grounds excavated by MOLA, such as the City Bunhill burial ground (1833–53), Golden Lane, London borough of Islington (Connell and Miles 2010); the burial ground of the Catholic Mission of St Mary and St Michael (1843–54), Commercial Road, Whitechapel, London borough of Tower Hamlets (Henderson et al in prep); and St Marylebone churchyard (1750–1850), Marylebone High Street, London borough of Westminster (Miles et al 2008). At these grounds stacks of up to nine coffins were found within individual graves.

Sixty-eight primary inhumations originated from this group,

including eight females, 31 males and four subadults (Table 8). There were a further 241 portions of articulated individuals, whilst the 74 contexts of disarticulated bone contained the remains from a minimum of 42 individuals. The majority of articulated contexts in this group (208/309: 67.3%) were well preserved.

Animal remains were recovered from 43 of the graves. The majority of the graves (30) produced small assemblages of 20 fragments or fewer, with sheep/goat and cattle elements dominating. Cattle-size and sheep-size rib and long-bone fragments were also common. The make-up of the cattle and sheep/goat assemblages suggests that here the majority represent

29

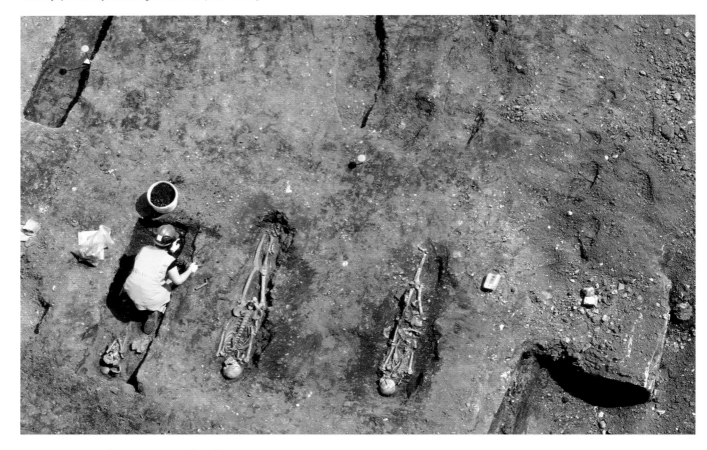

Fig 23 Excavation of graves in group 20 (OA6)

Table 8 Demographic summary of the group 20 primary inhumations (OA6)

Age	Subadult	Female	Male	Intermediate	Undetermined	Total
<4 weeks	3	0	0	0	0	3
1–6 months	0	0	0	0	0	0
7–11 months	0	0	0	0	0	0
1–5 years	0	0	0	0	0	0
6–11 years	1	0	0	0	0	1
12–17 years	0	0	0	0	0	0
Subadult	0	0	0	0	0	0
18–25 years	0	1	4	2	1	8
26–35 years	0	2	9	0	0	11
36–45 years	0	2	10	0	2	14
≥46 years	0	2	3	0	0	5
Adult	0	1	5	0	20	26
Total	4	8	31	2	23	68

kitchen waste. Although individual elements with evidence for dissection were present (Chapter 7.7), the majority of the cattle and sheep remains displayed evidence for having been intensively butchered.

Graves [332] and [447] produced 35% of the animal assemblage, owing to the large number of dog and rabbit remains recovered. However, the majority of these remains came from complete or partial associated bone group (ABG) deposits, recovered from a number of the graves in this group (Chapter

7.9; Table 82). Dogs were associated with seven graves, with two animals recovered from [470]. Rabbit ABGs were present in three graves, two individual specimens being identified from [332]. The last human burials in [332] and [447] had both dog and rabbit deposits associated within them.

Group 21

To the east of group 20 and the projected line of the first-phase cemetery wall (S3), in the area between East Mount Terrace and the wall of the cemetery shown in Oatley's plan of the *c* 1830 hospital, was a group of 16 graves containing 74 burials (Fig 24). The group of burials extended to the limit of excavation in the north, and was bounded to the west by the group 20 graves, to the east by East Mount Terrace, and to the south by the group 22 graves.

The group 21 graves were arranged in ordered rows in the same way as the group 20 graves, but they were deeper and more closely packed, and contained a larger number of burials than those further to the west. Six of the graves were dug end to end. The relationship between the graves suggests that they were near-contemporary in date and that the later grave of each pair was dug immediately after the earlier grave had been backfilled, possibly exposing the ends of the coffins in the first stack, and creating in effect one double-length grave.

The bases of the deeper graves were inundated with water, leading to some disturbance of the remains. This factor,

N

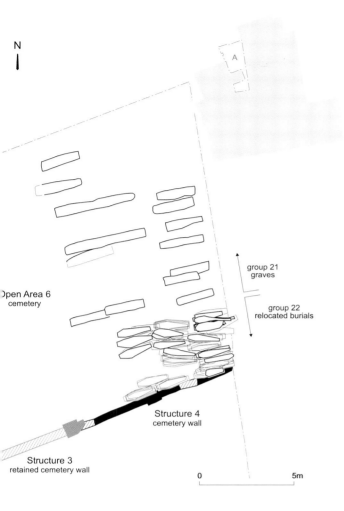

Open Area 6
cemetery

group 21
graves

group 22
relocated burials

Structure 4
cemetery wall

Structure 3
retained cemetery wall

0   5m

Fig 24 Plan of the secondary phase of the cemetery (OA6, period 4): group 21 graves and group 22 relocated burials (scale 1:200); inset (top right) locates area A within the overall area of phase 1 works (see Fig 3)

Table 9 Demographic summary of the group 21 primary inhumations (OA6)

Age	Subadult	Female	Male	Intermediate	Undetermined	Total
<4 weeks	2	0	0	0	0	2
1–6 months	0	0	0	0	0	0
7–11 months	0	0	0	0	0	0
1–5 years	2	0	0	0	0	2
6–11 years	0	0	0	0	0	0
12–17 years	2	0	0	0	0	2
Subadult	6	0	0	0	0	0
18–25 years	0	0	1	1	0	2
26–35 years	0	4	6	0	1	11
36–45 years	0	1	5	0	0	6
≥46 years	0	1	3	0	0	4
Adult	0	3	6	0	17	26
Total	6	9	21	1	18	55

There were 55 primary inhumations in this group, including 21 males, nine females and six subadults (Table 9). There were 132 portions of articulated individuals and 51 contexts of disarticulated bone containing the remains of a minimum of 41 individuals. Preservation was more evenly distributed between contexts that were moderately well preserved (92/187: 49.2%) and those with good preservation (80/187: 42.8%) (see Table 16).

Animal remains were recovered from all the graves apart from [141] and [293], the latter having no human remains, owing to truncation. The majority (89%) of the remains came from just four graves: [207], [220], [251] and [458]. This is not surprising as each of these graves contained a number of ABG deposits. Group 21 produced an assemblage similar in size to group 20 (see above), with the majority of deposits yielding only small assemblages of mainly cattle and sheep/goat remains derived from the hospital's kitchens. Individual specimens, such as the dissected cow periodic bone, have been identified as possible anatomy school deposits (Chapter 7.7, 7.9; Table 82). Although the majority of the ABGs were from dogs, the graves in this group also contained a number of non-native species, including tortoise and monkey.

Group 22 (relocated burials)

Abutting the east–west cemetery wall (S4) was a group of tightly packed burials arranged in stacks and covered with rubble backfill (Fig 25). Seventy burials were recorded in this area, stacked up to five deep and including 50 primary inhumations. Traces of decayed wooden coffins were associated with 20 of the burials. The level of the ground surface below the graves lay at 10.49–10.69m OD.

The burial of these remains was substantially different from those in the graves in group 20 and group 21, being extremely closely packed and apparently contemporary. Similar tightly packed graves and burial trenches are known from other burial grounds of similar date, such as St Pancras church burial ground (1793–1854), York Way, London borough of Islington (Emery and Wooldridge 2011) and St Marylebone churchyard (above,

together with the presence of burials containing multiple body parts and the near-complete decay of the coffins, contributed to difficulties in identifying the number of burials within each grave. It was estimated that the deepest graves originally contained as many as eight burials, but all the graves in the area contained in excess of four burials.

The utilisation of an area outside the original confines of the burial ground, together with the greater depth of the graves in this area and the digging of the graves end to end, suggests an increasing pressure on space within the burial ground. Greater horizontal truncation had occurred in the area of the group 21 graves, and the graves were encountered at c 10.65–11.26m OD, in comparison to the group 20 graves, which were encountered at an average height of c 11.17–11.43m OD. The bases of the group 20 graves lay at 10.63–11.37m OD, but there was no indication that the earlier burials had originally extended further to the east into the area of the group 21 graves. If the ground level contemporary with the use of the group 21 graves was originally comparable to the level at which the group 20 graves were encountered, the greater depth of the group 21 graves is even more striking.

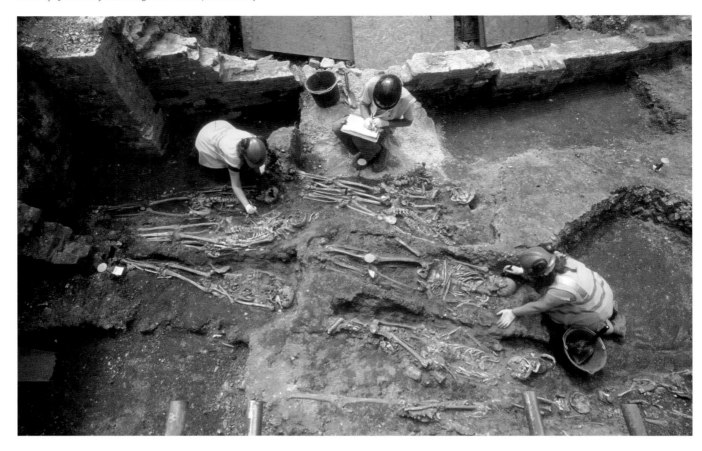

Fig 25 Excavation of burials in group 22 (OA6, period 4), looking south, with the south cemetery wall (S4) to the top

'Group 20'). However, the practice is unlike other burials within the hospital cemetery, where a clear attempt was made to bury the remains in regularly laid out graves. The rubble fill sealing the burials appeared to indicate that all the remains were deposited in one episode.

These burials were probably moved to this location during the building of the extension to the east wing of the hospital in 1841, when the house committee ordered in October the construction of a wall from the south-east corner of the cemetery to East Mount Terrace (RLH, LH/A/5/23, 142). This description fits the excavated wall (S4) and at the same time as the house committee ordered the construction of this wall, they ordered that coffins disturbed during the building of the new extension to the east wing be buried in the 'new enclosure'. Presumably they meant the new burial ground further to the south, but it appears more likely that they were instead reinterred in the area enclosed to the north of the newly constructed wall (S4).

Although the poor preservation of the coffins and the tight packing of the burials in this group made distinguishing between separate burials difficult, some of the deposits of portions and disarticulated material within this group appeared not to be within standard coffins. It is unclear whether the material was originally interred in this way, or whether it was disturbed during the construction work.

The rubble sealing the relocated burials yielded ceramics used in the hospital during the second and third quarters of the 19th century, including a range of items such as sanitary wares and items used for serving food and drink, produced for the hospital and bearing its image (Chapter 5.10).

Of the 50 primary inhumations in this group, 28 were male, 13 female and three subadult (Table 10). Ninety portions of articulated individual were recovered together with 47 contexts of disarticulated bone containing parts of a minimum of 47 individuals. In total 51.4% of the articulated sample was well preserved (72/140) (see Table 16).

This group produced a much smaller assemblage of animal remains than groups 20 or 21 (below and Table 19). Eighteen of the stacks contained animal bones but the majority (12) contained fewer than ten bones. Nearly half the remains (46%) were recovered in association with human burials [229] and [431], both of which contained ABG deposits. There was also a much smaller number of ABG deposits in this group and the majority consisted of small partial deposits of head and vertebra elements (Chapter 7.9; Table 82). The exception is the almost complete hedgehog from a lower burial in [229]. It is possible that this represents an accidental deposit (an animal that fell or burrowed into the grave whist it was still open). The hedgehog's feet were missing but there was no evidence of dissection marks on the elements present. It was, however, in close association with dissected human remains and it is possible therefore that the hedgehog also came from the anatomy school.

Overall this group contained a large proportion of kitchen waste. Sheep/goat was the most common species, with vertebral

Table 10 Demographic summary of the group 22 primary inhumations (OA6)

Age	Subadult	Female	Male	Intermediate	Undetermined	Total
<4 weeks	0	0	0	0	0	0
1–6 months	0	0	0	0	0	0
7–11 months	0	0	0	0	0	0
1–5 years	1	0	0	0	0	1
6–11 years	0	0	0	0	0	0
12–17 years	2	0	0	0	0	2
Subadult	0	0	0	0	0	0
18–25 years	0	3	1	0	0	4
26–35 years	0	4	10	1	1	16
36–45 years	0	6	12	0	0	18
≥46 years	0	0	3	0	0	3
Adult	0	0	2	1	3	6
Total	3	13	28	2	4	50

and pelvis elements predominating. Many of these elements had been butchered and appeared to represent particular cuts of meat (Chapter 5.10).

Coffins

Traces of timber and staining from decayed wooden coffins were recorded with 111 of the burials within all three groups, but it is probable that all the remains from the burial ground were originally interred in coffins. The recorded coffins were very plain and had no plates or grips, with the sole exception of a single coffin with three iron grips. Similar crudely constructed paupers' coffins in a better state of preservation have been excavated at the Cross Bones burial ground in Southwark, the burial ground for the poor of St Saviour's parish (Brickley and Miles 1999, 26–7). The coffins in the hospital ground, where it was possible to discern this, were kite-shaped. Iron coffin nails were recorded with 33 of the coffins (29.7%); the remainder would have been constructed with wooden joints. In 11 cases (9.9%) there were traces of a brown resin, probably the remnants of pitch used for sealing the joints. This characteristic was confined to coffins in group 21, perhaps suggesting a change in the supply of coffins to the hospital.

In February 1833 the house committee received a letter from Messrs Chessell & Co offering to supply the hospital with coffins and shrouds for 7s each (RLH, LH/A/5/20, 27–8). By 1841 the hospital used coffins supplied by Mr Scotcher, a furnishing undertaker based in Ratcliff Highway who also supplied the Whitechapel Union with coffins for paupers. The hospital specified coffins of the same quality and description as those supplied to the Union and at the same price, namely 8d per foot above four feet in length, and 5d per foot under four feet in length, with an additional shilling to cover the cost of pitching the joints (RLH, LH/A/5/23, 64). A coffin five feet in length would have cost the hospital 4s 4d; one six feet in length would have cost 5s. This is slightly more expensive than the 3s 6d quoted by the Southwark undertaker Mr Wild as the cost of an 'adult pauper's coffin with a shroud, but with no cloth or

nails, or name-plate or handles' in 1843, although he qualified this price with the comment that 'the contract is usually for deal, inch thick, but they never are; if they were, they could not be supplied under 4s; they often break when taken to the grave' (Chadwick 1843, 108–9).

Finds associated with the burials

Very few finds (Table 7) were associated with the burials, which were generally stripped of personal possessions prior to burial; clothing was removed by the surgery beadle (RLH, LH/A/5/18, 4 March 1828, 201). Most finds and ceramics were found in the overlying soils (Chapter 5.8, 5.10, 5.11). However, one plain copper-alloy finger ring (<9>) was found on the left hand of female skeleton [259]. Three further small copper-alloy rings (<10>, <11> and <89>), found closely associated with burials [282], [411] and [365], may be fabric button supports. Buttons were found closely associated with five of the burials. They are made of bone and pearl oyster shell (<S2>–<S6>, <S7>, not illustrated) and are small, ranging from 11mm to 17mm, with between one and five thread-holes. Buttons of this type were ubiquitous in the 19th century on both male and female clothing (outer and underwear). Two of the buttons were found by the pelvis and may be from clothing, but it is also possible that they were casual losses. Two pins (<S8> and <S9>, not illustrated) found closely associated with two of the burials are small 'dressmaker' pins with solid socketed heads and tinned shanks; again these are commonly found in 19th-century rubbish but could have derived from hospital use. Pins may also have been used to secure reflected soft tissue during dissection (Henderson et al 1996, 937).

A numbered bone label (<S36>, Fig 193) may have come from a numbered prosection disposed of by the medical college (Chapter 7.8). The rest of the identifiable finds in the burial group consist of small fittings and structural fragments, some of which may also have come from prosections, although some may be background refuse material. A piece from a circular moulded copper-alloy fitting with a decorative beaded edge and a curtain ring with a hook (<8>, <23>) are domestic or institutional fittings. The function of a strip of lead, folded at one end and tapering to a hook at the other is not known (<S10>, not illustrated).

Two pipe bowls and two stem fragments found in the cemetery soil are widely separated in date and derive from background refuse. One pipe bowl was made c 1780–1820 (<84>; AO27) and marked with the initials S (reversed) B.

Osteological sample size and demographic profile

In total, 636 articulated contexts were recovered from area A (Table 11): 173 primary inhumations (Table 12) and 463 portions. For the purposes of analysis, adults assigned as probable male or probable female were added to the male and female totals respectively. A total of 175 contexts contained disarticulated bone (ie, elements that could not be associated with an articulated individual or body portion).

Table 11 Demographic profile of the articulated human remains (636 contexts); NB, this does not represent a total sample population size

Age	Subadult	Male	Probable male	Intermediate	Probable female	Female	Undetermined	Total
<4 weeks	8	0	0	0	0	0	0	8
1–6 months	0	0	0	0	0	0	0	0
7–11 months	0	0	0	0	0	0	0	0
1–5 years	3	0	0	0	0	0	0	3
6–11 years	4	0	0	0	0	0	0	4
12–17 years	11	0	0	0	0	0	0	11
Subadult	7	0	0	0	0	0	0	7
18–25 years	0	15	6	4	3	6	6	40
26–35 years	0	30	8	2	2	14	4	60
36–45 years	0	34	13	0	4	10	3	64
≥46 years	0	10	2	0	1	4	0	17
Adult	0	11	23	1	8	5	374	422
Total	33	100	52	7	18	39	387	636

Table 12 Demographic profile of the 173 primary inhumations

Age	Subadult	Female	Male	Intermediate	Undetermined	Total
<4 weeks	5	0	0	0	0	5
1–6 months	0	0	0	0	0	0
7–11 months	0	0	0	0	0	0
1–5 years	3	0	0	0	0	3
6–11 years	1	0	0	0	0	1
12–17 years	4	0	0	0	0	4
Subadult	0	0	0	0	0	0
18–25 years	0	4	6	3	1	14
26–35 years	0	10	25	1	2	38
36–45 years	0	9	27	0	2	38
≥46 years	0	3	9	0	0	12
Adult	0	4	13	1	40	58
Total	13	30	80	5	45	173

one aged 7–11 months, three aged 6–11 years and two aged 12–17 years); cranial remains from a minimum of 39 males and 15 females; and pelvic remains from 29 males and 12 females. Thus 71.6% of the 95 elements for which sex could be estimated were male.

At least 259 individuals were excavated from Open Area 6, based on the greatest number of repeated elements (right distal femur and left distal humerus), though the actual number of individuals present is likely to be rather higher since many individuals may have been incomplete when they were interred (Chapter 7.8).

The mortality profile of the 173 primary inhumations reveals a low proportion of subadults and a peak in mortality in the 26–45-year age group (Fig 26). To some extent these results have been distorted by the large proportion of adults (58/160: 36.3%) that could not be placed in specific age categories. Amongst the subadults, the perinatal (interuterine/neonate, <4 weeks) category contained the largest proportion of individuals (Figs 26–7). This was, however, based on a small sample size (13).

Forty-nine contexts from the articulated sample (49/636: 7.7%) had suffered truncation, largely as a result of building work and ground reduction. Primary inhumations (43/173: 24.9%) were more frequently affected than portions (6/463: 1.3%). As portions are by their nature incomplete, no significance should be ascribed to this difference.

Whilst preservation was generally good, the completeness of the primary inhumations was varied and widely distributed (Fig 28): 48% of adults were less than 50% complete. This was partly caused by truncation but also resulted from the deliberate removal of elements by amputation, autopsy or dissection and is thus a reflection of the origins of the assemblage. The high percentage peaks for subadult completeness reflect the small sample size (13).

By their very definition, the pattern of skeletal completeness in the portions varied significantly from that of primary inhumations: 78.2% of all portions were between 0% and 10% complete (Fig 29). The most intact 'portion', [22801], was 70–75% complete and was reassembled from a number of separated

In all, 7571 elements (a complete long bone being three elements) were recorded within the disarticulated bone. It is likely that much of this represented the disturbance of articulated material within each grave because although some bone was considered as intrusive within graves there was no evidence of the intercutting of graves, which, in other cemeteries of post-medieval date, is often the explanation for such deposits. It is also likely that some bone was deposited as single, disarticulated elements following surgical removal or dissection (Chapter 7.8); 167 contexts from the articulated sample (167/636: 26.3%), including 69.9% of the primary inhumations (121/173), contained intrusive human bone, which was catalogued as disarticulated.

To prevent the double counting of midshaft elements where a limb had been sawn precisely at the midpoint, the midshaft was not used to calculate the minimum number of individuals (MNI) represented by the disarticulated sample. Based on a count of the maximum number of repeated elements (discounting demographic information), the MNI for the disarticulated assemblage was 79 (right proximal tibia). This included a minimum of seven subadults (comprising at least one neonate,

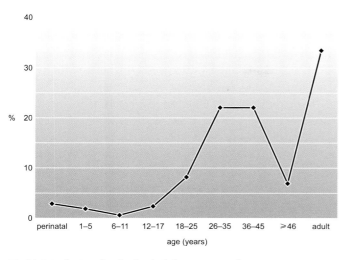

Fig 26 Distribution of aged individuals from primary inhumations

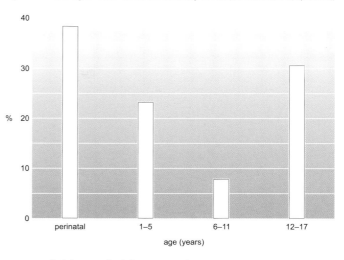

Fig 27 Subadult age at death for primary inhumations

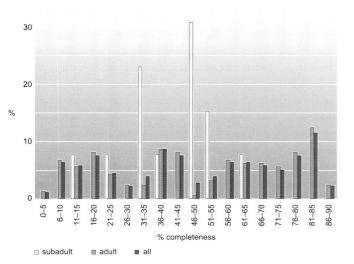

Fig 28 Skeletal completeness of primary inhumations

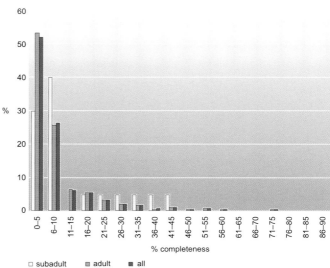

Fig 29 Skeletal completeness of portions

segments found within the same grave that could be securely identified as being from the same individual. It is possible that other graves with sawn and cut remains contained similarly large proportions of specific individuals, but there was insufficient evidence to permit the secure matching of skeletal elements.

Morphology and non-metric traits

Data from primary inhumations and portions were combined to calculate cranial, femoral (platymeric) and tibial (platycnemic) indices for the burial ground as a whole. These indices are used to establish the shape of the cranium, anteroposterior flattening of the femoral shaft at the proximal end and mediolateral flattening of the tibial shaft. The majority of males were dolichocranic (ie, long-headed) while most females were mesocranic (middle-headed); considerably fewer adults were brachycranic (broad-headed) (Fig 30). Males had a mean index of 75.0 (range 70.6–81.0, n=14) and females a mean of 76.5 (range 73.5–80.2, n=6). The total range for the adult sample was 70.6–81.0 with a mean value of 75.5.

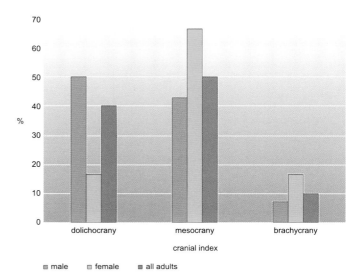

Fig 30 Cranial index

The platymeric index reflects the level of anteroposterior flattening in the subtrochanteric femur (Table 13). The mean measurements cluster around the platymeric/eurymeric border. The platycnemic index expresses the degree of transverse flattening to the tibia at the level of the nutrient foramen, with mean mesocnemic and eurycnemic values in this case (Brothwell 1981, 89) (Table 13).

Biodistance studies employ non-metric variations in skeletal morphology by measuring the similarity or presence of relationships between skeletal samples. However, only brief note is made of them here, as their polymorphic nature together with uncertainty over the environmental contribution to expression compromises such studies (Tyrrell 2000, 301).

The most frequently observed cranial traits were the presence of the posterior condylar canal, the parietal and extrasutural

mastoid foramen, supraorbital groove, supraorbital foramen and the lambdoid wormian bones (Table 14). There was a particularly low prevalence rate of bregmatic, epipteric and parietal notch bones, sagittal and coronal wormians, torus auditivi and multiple mental foramina.

The most frequently observed post-cranial traits within the burial ground were double facets on the calcaneus and talus, lateral squatting facets on the tibia and talus, third trochanters and hypotrochanteric fossae on the femur and vastus notches on the patella (Table 15). There were low prevalence rates of the supracondylar process of the distal humerus, bipartite transverse foramen of the atlas, bipartite patella, medial squatting facets on the tibia and os trigonum of the talus.

An example of inca bones (large ossicles in the occipital) was found in the disarticulated assemblage, as were a sternum with a midline foramen and an example of os acromiale in a right scapula.

Comparison of the groups of burials

Skeletal preservation was superior in the group 20 graves from the western part of the surviving burial ground when compared particularly to group 21 (Table 16). This may be a result of differences in the burial environment between the groups, caused by the greater depth and number of burials in the graves in group 21, and, to a lesser extent, the disturbance of the group 22 burials during their relocation.

The primary inhumations from group 22 revealed a large proportion of middle-aged adults (Fig 31), probably resulting from the small number of unaged adults in comparison with the

Table 13 Post-cranial indices (mean values)

Index	Sex	n	Element	
			Left femur	Right femur
Platymeric	male	141	83.7	86.1
	female	56	80.7	86.2
	all adults	253	83.3	86.1
			Left tibia	Right tibia
Platycnemic	male	93	69.4	69.1
	female	39	68.2	70.8
	all adults	224	70.2	71.1

Table 14 Cranial non-metric traits

	Present		Absent		Total observable		% prevalence	
Cranial trait								
Metopism	6		87		93		6.5	
Lambdoid bone	4		49		53		7.5	
Inca bone	2		78		80		2.5	
Bregmatic bone	1		65		66		1.5	
Sagittal wormians	0		29		29		-	
	R	L	R	L	R	L	R	L
Asterionic bone	2	1	56	53	58	54	3.4	1.9
Epipteric bone	0	0	27	25	27	25	-	-
Coronal wormians	0	1	58	51	58	52	-	1.9
Lambdoid wormians	15	9	25	25	40	34	37.5	26.5
Squamo-parietal wormians	1	1	30	29	31	30	3.2	3.3
Parietal notch bone	0	1	61	60	61	61	-	1.6
Torus auditivi	0	0	88	91	88	91	-	-
Torus maxillaris	1	1	83	80	84	81	1.2	1.2
Torus palatinus	1	2	76	77	77	79	1.3	2.5
Supraorbital foramen	8	13	66	61	74	74	10.8	17.6
Supraorbital groove	7	15	63	54	70	69	10.0	21.7
Mastoid foramen	37	35	40	41	77	76	48.1	46.1
Foramen of Huschke	5	8	83	83	88	91	5.7	8.8
Parietal foramen	46	34	31	44	77	78	59.7	43.6
Accessory infraorbital foramen	3	3	27	29	30	32	10.0	9.4
Posterior condylar canal	30	35	22	16	52	51	57.7	68.6
Multiple mental foramen	0	1	86	87	86	88	-	1.1
Torus mandibularis	2	3	87	85	89	88	2.2	3.4
Mylohyoid bridge	9	6	73	71	82	77	11.0	7.8

Table 15 Post-cranial non-metric traits

Post-cranial trait	Present		Absent		Total observable		% prevalence	
Sternal foramen	2		40		42		4.8	
Manubrio-corpal synostosis	9		89		98		9.2	
	R	L	R	L	R	L	R	L
Os acromiale	6	11	86	90	92	101	6.5	10.9
Acromial articular facet	5	5	81	86	86	91	5.8	5.5
Septal aperture	7	6	130	143	137	149	5.1	4.0
Supracondylar process	2	3	151	160	153	163	1.3	1.8
Atlas posterior bridge	9	9	72	72	81	81	11.1	11.1
Atlas lateral bridge	4	2	74	81	78	83	5.1	2.4
Atlas transverse foramen bipartite	1	1	65	69	66	70	1.5	1.4
Atlas double facet	13	19	90	87	103	106	12.6	17.9
Accessory sacral/iliac facets	9	8	61	56	70	64	12.9	12.5
Acetabular crease	16	21	127	120	143	141	11.2	14.9
3rd trochanter	31	40	106	89	137	129	22.6	31.0
Allen's fossa	11	7	103	103	114	110	9.6	6.4
Hypotrochanteric fossa	41	33	125	118	166	151	24.7	21.9
Patella vastus notch	29	28	70	76	99	104	29.3	26.9
Bipartite patella	0	1	102	103	102	104	-	1.0
Tibia medial squatting facet	0	0	117	108	117	108	-	-
Tibia lateral squatting facet	34	31	83	72	117	103	29.1	30.1
Calcaneus facet absent	5	4	107	100	112	104	4.5	3.8
Calcaneus facet double	54	56	57	47	111	103	48.6	54.4
Talus os trigonum	1	2	118	113	119	115	0.8	1.7
Talus facet double	30	27	64	61	94	88	31.9	30.7
Talus squatting facet	25	23	87	85	112	108	22.3	21.3

Table 16 Preservation by land use

Preservation grade/sample	Group 20		Group 21		Group 22	
	n	%	n	%	n	%
Primary inhumations						
Good	41	60.3	11	20.0	22	44.0
Moderate	21	30.9	37	67.3	25	50.0
Poor	6	8.8	7	12.7	3	6.0
Portions						
Good	167	69.3	69	52.3	50	55.6
Moderate	70	29.0	55	41.7	32	35.6
Poor	4	1.7	8	6.1	8	8.9

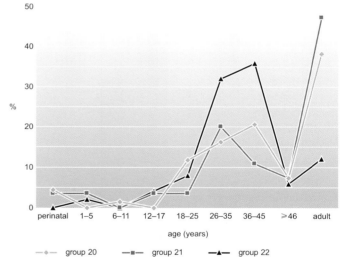

Fig 31 Primary inhumation distribution of aged individuals by land use

other groups, and reflecting skeletal completeness rather than variations in mortality. In group 22 there were fewer adults of undetermined sex and a higher proportion of males and females when compared to the other two groups (Fig 32).

The primary inhumations from group 21 had a higher ratio of subadults to adults when compared to the other groups, although not to a statistically significant extent (Table 17). The similarity of the demography in groups 20 and 22 supports the hypothesis that they were originally part of the same burial ground.

The male:female sex ratio for primary inhumations was 2.7:1, far beyond the expected birth ratio (Rousham and Humphrey 2002, 128), although in 45 individuals there were insufficient skeletal elements remaining to allow sex estimation to take place (45/160: 28.1%). This very high proportion of males contrasts with the ratios from near-contemporary sites in east

London (London borough of Tower Hamlets): St Mary and St Michael (1.4:1), Bow Baptist and Sheen's burial ground (0.7:1) (Henderson et al in prep). The comparative age distributions suggest that most females died younger than males (Fig 33).

A very large section of adult portions could not be placed into specific age categories and this, together with the aforementioned problems in identifying the number of individuals, prevented the building of a mortality profile. However, individual portions were assigned an age and sex estimate where possible (Table 18).

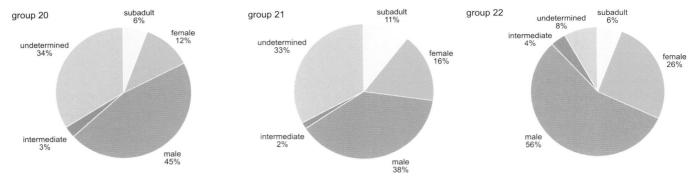

Fig 32 *Demographic profile of primary inhumations from groups 20, 21 and 22*

Table 18 *Demographic data for the articulated body portions*

Table 17 *Primary inhumation adult:subadult ratio by land use*

Group	Adults	Subadults	Ratio
20	64	4	16:1
21	49	6	8:1
22	47	3	16:1

Age	Subadult	Female	Male	Intermediate	Undetermined	Total
<4 weeks	3	0	0	0	0	3
1–6 months	0	0	0	0	0	0
7–11 months	0	0	0	0	0	0
1–5 years	0	0	0	0	0	0
6–11 years	3	0	0	0	0	3
12–17 years	7	0	0	0	0	7
Subadult	7	0	0	0	0	7
18–25 years	0	5	15	1	5	26
26–35 years	0	6	13	1	2	22
36–45 years	0	5	20	0	1	26
≥46 years	0	2	3	0	0	5
Adult	0	9	21	0	334	364
Total	20	27	72	2	342	463

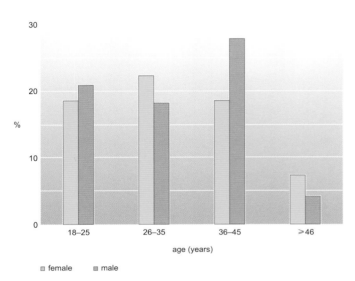

Fig 33 *Adult age distribution by sex*

The faunal assemblage

The unique nature of the animal bone assemblage is highlighted when the species proportions are considered. The most commonly recovered elements from the grave contexts are those of dog followed by rabbit. The usually more common sheep/goat and cattle are the third and fourth most common species. The large number of dog and rabbit elements is due to the high number of ABGs; however, when minimum numbers of individuals are calculated, dog is still the most common with 19 individual animals represented. Sheep/goat is the second most common species with 13 individuals represented, followed by rabbit with nine.

Thirty-two ABGs were identified during excavation and post-excavation and all but one (a wired cat hindlimb from

[100]) were found in grave contexts. ABGs account for just over half of all the animal remains recovered from grave contexts (Table 19). It is also likely that some of the other animal remains came from ABG deposits that became disassociated owing to slumping and disturbance of the graves. Evidence of the use of animals in the teaching of anatomy is discussed in detail in Chapter 7.7, but a large proportion of the remains appears to have come from the hospital's anatomy school.

3.5 The post-1841 cemetery (OA7) (period 4)

Twenty-nine grave cuts were recorded in area B (on the north-eastern edge of the area of phase 1 works), regularly spaced in up to four rows (Fig 34). Three contexts of human bone were recorded at assessment level only: [850], [859] and [863]. They contained portions from three males and, in total, eight body portions and three bags of mixed bone fragments were recorded, all of which had evidence of dissection. One dentition was present – the male in question had lost a number of teeth during life. A right radius with a healed transverse fracture and healed osteomyelitis (infection) was recorded in burial [850].

Table 19 Summary of the animal remains recovered from graves in groups 20, 21 and 22: count of the number of individual specimens present (NISP) with count of how many of the bones came from ABG deposits in parentheses

Taxon	Group 20	Group 21	Group 22	Total
Mammal				
Cattle	69	39	19 (5)	**127 (5)**
Sheep/goat	117 (7)	78	44 (6)	**239 (13)**
Goat	1	0	0	**1**
Pig	17	14 (4)	4	**35 (4)**
Horse	6	6 (4)	0	**12 (4)**
Dog	499 (448)	254 (237)	5 (4)	**758 (689)**
Cat	11 (8)	30	31 (24)	**72 (32)**
Primate, *Cercopithecus*	0	118 (118)	0	**118 (118)**
Primate	1	2	0	**3**
Hare	3 (2)	0	0	**3 (2)**
Rabbit	134 (91)	191 (167)	3	**328 (258)**
Hedgehog	0	0	37 (37)	**37 (37)**
Rat	2	0	1	**3**
Bird				
Chicken	11	4	1	**16**
Goose	1	2	1	**4**
Mallard	0	0	1	**1**
Passerine	0	1	0	**1**
Fish				
Gadid sp	1	0	1	**2**
Conger eel	0	12 (12)	0	**12 (12)**
Mackerel	1	0	0	**1**
Plaice	0	39 (39)	0	**39 (39)**
Plaice/flounder	0	1	0	**1**
Amphibian/reptile				
Frog/toad	1	0	0	**1**
Tortoise	0	19 (18)	0	**19 (18)**
Unidentified				
Cattle-size	99	57	10	**166**
Sheep-size	113	52	18	**183**
Mammal		1	3	**4**
Bird	2	1	2	**5**
Fish	1	1	0	**2**
Total	**1090 (556)**	**922 (599)**	**181 (76)**	**2193 (1227)**

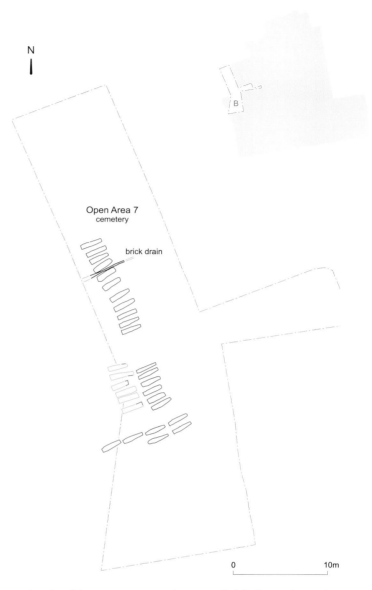

Fig 34 Plan of the post-1841 cemetery (OA7, period 4) (scale 1:400); inset (top right) locates area B within the overall area of phase 1 works (see Fig 3)

A single pipe bowl (<75>; AO27) was recovered from one of the graves, decorated with moulded wheatsheaf seams and marked IF in relief on the sides of the heel. A brick drain aligned east–west ran between two of the recorded graves and may have been contemporary with the use of the area as a burial ground.

3.6 Machined deposits (OA8) (period 5)

Across the site deposits overlying the excavated archaeological remains were removed by machine but screened for archaeological finds and skeletal remains. The assemblage recovered consisted of both rubbish from the hospital and remains that probably originated from disturbed burials. These deposits (not recorded in detail) included 19th-century and later make-up deposits and dumps. Wall foundations relating to later buildings constructed over the burial ground were recorded in area A (not illustrated).

Human bone was recovered from three contexts overlying the earlier hospital burial grounds: [100], [650] and [660]. As outlined in Chapter 1.7, these remains were screened by a team of osteologists during excavation and are biased to those elements that showed signs of surgical intervention. The proportions of different elements recovered can therefore be seen as representative of the areas of the body that had undergone surgical investigation, whether in life or after death.

Context [100] contained elements from at least two males, two probable males, two females and one subadult; [650] a small amount of bone from a minimum of two adults of undetermined sex; and [660] the remains of a minimum of 58 individuals, including 16 males, 11 probable males, two adults with

Table 20 Demographic profile of the disarticulated human remains from machined deposits (OA8)

	Male (MNI)	Probable male (MNI)	Intermediate (MNI)	Probable female (MNI)	Female (MNI)	Subadult (MNI)
Skull	18	13	2	6	2	3
Axial (ribs & vertebrae)	0	0	0	0	0	1
Upper limbs	0	0	0	0	0	2
Lower limbs	4	2	1	0	2	4
Total (MNI)	22	15	3	6	4	10

MNI = minimum number of individuals

Table 21 Number of catalogued bone elements (excluding ribs and sternabrae) from machined deposits (OA8)

Context no.	Cranium	Vertebrae	Upper limb	Lower limb
[100]	42	25	104	101
[650]	3	0	3	5
[660]	512	131	302	636
Total	557	156	409	742

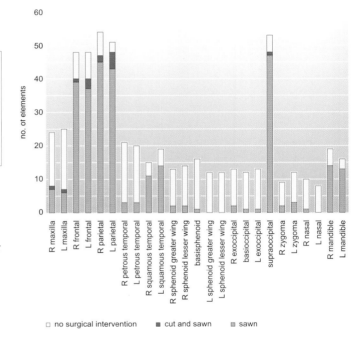

Fig 35 Proportion of cranial elements with evidence of surgical intervention

intermediate sexual characteristics, four probable females, two females and four subadults. When the information from all three contexts is combined, and based on the maximum number of repeated elements (distal femur), a minimum of 70 individuals is represented by this collection of disarticulated bone. The demographic profile can be seen in Table 20. As with the burials in Open Area 7, there is a significant male bias (3.7:1).

In total, 1864 bone elements were catalogued (Table 21) and 965 associated bones or bone elements (eg, paired long bones, associated tibiae and fibulae) were noted. This does not preclude other possible associations that were not made, so the MNI remains the most accurate measure of the number of individuals present.

Hand collection from machine-excavated deposits also accounts for the under-representation of the small elements of the hands (six metacarpals) and feet and the smaller thoracic elements: just two left ribs (one sawn), 11 sterna (seven sawn) and four sawn manubria were recovered.

A significant proportion of the material showed cut (scalpel) and saw marks (Fig 35). The high proportion of frontal, parietal and occipital elements (and the high proportion of these with marks of surgical intervention) is an indication of individuals who had undergone craniotomy, though a large percentage of the mandibles that were recovered had also been subject to (post-mortem) intervention. One discarded prepared specimen was also noted – a bisected adult cranium with indications of fixings for suspension ([660], Fig 36).

The distribution of recovered vertebrae showed a focus on the lower part of the spine, with the first lumbar and first and second sacral vertebrae most numerous (Fig 37). Only saw cuts were present and these all appeared to be related to the post-

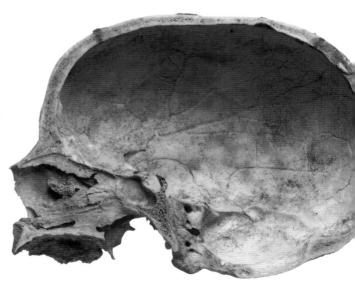

Fig 36 Bisected adult cranium from [660] (OA8) with evidence of having been suspended (scale c 1:2)

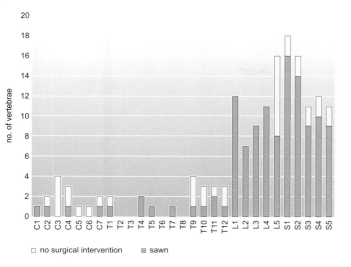

Fig 37 Number of vertebrae present (OA8) and proportion in which evidence of surgical intervention was noted

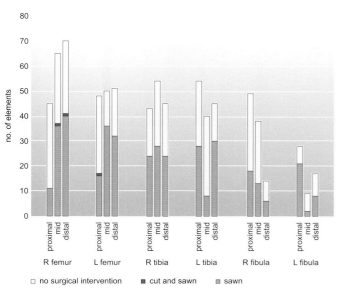

Fig 39 Number of elements from the long bones of the lower limb (OA8) and number with evidence of surgical intervention

mortem division of the body (Chapter 7.8).

Amongst the major long bones of the upper limbs, the humerus was found in greatest numbers (Fig 38). The long bones of the lower limbs were more numerous, with particularly large numbers of femoral elements collected (Fig 39). Given that collection was undertaken by a skilled and experienced team it seems likely that this reflects a genuine pattern with surgical intervention more frequent in the thigh. One left patella, two left tali, two tarsals, five metatarsals and one foot phalanx were also recovered, with surgical saw cuts noted in a right medial cuneiform and the left patella. In contrast to the articulated assemblage (burials and portions) only a small number of pelvic elements were collected: 27 elements were catalogued and of these 18 (66.7%) showed signs of surgical intervention.

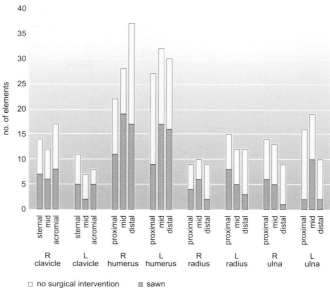

Fig 38 Number of elements from the long bones of the upper limb (OA8) and number with evidence of surgical intervention

The presence of many associated elements argues for the majority of the remains having originated from anatomical teaching rather than surgery. Evidence of dental and skeletal pathology – including infection, trauma, joint disease and congenital – abnormalities were seen, notably an adult male temporal with evidence of mastoiditis, a cranial vault with healed stellate lesions, limb-bone changes indicative of venereal syphilis and 20 healed long-bone fractures and a healed fracture of the ilium.

Deposits overlying the graves also produced small assemblages of animal bone (Table 22). The majority of the remains consisted

Table 22 Summary of the animal remains recovered from layers overlying the burials (OA8); figures indicate the number of individual specimens present (NISP)

Taxon	Area A	Area B	Total
Mammal			
Cattle	6	59	65
Sheep/goat	10	125	135
Pig	1	3	4
Horse	0	3	3
Dog	12	17	29
Cat	6	13	19
Rabbit	0	2	2
Rat	1	0	1
Primate	1	0	1
Guinea pig	1	0	1
Bird			
Chicken	4	0	4
Goose	1	0	1
Turkey	3	0	3
Unidentified			
Cattle-size	3	45	48
Sheep-size	1	27	28
Bird	1	0	1
Total	51	294	345

of individual fragments but one ABG was noted from [100] – a complete cat pelvis and femur that had been wired together. A dissected sheep/goat mandible, also with evidence of having once been part of a wired skeleton, was recovered from [650] (Chapter 7.7). The skull and maxilla of a guinea pig (*Cavia porcellus*) were present in [100] (Fig 40), along with a complete juvenile *Cercopithecus* humerus, which was recovered with cut marks on the distal shaft (Chapter 7.7). It is possible that a number of the dog and cat elements also originated from the hospital's anatomy school. These remains may represent the mixing and redeposition of material previously disposed of within the graves or may represent material 'dumped' once the anatomy school moved in 1852.

Kitchen waste was present, with butchered vertebral, pelvic and long-bone elements from sheep/goat and cattle indicating specific cuts of meat. A small number of bird long-bone elements were also present. Of particular note were three complete turkey (*Meleagris gallopavo*) tibiotarsi, all with exostoses on the proximal ends and bowing of the shaft. They were from very large birds, the equivalent of modern-day Norfolk Blacks and the pathological changes are suggestive of avian tibial dyschondroplasia (Fothergill et al in prep).

A number of animal remains were recovered from [660] and

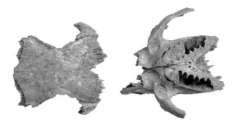

Fig 40 Skull and maxilla of a guinea pig recovered from [100] (OA8) (scale c 1:1)

[850]. Two cattle and two horse elements were recorded from [850]; the rest of the assemblage came from [660]. This assemblage is larger than the one recovered from the cemetery in Open Area 6 (above, 3.4) and has a different composition, dominated by the remains from sheep/goat and cattle, in particular sheep/goat lumbar vertebra and pelvis fragments. These remains have all been butchered and represent the purchase and consumption of particular cuts of meat by the hospital's kitchens (Chapter 5.10). A small number of dog, cat and rabbit remains were present and, although none showed signs of dissection, it is possible they originated from the anatomy school.

4

Health and disease

Ever the same tale, disease, disease, disease. Well, there are hospitals; we pay well to them, and – it's no affair of ours. But … one thing is certain enough … that the fiend of pestilence is no respecter of persons; and the same power that to-day has made a 'slovenly, unhandsome corpse' of poor Pat, the labourer, tomorrow may strike into genteel nothingness the most aristocratic of lords. (Phillips 1855, 8–9)

4.1 Historical evidence of health and disease in the 19th century

Responsibility for public health

The house committee felt a keen responsibility towards the health of the general public and the records of the response to outbreaks of contagion, such as cholera (below), provide us with first-hand accounts of the perceived health risks of the time. Clearly the governors and staff did not view their responsibilities as beginning and ending at the hospital door, but rather saw their role extending to research, prevention and education in matters of public health.

Rabies was of major concern in the early 1800s and by the 1830s had become a class issue, perceived to be linked to the way in which the poor treated their dogs (Pemberton and Worboys 2007, 6, 26). Outbreaks of rabies occurred in 1810 and the summer of 1825 (Fig 41). At the time of the latter episode, the minute books recorded that a number of stray dogs with suspected rabies had been identified in the neighbourhood of the hospital. One person had died from their wounds, another had been admitted to the hospital with 'hydrophobia' and a further six patients had been admitted with dog bites. As well as treating those immediately affected, the surgeons wrote a report that they asked should be passed to the Secretary of State (RLH, LH/A/5/18, 39–40).

The confinement of people in close quarters inevitably creates an increased risk of disease transmission. Whilst the admissions policy of the London Hospital was designed to mitigate against such risks (Chapter 5.3), the possibility of fever epidemics was a very real fear for the institutions of the 19th century. Typhus fever was a continual threat to public health as it is spread by lice and thrives in crowded conditions such as those provided in prisons (it was also known as gaol fever) and hospitals (Lane 2001, 143–4). A report of an inquest held in June 1820 notes that the victim, Antonio Dosser, was brought in to the London Hospital with a wound to his nose (inflicted by Sophia Brandy). Having apparently recovered from the wound and a resultant fever, he later died of typhus fever, presumably contracted on the wards (*Old Bailey Proc*, June 1820, Sophia Brandy (t18200628-39)). The hospital was well aware of the problems of disease and had measures in place to deal with the threat of epidemics, specifically the isolation of patients.

Concern for public health was not limited to infectious disease. In February 1830 the committee 'ordered that the overseer of Walthamstow be informed that an Apprentice from his Parish had been sent to the Hospital with diseased legs and had stated that he had suffered very cruel usage from his master' (RLH, LH/A/5/18, 307). Drug and alcohol addiction and misuse were also of concern and when in 1832 a Mr Gordon wrote to the committee regarding a patient named Harriet Sims, who had been admitted with (presumably deliberate and self-inflicted) arsenic poisoning, having bought the drug whilst 'intoxicated', the committee decided to pass his letter, expressing concern that the druggists in Lambeth were prepared

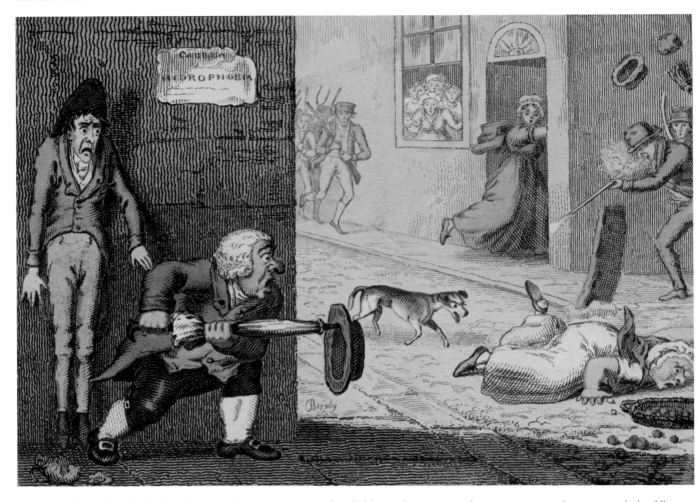

Fig 41 Mad dog, *coloured etching by Thomas L Busby, 1826; citizens attack a rabid dog, on the run in a London street, as it approaches a woman who has fallen over* (Wellcome Library, London, L0048997)

to sell poisons to someone in such a state, to the Lambeth police (RLH, LH/A/5/19, 427–8). The hospital also took a lead in matters of public health when on 9 December 1830 they resolved to use sweeps only from the Society for the Prevention of the use of Climbing Boys (RLH, LH/A/5/18, 393).

The cholera epidemic of 1832

Perhaps the greatest threat to British public health in the early 19th century was the introduction of cholera, and as the first epidemic unfolded the London Hospital played a key role. When the disease arrived on British shores it was poorly understood. Some even doubted its existence, believing that it was a creation of the authorities to frighten the poor into hospitals, where they could be experimented on in life or after death (Richardson 2001, 227).

Cholera reached England for the first time in 1831 (Allen 2008, 10), and the danger was recognised early on by those at the London Hospital. On 27 October 1831 William Blizard wrote a paper recommending a course of action should cholera morbus reach England (RLH, LH/A/5/19, 133). The state was also keenly aware of the impending disaster and on 12 November Charles Greville, clerk of the Privy Council,

requested that the hospital should tell the Lords of the Privy Council what provision they had made to cope with a cholera outbreak. The hospital was also to notify Privy Council of any suspicious illness. The hospital responded by deciding that extra cases (with the exception of accidents) should be examined in the waiting hall, to provide a method of screening before admission (ibid, 145–6). In January 1832 the resolution was made that cholera patients could not be admitted (reinforcing the statement in the existing by-laws) and that this information was to be passed to the local authorities (ibid, 186). The hospital again wrote to the surrounding parishes to ask where cholera cases should be sent. Some replied to say that arrangements had been made at parish workhouses (Clark-Kennedy 1962, 234–5).

On 5 January 1832 a letter was received from Dr Frederic(k) Cobb, a physician at the London Hospital, remarking that the information on cholera in Newcastle was not sufficient. The committee resolved to send Cobb north and to write to the Board of Health requesting assistance (RLH, LH/A/5/19, 168–9). Cobb returned to report back to the hospital on 26 January and the hospital decided to print 250 copies of his report (ibid, 180). Following Cobb's report, the hospital resolved to dedicate a separate, isolation ward for cholera cases to mitigate against the accidental introduction of the disease (ibid, 196). If a case of cholera were to be identified, infected patients would be moved to the attic above Harrison ward and, if necessary, the east end of the room that was formerly the library (ibid, 199, 204, 208). On 21 June 1832, the apothecary was charged with the duty of visiting the wards twice a day (at 10am and 8–10pm) and reporting immediately to the house governor, William Valentine, should any disease resembling cholera appear, so that 'persons so affected may be at once removed to the ward which has … been appointed to the reception of such cases' (ibid, 266–7). In September 1832, the committee also wrote to Tower Hamlets Commission of Sewers asking for a new main drain to be constructed in Whitechapel High Street on the grounds of the current prevalence of disease (ibid, 310).

The response to the threat of a cholera epidemic provides us with evidence of the perceived catchment area of the London Hospital, the governors requesting in January 1832 that the information on the changes to their admissions policy be passed to the authorities in Tower Hamlets and east of a line from London bridge to Shoreditch church and to Stratford (RLH, LH/A/5/19, 186). A list of churches to whom the cholera circular was to be sent stretched from St Magnus London bridge, to St Mary Haggerston and St Martin Wanstead, though the majority lay in the East End (ibid, 199–200). Part of Whitechapel workhouse had been set aside for cholera patients. The hospital wished to send their afflicted patients to the workhouse, but was reminded that only people from the parish of Whitechapel would be accepted (ibid, 201). Accommodation was also provided at Wapping, Leyton, Walthamstow and Stratford workhouses and, in March 1832, the parish authorities of Barking, Shoreditch and Spitalfields wrote to inform the hospital to say that they were also able to provide space for cholera patients from their parishes (ibid, 203, 210).

In spite of the resolution forbidding the admission of patients suffering from cholera, it is likely that many were in fact admitted with the disease. In 1832 there was a sharp rise in the number of extra cases admitted by the physicians: 322 extra compared with 162 in 1831 and 158 in 1833 (RLH, LH/A/15/1–21) (Chapter 5.3). The mortality rate within the hospital also rose to 13.5% (Fig 42), and there was an accompanying rise in the cost incurred by the hospital for burying patients unclaimed by relatives or friends (Fig 16).

In the end over 11,000 cases were reported in London, of which half were fatal (Clark-Kennedy 1962, 235), but it seems that the preparations paid off. On 15 November 1832, the committee recorded that cholera had 'disappeared' (RLH, LH/A/5/19, 365). Meanwhile the hospital had received a letter from the Board of Health suggesting that as long as the house was kept clean, cholera cases could be admitted, as the precautions already in use to stop the spread of typhus would be sufficient (ibid, 367).

The archaeological excavations found no evidence of the mass burial of fever victims. Deposits of lime were found (Chapter 3.1), perhaps connected to the belief in 'bad airs' as methods of disease transmission, but they do not directly relate

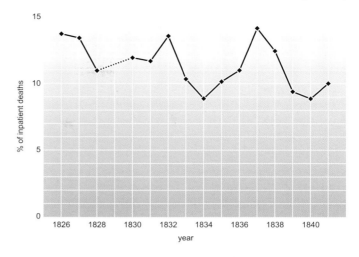

Fig 42 *Mortality rate for inpatients, compiled from the figures published in the annual reports (RLH, LH/A/15/1–21) (data for 1829 not available)*

to cholera prevention; lime and limewashes were also used as a precautionary measure during times of epidemic (Hempel 2006, 40). However, fear of the disease did affect the way in which the dead were treated. In February 1832, in the wake of concerns about cholera, Dr Archibald Billing requested better regulations for post-mortem examination, adding a clause to the standing order that stated that no body should be removed within 24 hours and that the permission of the medical officer in charge of the patient was needed (RLH, LH/A/5/19, 197, 205, 208).

In 1848 there was another outbreak of cholera. In common with other hospitals, the London made provision for admitting cases and ordered first that the attics, followed by two other wards, be made ready. It was soon realised that if all cholera cases were admitted they would take over the hospital, and so it was decided that when 10% of all the patients were cholera patients (*c* 40 cases) no more should be admitted. There were 6644 fatal cases in London during this epidemic (Clark-Kennedy 1963, 20).

During the 1866 cholera epidemic, which killed *c* 8000 Londoners, the London Hospital accepted 586 cases of cholera and 279 of choleratic diarrhoea, of which 301 and 26 respectively died. Others were treated as outpatients (Clark-Kennedy 1963, 47). The staff of the hospital experimented with numerous noxious treatments, none of which proved effective (Hempel 2006, 269).

Typhus

As deadly as the 1832 cholera epidemic, typhus fever is thought to have caused in the region of 28,000 deaths in England and Wales between 1837 and 1838, with several thousand of these occurring in London (Kohn 2008, 107). In June 1837 *The Times* reported that owing to the prevalence of typhus fever amongst the poor in several areas of London, the London Fever Hospital at King's Cross was now so full that it had been compelled to turn patients away (*The Times*, 10 June

1837, issue 16439, p 6, col A).

Although the London Hospital generally excluded patients suffering from infectious disease (Chapter 5.5), a peak in the number of deaths and burials during 1837 (Fig 16), together with circumstantial evidence from the minutes of the house committee for the presence of cases of typhus within the hospital, suggests that an outbreak of typhus at the London had more devastating effects than the cholera epidemic of 1832. In December 1837 three of the physicians wrote to ask the house committee for some remuneration for Catherine Briggs, the assistant nurse in the attic – the location of the fever wards (RLH, LH/A/5/19, 324) – for her good conduct under circumstances of extra fatigue and responsibility. The matron was asked to give her £1 or £2 (RLH, LH/A/5/22, 36), and a payment of £5 was also made to Jane Holloway, the widow of the hospital's labourer, who had died of a fever after a few days' illness (ibid, 37).

Unlike the cholera epidemic of 1832, there was only a small rise in the number of extra cases admitted by the physicians during 1837, but there were many more deaths and the mortality rate rose to 14.1%. This may indicate that in contrast to the cholera epidemic, many patients contracted typhus after admission. Given that the disease is spread by lice (Roberts and Cox 2003, 338), and the hospital had a problem with sanitation of the beds (Chapter 5.8), this is perhaps not surprising. It would also explain why in December 1837 Dr Frampton Jr was asked to attend the committee in order to be questioned about a case of his who had been admitted suffering from rheumatism, but had died several days later of typhus fever (RLH, LH/A/5/22, 39).

4.2 Osteological evidence of health and disease in the buried population

Natasha Powers and Don Walker

The detailed examination of the human remains revealed evidence of the ailments and injuries suffered by those people when alive. This chapter presents the results of analysis in comparison to other contemporary groups and hospital

assemblages and discusses the implications of the patterns seen. Further discussion of specific aspects of the health of the assemblage can be found in subsequent chapters (eg, Chapters 5.7, 5.11, 7.8). Crude prevalence rates of disease (number of individuals affected as a percentage of the total individuals) were applied to the primary inhumation sample only (Table 12). This prevented the potential for 'double counting' of a condition where an individual might have been divided into several portions that were interred in separate graves, or could not be confidently reassociated.

Dental health

Dental disease affected 51 male (51/80: 63.8%), 19 female (19/30: 63.3%) and four subadult (4/13: 30.8%) primary inhumations – 45.7% of the primary inhumations in total (79/173) (Table 23). All three dentitions containing deciduous teeth (all primary inhumations) were affected: two by calculus (7/32 deciduous teeth; 21.9%) and caries (9/32: 28.1%) and one tooth position with periodontal disease (1/50 tooth positions; 2.0%). The periodontal disease and one instance of calculus were in retained teeth in the mandible of adult female [386]. All deciduous teeth have been included in calculations of prevalence rates in this section.

True prevalence rates for the articulated assemblage (calculated by tooth or tooth socket as appropriate) can be seen in Table 24. For all conditions, overall differences between males and females in both true and crude prevalence rates were small, with the exception of the crude prevalence of caries and periapical lesions.

Ante-mortem tooth loss affected 24.7% of tooth positions with a crude prevalence rate of 38.2% of the primary inhumations, somewhat lower than the crude prevalence rate of 57.3% (51/89) reported for the articulated burials at Newcastle Infirmary (Boulter et al 1998, 69). Elderly males [408] and [492] and 26–35-year-old female [452] were edentulous.

In common with most skeletal assemblages, all dental disease showed an increased true prevalence rate with age, up to 36–45 years, with a subsequent decline largely a product of the great increase in ante-mortem tooth loss (Fig 43).

In total, 39.9% of the primary inhumations from the London had suffered caries, compared to 57.3% of the articulated burials from Newcastle Infirmary (51/89) (Boulter et al 1998, 66).

Table 23 Crude prevalence rate of dental disease in the primary inhumations

	n	Ante-mortem tooth loss	%	Caries	%	Calculus	%	Periodontal disease	%	Periapical lesions	%	Enamel hypoplasia	%
Male	80	45	56.3	43	53.8	50	62.5	47	58.8	10	12.5	31	38.8
Female	30	18	60.0	19	63.3	18	60.0	19	63.3	1	3.3	11	36.7
Subadult	13	0	-	4	30.8	3	23.1	1	7.7	0	-	1	7.7
All adult	160	66	41.3	65	40.6	73	45.6	70	43.8	12	7.5	47	29.4
All primary inhumations	173	66	38.2	69	39.9	76	43.9	71	41.0	12	6.9	48	27.7

Table 24 True prevalence rate of dental disease in the articulated assemblage

	No. of teeth	No. of sockets	Ante-mortem tooth loss	%	Caries	%	Calculus	%	Periodontal disease	%	Periapical lesions	%	Enamel hypoplasia	%
Primary inhumations														
Male	1049	1593	354	22.2	176	16.8	879	83.8	667	41.9	15	0.9	168	16.0
Female	367	596	175	29.4	80	21.8	307	83.7	230	38.6	1	0.2	52	14.2
Subadult	75	116	0	-	18	24.0	14	18.7	2	1.7	0	-	6	8.0
All adult	1483	2314	559	24.2	262	17.7	1241	83.7	914	39.5	18	0.8	235	15.8
Total	1558	2430	559	23.0	280	18.0	1255	80.6	916	37.7	18	0.7	241	15.5
Portions														
Male	99	280	111	39.6	18	18.2	65	65.7	51	18.2	1	0.4	21	21.2
Female	71	172	66	38.4	17	23.9	57	80.3	60	34.9	3	1.7	13	18.3
Subadult	1	29	0	-	0	-	0	-	0	-	0	-	0	-
All adult	243	572	191	33.4	47	19.3	178	73.3	143	25.0	4	0.7	53	21.8
Total	244	601	191	31.8	47	19.3	178	73.0	143	23.8	4	0.7	53	21.7
Total														
Male	1148	1873	465	24.8	194	16.9	944	82.2	718	38.3	16	0.9	189	16.5
Female	438	768	241	31.4	97	22.1	364	83.1	290	37.8	4	0.5	65	14.8
Subadult	76	145	0	-	18	23.7	14	18.4	2	1.4	0	-	6	7.9
All adult	1726	2886	750	26.0	309	17.9	1419	82.2	1057	36.6	22	0.8	288	16.7
Grand total	1802	3031	750	24.7	327	18.1	1433	79.5	1059	34.9	22	0.7	294	16.3

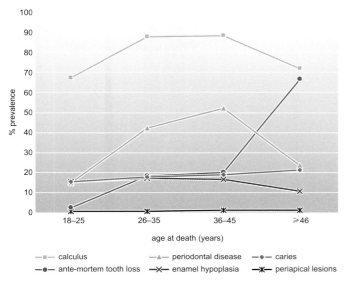

Fig 43 True prevalence rate of dental disease by adult age at death in the articulated assemblage

Twelve male portions, eight female portions and one subadult portion were also affected. Buccal and root caries affected the molar and premolar teeth of 36–45-year-old male [147] and may indicate that he practised a particularly abrasive regime of dental hygiene. The overall true prevalence rate of dental caries was 18.1%; 17.9% of the adult teeth and 23.7% of subadult teeth were affected. In comparison, adult caries rates of 12.2% (true prevalence rate) and subadult rates of 8.9% were reported at the Greenwich Naval Hospital cemetery, with a total true prevalence rate of 11.7% (Boston et al 2008).

Severe carious lesions were present in the maxillary incisors of 1–5-year-old [454]. Destruction focused on the centre of the buccal crowns and the symmetrical distribution suggests that they may have been caused by the use of a comforter or nursing bottle containing sweetened, erosive or sugar-rich foods (Julia Beaumont, pers comm).

Calculus, deposits of mineralised plaque, affected 43.9% of the primary inhumations, again a smaller proportion than seen at Newcastle (61/89: 68.5%) (Boulter et al 1998, 72). A large proportion of calculus deposits (1178/1433: 82.2%) were located below the gum line (subgingival). Such deposits have a clear relationship to rates of periodontal disease (Hillson 1996, 260), but a comparatively low number (34.9%) of tooth positions were affected by this latter condition.

Enamel hypoplasia affected 47 adult primary inhumations and one subadult (Table 23). Of the 294 affected teeth, 17.3% of the enamel defects were located in the cusp third of the tooth, 51.4% in the middle third and 31.3% in the neck third. 12–17-year-old [122] had grey discoloration of the occlusal half of the crowns of the molars and premolars and some of the other teeth. The molar teeth were all badly affected by caries. It is possible, therefore, that the discoloration was due to enamel that was poorly formed as a result of illness and/or malnourishment during growth. Alternatively, the enamel may have been weakened by regular immersion in an acidic environment such as would be created by particular feeding practices or food or by persistent vomiting. The crude prevalence rate of enamel hypoplasia (27.7%) was once again considerably lower than that found in the articulated burials at Newcastle Infirmary (42/89: 47.2%) (Boulter et al 1998, 75). In contrast, 41.0% of the primary inhumations at the London had suffered from periodontal disease whereas this figure was only 10.1% (9/89) for the articulated individuals from Newcastle (ibid, 74).

Just 0.7% of tooth positions (a crude prevalence rate of 6.9%

Table 25 Dental disease in the disarticulated assemblage

	Total present	Caries n	Caries %	Calculus n	Calculus %	Periodontal disease n	Periodontal disease %	Enamel hypoplasia n	Enamel hypoplasia %	Periapical lesion n	Periapical lesion %	Ante-mortem tooth loss n	Ante-mortem tooth loss %
Male	80	45	56.3	43	53.8	50	62.5	47	58.8	10	12.5	31	38.8
R mandible	93	22	23.7	18	19.4	13	14.0	10	10.8	4	4.3	15	16.1
L mandible	95	24	25.3	22	23.2	16	16.8	10	10.5	4	4.2	17	17.9
R maxilla	63	10	15.9	9	14.3	11	17.5	5	7.9	2	3.2	11	17.5
L maxilla	73	15	20.5	9	12.3	10	13.7	5	6.8	3	4.1	11	15.1
Total elements	324	71	21.9	58	17.9	50	15.4	30	9.3	13	4.0	54	16.7

of primary inhumations) had periapical lesions, a surprisingly low figure considering the relatively high rate of caries and, once again, lower than the crude prevalence rate for the articulated burials at Newcastle (15/89: 16.9%) (Boulter et al 1998, 70). As the result of the formation of an abscess, a deep periodontal pocket (maximum 15.1mm) was present alongside the left mandibular premolars of 36–45-year-old male [340].

Loose and unassociated teeth from the disarticulated sample were not catalogued. Dental disease was instead quantified by bone element affected (Table 25). Although this method does not allow direct comparison with the true or crude prevalence rates from the remaining assemblage, the rates of dental disease were consistently high. Caries affected 30 groups of associated disarticulated elements (eg, a complete mandible), including eight males and two females and an example of rampant caries in an adult mandible from [568]; calculus affected 32 (five male); periodontal disease 26 (nine male, one female); enamel hypoplasia 16 (five male, one intermediate adult and one 12–17-year-old); periapical lesions six (one female); and ante-mortem tooth loss 35 (17 male, 3 female and one intermediate adult). Two impacted molars, one maxillary and one mandibular, were also noted and a fracture noted in the right third mandibular molar of remains from [225].

Although no evidence of dental treatment and no dental prostheses were found in the assemblage, 18–25-year-old male portion [542], in which the right maxilla had been sawn, had an unusual horizontal groove in the buccal and distal cementoenamel junction (CEJ) of the first right mandibular premolar and wear on the adjacent canine. It is possible that this was caused by the wearing of a bridge with a false tooth in the position of the first molar (Fig 44).

Pipe facets

Rounded facets form in the teeth as a result of the habitual clamping of clay pipe stems between the jaws; tobacco may also stain the teeth. Previous work on the 19th-century east London burial ground of the Catholic Mission of St Mary and St Michael, Whitechapel (London borough of Tower Hamlets), explored methods of recording and analysing smoking in skeletal human remains (Walker and Henderson 2010) and these methods were repeated here. Pipe facets or notches were identified in

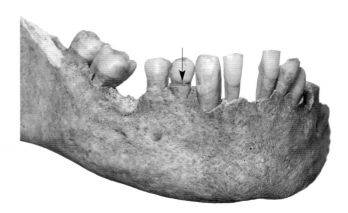

Fig 44 Groove (arrowed) in the mandibular premolar of 18–25-year-old male portion [542] (scale c 1:1)

15.6% (25/160) of adult primary inhumations, while brown staining on the lingual aspects of the teeth, possibly the result of smoking, was found in 27 (16.9%) (Table 26). Only adults were affected, with a male:female ratio of 5.3:1.

Four further examples (two male) were identified from the disarticulated assemblage and originated from contexts [372], [494], [257] and [402].

Individuals with pipe facets and staining were combined in an attempt to identify smokers, and thus facilitate comparison with non-smokers from the London, as well as from the St Mary and St Michael sample (Table 27). A greater number of individuals, and particularly males, were affected at St Mary and St Michael.

When mortality rates were compared (Fig 45), male smokers

Table 26 Crude prevalence rate of pipe facet and dental (lingual) staining in the primary inhumations

	n	Pipe facet n	Pipe facet %	Lingual stain n	Lingual stain %	Facets & stains n	Facets & stains %
Adults	160	25	15.6	27	16.9	22	13.8
Females	30	4	13.3	4	13.3	3	10.0
Males	80	19	23.8	21	26.3	17	21.3

Table 27 Crude prevalence rate of smokers at the London Hospital and at St Mary and St Michael

| | London Hospital | | | St Mary & St Michael | | |
	n	Smokers	%	n	Smokers	%
Adults	160	30	18.8	268	65	24.3
Females	30	5	16.7	105	6	5.7
Males	80	23	28.8	143	59	41.3
Total	173	30	17.3	705	65	9.2

died more frequently between the ages of 26 and 35 years than non-smokers (χ^2 = 3.81, df = 1, p≤ 0.05). When all aged adults were considered, the same was true between 26 and 45 years of age (χ^2 = 13.25, df = 1, p≤ 0.000).

Evidence of smoking was also seen in the disarticulated material, with the dentitions from four individuals (including two males) displaying pipe notches and one female with lingual staining ([284]).

Infectious disease

Periosteal lesions

Periosteal lesions result from inflammation of the soft-tissue layer of periosteum encasing the shafts of long bones (periostitis). In many cases there is insufficient evidence to assign such changes to a specific disease. Although frequently identified as a reaction to infection and hence included in this section of the text, periosteal lesions can also be associated with neoplastic disease, trauma, scurvy, venous stasis and secondary hypertrophic osteoarthropathy (Resnick 2002, 4884; Ortner 2003, 88).

The crude prevalence rate of primary inhumations affected

by non-specific periosteal changes was 32.9% (57/173). This included 23.1% (3/13) of subadults and 33.8% (54/160) of adults: 35% of males (28/80), 33% of females (10/30). There was no significant difference observed between the sexes. All cases involved periosteal lesions only. When compared with other near-contemporary sites in east London, the adult sample from the London Hospital was found to have a similar crude prevalence rate to Bow Baptist church but a statistically lower rate than the burial ground of the Catholic Mission of St Mary and St Michael, Whitechapel (χ^2 = 4.41, df = 1, p≤ 0.04) (Henderson et al in prep) (Table 28). The crude prevalence rate of non-specific periosteal change at the London Hospital was twice that seen amongst the articulated burials at Newcastle Infirmary (35/210: 16.7%) (Boulter et al 1998, 87).

True prevalence rates of periosteal lesions for the entire articulated assemblage (primary inhumations and portions) can be seen in Tables 29–31. While extensive variation between the

Table 28 Comparison of the crude prevalence rate of periosteal lesions in the primary inhumations with two other excavated east London samples

| | | Periosteal lesions | |
	n	n	%
London Hospital			
Subadults	13	3	23.1
Adults	160	54	33.8
Total	173	57	32.9
St Mary & St Michael			
Subadults	437	49	11.2
Adults	268	118	44.0
Total	705	167	23.7
Bow Baptist church			
Subadults	202	21	10.4
Adults	214	63	29.4
Total	416	84	20.2

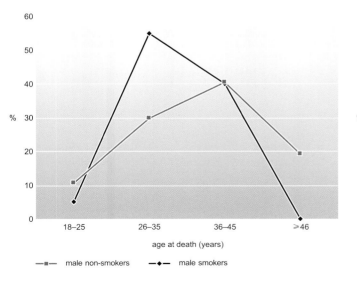

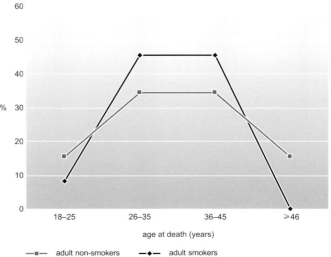

Fig 45 Mortality profiles of (left) males and (right) all adults with evidence of smoking compared to those with no evidence of smoking

Table 29 True prevalence rate of cranial non-specific periostitis in the articulated assemblage

		Female			Male			Adult			Subadult			All individuals		
		n	Affected	%	n	Affected	%	n	Affected	%	n	Affected	%	n	Affected	%
Primary inhumations																
Parietal	R	19	0	-	55	0	-	79	0	-	6	0	-	85	0	-
	L	19	0	-	56	0	-	80	I	1.3	6	0	-	86	I	1.2
	total	38	0	-	111	0	-	159	I	0.6	12	0	-	171	I	0.6
Petrous temporal	R	20	0	-	53	0	-	78	0	-	5	0	-	83	0	-
	L	19	0	-	52	I	1.9	75	0	-	5	0	-	80	0	-
	total	39	0	-	105	I	1.0	153	0	-	10	0	-	163	0	-
Zygomatic	R	18	0	-	49	I	2.0	71	I	1.4	4	0	-	75	I	1.3
	L	18	0	-	50	0	-	72	0	-	2	0	-	74	0	-
	total	36	0	-	99	I	1.0	143	I	0.7	6	0	-	149	I	0.7
Maxilla	R	18	I	5.6	49	2	4.1	72	3	4.2	2	0	-	74	3	4.1
	L	19	I	5.3	50	4	8.0	73	5	6.8	3	0	-	76	5	6.6
	total	37	2	5.4	99	6	6.1	145	8	5.5	5	0	-	150	8	5.3
Mandible	R	20	0	-	54	0	-	79	0	-	5	0	-	84	0	-
	L	20	I	5.0	51	0	-	76	I	1.3	6	0	-	82	I	1.2
	total	40	I	2.5	105	0	-	155	I	0.6	11	0	-	166	I	0.6
Portions																
Mandible	R	6	0	-	7	2	28.6	17	2	11.8	2	0	-	19	2	10.5
	L	7	I	14.3	10	0	-	22	I	4.5	I	0	-	23	I	4.3
	total	13	I	7.7	17	2	11.8	39	3	7.7	3	0	-	42	3	7.1

Table 30 True prevalence rate of long-bone non-specific periostitis in the articulated assemblage

		Female			Male			Adult			Subadult			All individuals		
		n	Affected	%	n	Affected	%	n	Affected	%	n	Affected	%	n	Affected	%
Primary inhumations																
Clavicle	R	21	0	-	58	I	1.7	99	I	1.0	11	0	-	110	I	0.9
	L	22	0	-	63	I	1.6	106	I	0.9	10	I	10.0	116	2	1.7
	total	43	0	-	121	2	1.7	205	2	1.0	21	I	4.8	226	3	1.3
Humerus	R	24	0	-	58	I	1.7	104	2	1.9	11	2	18.2	115	4	3.5
	L	25	0	-	64	0	-	111	0	-	12	2	16.7	123	2	1.6
	total	49	0	-	122	I	0.8	215	2	0.9	23	4	17.4	238	6	2.5
Radius	R	23	0	-	62	I	1.6	101	I	1.0	7	0	-	108	I	0.9
	L	23	0	-	58	I	1.7	99	I	1.0	10	0	-	109	I	0.9
	total	46	0	-	120	2	1.7	200	2	1.0	17	0	-	217	2	0.9
Ulna	R	22	0	-	64	I	1.6	103	2	1.9	8	0	-	111	2	1.8
	L	23	0	-	57	I	1.8	99	2	2.0	11	I	9.1	110	3	2.7
	total	45	0	-	121	2	1.7	202	4	2.0	19	I	5.3	221	5	2.3
Femur	R	26	2	7.7	67	7	10.4	108	11	10.2	10	2	20.0	118	13	11.0
	L	25	I	4.0	64	7	10.9	106	11	10.4	9	0	-	115	11	9.6
	total	51	3	5.9	131	14	10.7	214	22	10.3	19	2	10.5	233	24	10.3
Tibia	R	25	4	16.0	55	15	27.3	105	28	26.7	11	I	9.1	116	29	25.0
	L	22	2	9.1	58	12	20.7	104	21	20.2	9	I	11.1	113	22	19.5
	total	47	6	12.8	113	27	23.9	209	49	23.4	20	2	10.0	229	51	22.3
Fibula	R	22	I	4.5	53	7	13.2	99	12	12.1	10	0	-	109	12	11.0
	L	22	2	9.1	52	8	15.4	98	14	14.3	7	0	-	105	14	13.3
	total	44	3	6.8	105	15	14.3	197	26	13.2	17	0	-	214	26	12.1
Portions																
Clavicle	R	3	0	-	13	0	-	39	I	2.6	3	0	-	42	I	2.4
	L	2	0	-	9	0	-	36	0	-	6	0	-	42	0	-
	total	5	0	-	22	0	-	75	I	1.3	9	0	-	84	I	1.2
Humerus	R	I	0	-	11	0	-	57	I	1.8	7	0	-	64	I	1.6
	L	2	0	-	8	0	-	63	0	-	6	0	-	69	0	-
	total	3	0	-	19	0	-	120	I	0.8	13	0	-	133	I	0.8
Radius	R	I	0	-	11	0	-	56	0	-	7	0	-	63	0	-
	L	2	0	-	8	0	-	65	I	1.5	5	0	-	70	I	1.4
	total	3	0	-	19	0	-	121	I	0.8	12	0	-	133	I	0.8
Ulna	R	I	0	-	11	0	-	58	2	3.4	6	0	-	64	2	3.1
	L	2	0	-	9	0	-	67	4	6.0	5	0	-	72	4	5.6
	total	3	0	-	20	0	-	125	6	4.8	11	0	-	136	6	4.4

Table 30 (cont)

		Female			Male			Adult			Subadult			All individuals		
		n	Affected	%	n	Affected	%	n	Affected	%	n	Affected	%	n	Affected	%
Femur	R	10	1	10.0	33	2	6.1	65	6	9.2	5	0	-	70	6	8.6
	L	5	0	-	27	3	11.1	51	5	9.8	4	0	-	55	5	9.1
	total	15	1	6.7	60	5	8.3	116	11	9.5	9	0	-	125	11	8.8
Tibia	R	1	0	-	15	5	33.3	60	20	33.3	3	1	33.3	63	21	33.3
	L	3	0	-	17	3	17.6	52	16	30.8	3	0	-	55	16	29.1
	total	4	0	-	32	8	25.0	112	36	32.1	6	1	16.7	118	37	31.4
Fibula	R	1	0	-	13	4	30.8	52	15	28.8	2	0	-	54	15	27.8
	L	2	0	-	17	2	11.8	50	11	22.0	2	0	-	52	11	21.2
	total	3	0	-	30	6	20.0	102	26	25.5	4	0	-	106	26	24.5

Table 31 True prevalence rate of appendages and other bones non-specific periostitis in the articulated assemblage

		Female			Male			Adult			Subadult			All individuals		
		n	Affected	%	n	Affected	%	n	Affected	%	n	Affected	%	n	Affected	%
Primary inhumations																
L scapula	R glenoid	20	0	-	57	2	3.5	95	0	-	9	0	-	78	0	-
	R coracoid	13	0	-	45	0	-	69	0	-	0	0	-	83	0	-
	R acromion	16	0	-	51	1	2.0	83	1	1.2	8	0	-	91	1	1.1
	R blade	21	0	-	57	1	1.8	99	2	2.0	9	0	-	108	2	1.9
	total	70	0	-	210	4	1.9	346	3	0.9	26	0	-	26	3	11.5
Sternum	manubrium	20	0	-	51	1	2.0	82	1	1.2	5	0	-	87	1	1.1
	sternal body	17	0	-	47	1	2.1	75	1	1.3	2	0	-	77	1	1.3
Ribs	R	239	6	2.5	647	35	5.4	1058	46	4.3	72	0	-	1130	46	4.1
	L	227	4	1.8	652	25	3.8	1065	29	2.7	89	0	-	1154	29	2.5
	unsided	2	0	-	7	0	-	13	0	-	11	0	-	24	0	-
	total	468	10	2.1	1306	60	4.6	2136	75	3.5	172	0	-	2308	75	3.2
Ilium	R	27	0	-	70	1	1.4	107	1	0.9	10	1	10.0	117	2	1.7
	L	27	0	-	69	0	-	108	0	-	11	1	9.1	119	1	0.8
Pubis	R	16	0	-	38	1	2.6	55	1	1.8	2	0	-	57	1	1.8
R hand	1st metacarpal	17	0	-	52	1	1.9	79	1	1.3	6	0	-	85	1	1.2
	2nd metacarpal	22	0	-	55	1	1.8	88	1	1.1	7	0	-	95	1	1.1
	3rd metacarpal	21	0	-	55	0	-	88	0	-	5	0	-	93	0	-
	4th metacarpal	21	0	-	51	0	-	85	0	-	5	0	-	90	0	-
	5th metacarpal	18	0	-	53	0	-	83	0	-	3	0	-	86	0	-
	total	99	0	-	266	2	0.8	423	2	0.5	26	0	-	449	2	0.4
R foot	R calcaneus	22	0	-	50	1	-	95	1	1.1	2	0	-	97	1	1.0
	1st metatarsal	18	0	-	42	0	-	82	0	-	7	0	-	89	1	1.1
	2nd metatarsal	19	1	5.3	44	0	-	82	1	1.2	8	0	-	90	0	-
	3rd metatarsal	18	0	-	41	0	-	78	0	-	5	0	-	83	1	1.2
	4th metatarsal	19	0	-	41	1	2.4	75	1	1.3	4	0	-	79	2	2.5
	5th metatarsal	22	0	-	44	1	2.3	87	2	2.3	6	0	-	93	0	-
	total	96	1	1.0	212	2	0.9	404	4	1.0	30	0	-	434	4	0.9
L foot	L calcaneus	17	0	-	45	1	2.2	83	1	1.2	4	0	-	87	1	1.1
	1st metatarsal	18	0	-	48	0	-	89	0	-	5	0	-	94	1	1.1
	2nd metatarsal	17	1	5.9	45	0	-	83	1	1.2	7	0	-	90	2	2.2
	3rd metatarsal	17	1	5.9	42	1	2.4	80	2	2.5	6	0	-	86	1	1.2
	4th metatarsal	16	0	-	45	1	2.2	81	1	1.2	4	0	-	85	3	3.5
	5th metatarsal	15	0	-	43	1	2.3	81	3	3.7	5	0	-	86	1	1.2
	total	83	2	2.4	223	3	1.3	414	7	1.7	27	0	-	441	8	1.8
Portions																
Sacrum	3	11	1	9.1	38	0	-	64	1	-	1	0	-	65	1	1.5
	4	10	1	10.0	34	0	-	55	1	-	1	0	-	56	1	1.8
	total	21	2	9.5	72	0	-	119	2	-	2	0	-	121	2	1.7
Ribs	R	62	5	8.1	146	26	17.8	522	38	7.3	63	0	-	585	38	6.5
	L	62	8	12.9	164	8	4.9	532	35	6.6	49	0	-	581	35	6.0
	unsided	0	0	-	1	0	-	55	0	-	7	0	-	62	0	-
	total	124	13	10.5	311	34	10.9	1109	73	6.6	119	0	-	1228	73	5.9
Ilium	R	13	1	7.7	42	0	-	63	1	1.6	4	0	-	67	1	1.5
	L	9	0	-	36	0	-	54	0	-	5	0	-	59	0	-
	total	22	1	4.5	78	0	-	117	1	0.9	9	0	-	126	1	0.8

Table 31 (cont)

		Female			Male			Adult			Subadult			All individuals		
		n	Affected	%	n	Affected	%	n	Affected	%	n	Affected	%	n	Affected	%
Pubis	R	8	1	12.5	28	0	-	38	1	2.6	0	0	-	38	1	2.6
L hand	1st metacarpal	1	0	-	3	0	-	25	0	-	2	0	-	27	0	-
	2nd metacarpal	2	1	50.0	4	0	-	35	1	2.9	2	0	-	37	1	2.7
	3rd metacarpal	1	0	-	5	0	-	37	0	-	2	0	-	39	0	-
	4th metacarpal	1	0	-	4	0	-	30	0	-	2	0	-	32	0	-
	5th metacarpal	1	0	-	4	0	-	29	0	-	2	0	-	31	0	-
	total	6	1	16.7	20	0	-	156	1	0.6	10	0	-	166	1	0.6

two samples was absent, where there was variation the portions revealed higher true prevalence rates. When right and left sides were combined, tibiae from the portions (37/118: 31.4%) were more frequently affected than those from the primary inhumations (51/229: 22.3%). The same difference was observed in the fibulae, and to a statistically significant extent – primary inhumations: 26/214, 12.1%; portions 26/106, 24.5%; χ^2 = 7.98, df = 1, p≤ 0.005. This pattern is discussed further in Chapter 7.8.

To test whether the nature of the assemblage, derived as it was from hospital patients, had resulted in a high rate of active non-specific periosteal change, the crude prevalence rate of active and healed bone lesions was compared. The results showed that healed lesions were more prevalent in all but subadult primary inhumations, where the sample size was extremely small (Table 32).

In the disarticulated assemblage, 4.1% (313/7571) of bone elements had lesions indicative of periosteal inflammation (including sinusitis and rib lesions). Only one subadult was affected (rib lesions, see below). In those where the nature of the bone formation could be observed, 73.8% (152/206) were noted as active at the time of death, 2.0% of the total number of disarticulated elements and a somewhat lower prevalence rate than the 5.8% noted at Worcester Royal Infirmary (Western 2010, 21).

SINUSITIS

Chronic upper respiratory infection may result in bone changes within the cranial sinuses (Roberts 2007). The data noted here were largely obtained from broken or dissected crania, and as

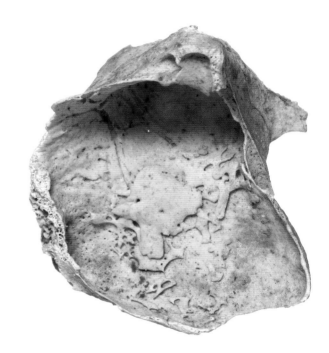

Fig 46 Maxillary sinusitis in 36–45-year-old female primary inhumation [424] (scale c 2:1)

such represent minimum prevalence rates. The crude prevalence rate of maxillary sinusitis (Fig 46) in the primary inhumation sample was 4.0% (7/173). Only sexed adults were affected – 5.4% of female maxillae (2/37) and 7.1% of male maxillae (7/99) (Table 33). In the disarticulated bone, 5.1% of maxillae were

Table 32 Crude prevalence rate of active and healed periosteal changes in the primary inhumations

		Active		Healed	
	n	n	%	n	%
Male	80	9	11.3	12	15.0
Female	30	2	6.7	6	20.0
Subadult	13	2	15.4	0	-
All adult	160	14	8.8	23	14.4
Total	173	16	9.2	23	13.3

Table 33 True prevalence rate of sinusitis in the primary inhumations

	Female			Male		
	n	Affected	%	n	Affected	%
R maxilla	18	1	5.6	49	2	4.1
L maxilla	19	1	5.3	50	4	8.0
Total	**37**	**2**	**5.4**	**99**	**6**	**6.1**
R zygomatic	18	0	-	49	1	2.0

affected (7/136); all were adult and in all instances the lesions were healed. When combined with the articulated material (9/193 maxillae; 4.7%), the overall true prevalence rate is 4.9% (16/329).

RIB LESIONS

New bone growth and/or lytic lesions on the visceral surfaces of the ribs represent non-specific pulmonary disease. Such lesions have been found in individuals with tuberculosis, neoplastic disease and secondary hypertrophic osteoarthropathy (Matos and Santos 2006, 196). They affected only adults in the articulated sample, with a crude prevalence rate for the primary inhumations of 11.3% (18/160) (Fig 47, Table 34). Four subadult ribs from the disarticulated sample were also affected and comprised remains from one individual (4/9 disarticulated subadult ribs, 44.4%) (Table 35). Of all the affected individuals, ten had active lesions (11 including the subadult), six had

mixed lesions (woven and lamellar bone) and two had healed lesions. The majority of affected disarticulated ribs also displayed woven or mixed bony lesions (62/107: 58.0%). This indicates that of those with pulmonary infections, the majority were suffering from an ongoing disease process at the time of death.

There was no statistically significant difference in true prevalence rates of rib lesions between the primary inhumations and the portions, and the higher rates seen in the disarticulated sample are a product of the smaller sample size.

The prevalence rates of rib lesions in adult primary inhumations (11.3% of individuals and 4.0% of ribs) and the overall true prevalence rate of 5.9% was low when compared to the population from St Mary and St Michael (26.5% and 8.9% respectively) but significantly higher than noted at the higher-status cemetery of St Marylebone (4.0% of adults (9/223) and 2.1% of adult ribs) (Miles et al 2008, 125) (see also Chapter 7.8).

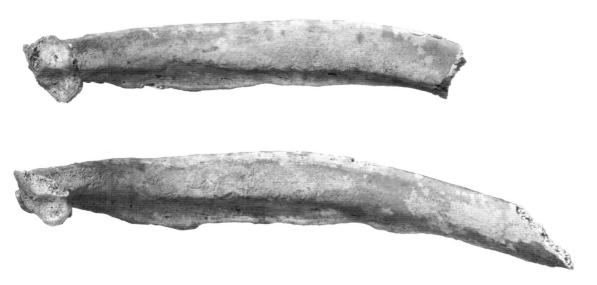

Fig 47 Woven new bone on the left ribs of 36–45-year-old probable male primary inhumation [138], indicating that a pulmonary infection was active at the time of death (scale c 1:1)

Table 34 Crude prevalence rate of rib lesions in the primary inhumations

Age	Female n	Affected	%	Male n	Affected	%	Intermediate n	Affected	%	Undetermined n	Affected	%	Subadults n	Affected	%	Adults n	Affected	%	All individuals n	Affected	%
<4 weeks	0	0	-	0	0	-	0	0	-	0	0	-	5	0	-	0	0	-	5	0	-
1–6 months	0	0	-	0	0	-	0	0	-	0	0	-	0	0	-	0	0	-	0	0	-
7–11 months	0	0	-	0	0	-	0	0	-	0	0	-	0	0	-	0	0	-	0	0	-
1–5 years	0	0	-	0	0	-	0	0	-	0	0	-	3	0	-	0	0	-	3	0	-
6–11 years	0	0	-	0	0	-	0	0	-	0	0	-	1	0	-	0	0	-	1	0	-
12–17 years	0	0	-	0	0	-	0	0	-	0	0	-	4	0	-	0	0	-	4	0	-
18–25 years	4	1	25.0	6	3	50.0	3	1	33.3	1	0	-	0	0	-	14	5	35.7	14	5	35.7
26–35 years	10	1	10.0	25	2	8.0	1	0	-	2	0	-	0	0	-	38	3	7.9	38	3	7.9
36–45 years	9	0	-	27	6	22.2	0	0	-	2	0	-	0	0	-	38	6	15.8	38	6	15.8
≥46 years	3	0	-	9	0	-	0	0	-	0	0	-	0	0	-	12	0	-	12	0	-
Adult	4	1	-	13	0	-	1	0	-	40	3	7.5	0	0	-	58	4	0	58	4	6.9
Total	30	3	10.0	80	11	13.8	5	1	20.0	45	3	6.7	13	0	-	160	18	11.3	173	18	10.4

Table 35 True prevalence rate of rib lesions

	Right			Left			Unsided			Total		
	n	Affected	%	n	Affected	%	n	Affected	%	n	Affected	%
Primary inhumations												
Adult	1058	48	4.5	1045	37	3.5	13	0	-	2116	85	4.0
Subadult	72	0	-	89	0	-	11	0	-	172	0	-
Total	1130	48	4.2	1134	37	3.3	24	0	-	2288	85	3.7
Portions												
Adult	522	38	7.3	532	35	6.6	55	0	-	1109	73	6.6
Subadult	63	0	-	49	0	-	7	0	-	119	0	-
Total	585	48	8.2	581	37	6.4	62	0	-	1228	85	6.9
Disarticulated bone												
Adult	365	45	12.3	328	50	15.2	117	8	6.8	810	103	12.7
Subadult	6	4	66.7	3	0	-	0	0	-	9	4	44.4
Total	371	48	12.9	331	37	11.2	117	8	6.8	819	85	10.4
Grand total	2086	144	6.9	2046	111	5.4	203	8	6.8	4335	255	5.9

Osteitis and osteomyelitis

Two contexts with periosteal lesions may also have had osteitis (infection of the cortical bone). The right tibia shaft of primary inhumation [423], a 36–45-year-old male, was covered by pitted and striated lamellar bone on its medial and lateral aspects, and was swollen at midshaft and along the anterior crest. The left femur of 26–35-year-old male portion [46501] was covered in a fully enclosing sleeve of mixed, pitted, woven and lamellar bone, which ended abruptly in the distal shaft, just above a sawn cut. The shaft was expanded mediolaterally and was unusually heavy.

A right femur, right mid femur and left mid and distal tibia, all from [457] in the disarticulated assemblage, also showed bony changes consistent with osteitis, affecting 0.3% of long-bone elements from the limbs (6/2090). This compares to a true prevalence rate of 11.0% noted for the long bones at Worcester Royal Infirmary (Western 2010, 21).

One primary inhumation, 36–45-year-old male [421], was affected by osteomyelitis. This was secondary to a probable compound fracture of the distal shaft of the left tibia. Both the fracture and the infection were healed, though a suboval sinus persisted in the lateral aspect of the bone. This represents 0.2% of all distal tibiae in the assemblage (1/439).

There were three examples of osteomyelitis amongst the portions. The first was from [62801], an adult of undetermined sex, and involved gross bony expansion and contour change to the proximal shaft and midshaft of a right proximal finger phalanx, possibly following an injury (1/2385 hand phalanges; <0.1%). A further adult of undetermined sex, [54802], had a healed suboval lytic lesion in the sternal end of a right rib surrounded by periosteal new bone growth (1/4148 ribs; <0.1%).

Adult male [52201], aged 18–25 years, had a grossly expanded proximal shaft of the right femur with a large, deep sub-circular pit (max Diam 13.1mm, max D 22.7mm) opening on the anterior aspect of the femoral neck and extending distally to terminate in a much smaller sub-circular opening (max Diam 6.3mm), again in the anterior proximal shaft (Figs 48–9). A further sub-circular pit was located on the inferior aspect of the anterior margin of the femoral head (max Diam 6.1mm, max D 5.1mm). The lesions were formed of mature bone and represent healed non-specific osteomyelitis with persisting cloacae. Femoral osteomyelitis can be found in cases of haematogenous spread of infection in subadults, causing fever, localised pain and swelling (De Groot et al n d). It can also follow bone fracture, but there was no evidence for this. In total 0.2% of proximal femora were affected (1/498).

Secondary osteomyelitis following a fracture was noted in a right clavicle from [343], again suggesting that the injury may have been a compound one.

Tuberculosis

Tuberculosis is an infectious disease which in humans is caused by *Mycobacterium tuberculosis* or *Mycobacterium bovis* (Aufderheide and Rodríguez-Martín 1998, 118). Symptoms, if they occur, can include weakness, breathlessness, chest pain and fever (Roberts and Buikstra 2003, 2). Tuberculosis was a significant killer in 19th-century London, thriving within malnourished communities in the crowded urban environment. It was spread from person to person either by infected sputum or from close contact with, or consumption of, infected animal products (Roberts and Cox 2003, 338). As bone changes occur in only 5–7% of sufferers, an apparently low rate of tuberculosis within a sample may reflect a much greater disease load within the living population (Aufderheide and Rodríguez-Martín 1998, 133), particularly since only a small proportion of those affected present with clearly diagnostic lesions

Amongst the primary inhumations three individuals were affected (3/173: 1.7%): one female (1/30: 3.3%) (see below) and two males (2/80: 2.5%), both of whom were in the 26–35-year age group. At Newcastle Infirmary a similar rate of just 1.0% (2/210) of the articulated individuals had indications of spinal tuberculosis, though a biomolecular study identified a further three cases (Boulter et al 1998, 91).

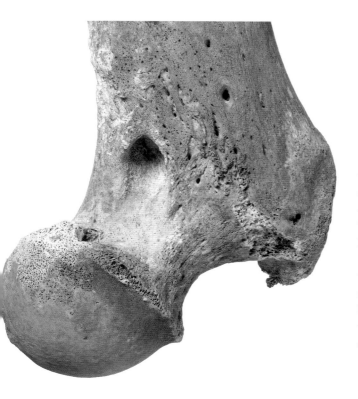

Fig 48 *Osteomyelitis in the right femur of 18–25-year-old male portion [52201] (scale c 1:1)*

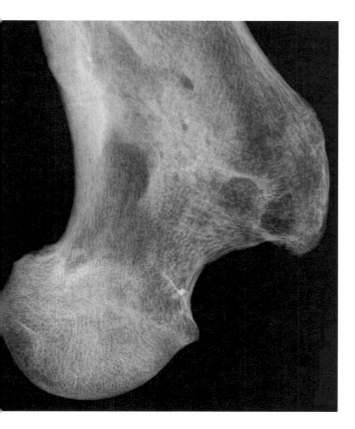

Fig 49 *Radiograph of osteomyelitis in the right femur of 18–25-year-old male portion [52201] (scale c 1:1)*

Female [582], aged 18–25 years at death, had a small sub-circular lytic lesion (max Diam 3.9mm, max D 3.6mm) with a remodelled, flat base on the left lateral margin of the articular surface of the inferior surface of the first thoracic vertebral centrum (Fig 50). There was a further sub-circular lytic lesion, with an irregular floor of remodelled trabeculae, on the right lateral margin of the superior surface of the body of the 12th thoracic vertebra. A sub-rectangular osteolytic lesion (33.5 × 14.9mm, max D 3.0mm), was evident on the anterior aspect of the inferior half of the first sacral vertebral body. The lesion was moderately well defined with sharp but remodelled undercut edges and a level floor consisting of remodelled trabecular bone. The remodelling and absence of fine porosity suggested that the lesion was healed at death.

Both thoracic lesions resembled Schmorl's nodes, but they were atypical in both form and location (Schmorl's nodes are normally centred on the midline sagittal plane of the vertebral bodies). The onset of infection may have occurred in childhood, when the disease is more likely to be multifocal (Aufderheide and Rodríguez-Martín 1998, 135).

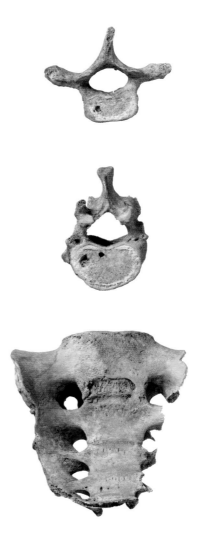

Fig 50 *Possible tuberculosis in the first (top) and 12th (middle) thoracic and sacral (bottom) vertebrae of 18–25-year-old female primary inhumation [582] (scale c 1:2)*

Adult portion [28509] had extensive destruction of the superior and inferior body of the third cervical vertebra. This is consistent with a probable diagnosis of tuberculosis but cannot be considered pathognomonic. Two vertebrae from the disarticulated assemblage also displayed scooped lytic lesions consistent with a diagnosis of tuberculosis (2/722 disarticulated vertebrae; 0.3%).

Septic arthritis

Male adult [212] had porosity and destruction of the right sacroiliac joint surface with remodelling of exposed trabeculae. In addition there were patches of healing new bone surrounding the articular surface. In the absence of the opposing surface and the spine, a diagnosis of septic arthritis, rather than tuberculosis, was appropriate (1/173 primary inhumations; 0.6%). No such changes were present in the portions or disarticulated assemblage, giving a true prevalence rate of 0.2% (1/472 ilia) for the entire assemblage.

Venereal syphilis

Venereal or acquired syphilis is one of four syndromes of bacterial infectious disease caused by spirochetes of the genus *Treponema*. It is the most widespread of the diseases, most commonly occuring in urbanised populations (Hackett 1975, 229; von Hunnius et al 2006, 559). Infection can progress through three different clinical stages, with bone changes predominantly the result of the tertiary stage (Resnick 2002, 2552; Ortner 2003, 279). Symptoms include fever, tenderness and pain in affected bones (Resnick 2002, 2555). Again, it was particularly prevalent in post-medieval London (Roberts and Cox 2003, 340).

Eight primary inhumations were found with lesions suggestive of venereal syphilis (8/173: 4.6%). Two females (2/30: 6.7%) and six males (6/80: 7.5%) were affected.

Adult male [398] was found with an interesting suite of bone changes, though unfortunately the majority of the cranium was absent. In the scapulae, the acromions appeared thickened, with mixed, pitted, woven and lamellar bone on their superior surfaces (Fig 51). Similar mixed lesions were observed on the anterior and medial aspects of the distal humeral shafts, the radial shafts and the proximal and midshafts of both ulnae. Both

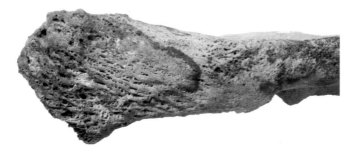

Fig 51 Superior view of right scapular acromion from adult male primary inhumation [398] with possible syphilis (scale c 2:1)

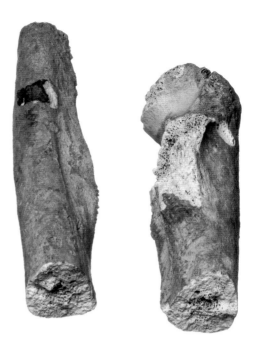

Fig 52 Cross-section view of left radial and ulnar shafts from adult male primary inhumation [398] with possible syphilis, showing infilling of medullary cavity with bone (scale c 1:1)

the forearm bones also exhibited fusiform expansion of their shafts. A post-mortem break in the left clavicle shaft revealed endosteal thickening, and similar bone changes were observed in the humeri, radii and ulnae (Fig 52). A peri-mortem fracture of the humeral surface of the right radial head revealed an irregular bone structure beneath, suggesting that there may have been a systemic underlying cause. The visceral surfaces of the ribs were covered with smooth, mature, new bone, with especially thick deposits on the left side.

The femora had gross fusiform expansion of the mid- and distal shafts, covered by plaques of compact lamellar bone on the medial and lateral aspects, and mixed woven and lamellar bone on the anterior and posterior aspects (Fig 53, top). The lesions were most severe on the distal shafts, where bony bridging was found above 'snail-track' grooves in the bone surface (Fig 53, middle). On the patellar facet of the left femur was a sharp-edged suboval depression (22.8 × 9.2mm, max D 1.9mm). Some healing was evident and the lesion appeared to be the result of osteochondritis dissecans, often linked to a trauma.

The proximal and midshafts of the left tibia were expanded medially, laterally and posteriorly. The entire shaft was covered in pitted and striated, mixed woven and lamellar bone. There was gross fusiform expansion of the right tibial shaft with a roughened irregular cortical surface consisting of striated and pitted, mixed woven and lamellar bone, with occasional smooth, raised plaques on the medial and lateral shafts, and smooth, dense but irregular lamellar bone overlying pitted mixed bone on the posterior shaft. The anterior crest was thickened. At the proximal end, within the anterior intercondylar area, was a healed teardrop-shaped lytic lesion (12.5 × 5.7mm) with steep undercutting sides and a remodelled

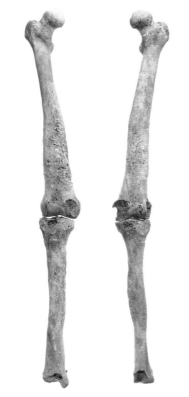

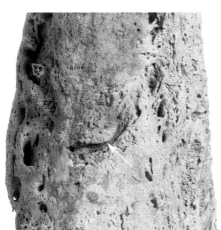

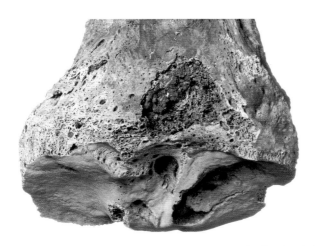

Fig 53 Femora and tibiae of adult male primary inhumation [398] with probable syphilis: top – anterior view of femora and tibiae (scale c 1:8); middle – medial view of right femur with 'snail-track' lesion (arrowed) (scale c 1:1); bottom – proximal view of right tibia (scale c 1:1)

sloping trabecular base (Fig 53, bottom). In addition, there was a suboval lytic lesion (25.5 × 14mm, max D 6.3mm) in the medial half of the lateral condyle with steep, irregular, undercutting sides containing small, dense, nodular excrescenses, and a trabecular base. The medial edge of the lesion was healed while the remainder was only slightly remodelled, suggesting the articular surface may have suffered at lease one phase of injury. There was also a sub-triangular (13.3 × 11.9mm) peri-mortem fissure fracture in the anteromedial corner of the medial condyle. On the distal articular facet there was an irregularly shaped (long and thin) smooth-edged pit (7.5 × 2.5mm, max D 2.2mm) with steep sides and a flat trabecular base. This lesion had similar qualities to those associated with osteochondritis dissecans, but was of a very unusual shape.

The fibular shafts, the medial surfaces of the calcanei and the plantar surfaces of the fifth metatarsals were covered in mixed, pitted, woven and lamellar bone.

The diffuse, bilateral and symmetrical, nongummatous periosteal lesions on the skeleton of this adult male, together with the cortical and endosteal thickening, and increased weight caused by new bone fusing to the cortex, are suggestive of venereal syphilis. The medullary cavity of the right ulna was almost completely closed, typical of late-stage nongummatous periostitis (Ortner 2003, 283–6). The majority of the cranium and both frontal bones were lost as a result of modern truncation, so the presence or absence of pathognomonic caries sicca could not be verified. However, the rough and hypervascular outer surface of the femora and tibia, together with the presence of bony bridging with some apparent 'snail tracks', suggests that the individual was suffering from the tertiary stage of venereal syphilis.

Erosive joint changes, such as that located in the interarticular area of the proximal right tibia, have been found in sufferers (Ortner 2003, 314–15). It is possible that the joints affected by the traumatic lesions eventually formed into Charcot's joints, a feature of tabes dorsalis in late-stage neurosyphilis (ibid, 585–6). In a Charcot joint, damage to nerves in the spinal cord by the syphilis infection means that the individual loses awareness of joint pain or joint position, which predisposes them to joint injury.This may have been responsible for the apparent refracturing within the knee joint and even possibly for the lesions resembling osteochondritis dissecans.

The surface of a sawn adult right humerus from portion [32908] was covered by a mixture of pitted, woven and lamellar bone with particularly florid changes on the posterior and a 'fluffy' appearance, increasing the circumference of the bone. The right ulna of the same portion was also covered with pitted and striated, mixed new bone. A recent break in the shaft revealed total obliteration of the endosteal space by poorly organised trabecular bone. Such changes are highly suggestive of venereal syphilis.

Further evidence of probable venereal syphilis was noted in the disarticulated assemblage, where three right tibiae (one with active changes), a left humerus and a left proximal and mid fibula with associated right femur displayed gummatous and sclerosing osteitis and/or periostitis and a right distal femur displayed gummatous osteomyelitis. Eighteen out of 7571 disarticulated bone elements (0.2%) were affected, though it should be cautioned that it is possible some of the infected elements originated from the same individuals as represented in the portions and primary inhumations.

Trauma

Evidence of trauma (bone and joint fractures, soft-tissue trauma and dislocations) was observed in 35.8% of individuals from the primary inhumation sample (62/173) – 38.1% of adults (61/160) and 7.7% of subadults (1/13).

Over half the males were affected (43/80: 53.8%) compared to 30.0% of females (9/30). Whilst the paucity of females hinders comparison between the sexes in each age category the overall crude prevalence rate demonstrates a significant male bias (χ^2 = 4.94, df = 1, p≤ 0.03) (Fig 54; Table 36). For the group as a whole, the prevalence rate of trauma increased with age, with those aged 46 years or over producing the highest crude

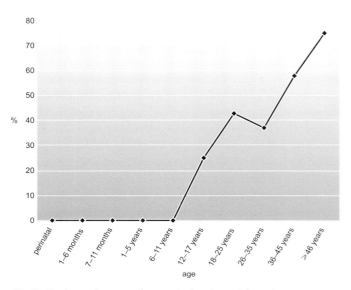

Fig 54 Crude prevalence rate of trauma in the primary inhumations

prevalence rate (9/12: 75.0%). The steep crude prevalence rise in trauma in the adolescent and young adult categories reflects the low number of subadults in the sample and may also have been affected by the rapid remodelling of lesions in subadults.

Primary inhumations from group 21 were less frequently affected by trauma than those from group 20 (χ^2 = 5.91, df = 1, p≤ 0.02) and group 22 (χ^2 = 13.29, df = 1, p≤ 0.000) (Table 37).

Forty portions (including ten male and two female portions) and 42 contexts of disarticulated remains also showed evidence of trauma.

A fracture to the right maxillary first premolar of portion [35401] was the only definite evidence of dental trauma (1/1802 teeth from the articulated assemblage; 0.1%). Small chips in the biting surfaces of teeth from males [365] and [299] probably resulted from accidental damage caused by biting a hard particle or object but indirect injury through the transfer of force from a blow to the head should also be considered.

Soft-tissue trauma

Soft-tissue trauma was identified in 8.1% (14/173) of primary inhumations. Only adults were affected (14/160: 8.8%), with a greater proportion of males (10/80: 12.5%) than females (2/30: 6.7%) affected; 4.4% (2/45) of adults of undetermined sex were also affected. The majority of cases presented as enthesopathies at sites of muscle attachments and may have been due to increased muscle development (Knusel 2000, 381) (Fig 55). An

Table 37 Crude prevalence rate of trauma in the primary inhumations by land use

Group	Subadult			Adult			All individuals		
	n	Affected	%	n	Affected	%	n	Affected	%
20	4	0	-	64	26	40.6	68	26	38.2
21	6	0	-	49	10	20.4	55	10	18.2
22	3	1	33.3	47	25	53.2	50	26	52.0

Table 36 Crude prevalence rate of trauma in the primary inhumations

Age	Female			Male			Intermediate			Undetermined			Subadults			Adults			All individuals		
	n	Affected	%	n	Affected	%	n	Affected	%	n	Affected	%	n	Affected	%	n	Affected	%	n	Affected	%
<4 weeks	0	0	-	0	0	-	0	0	-	0	0	-	5	0	-	0	0	-	5	0	-
1–6 months	0	0	-	0	0	-	0	0	-	0	0	-	0	0	-	0	0	-	0	0	-
7–11 months	0	0	-	0	0	-	0	0	-	0	0	-	0	0	-	0	0	-	0	0	-
1–5 years	0	0	-	0	0	-	0	0	-	0	0	-	3	0	-	0	0	-	3	0	-
6–11 years	0	0	-	0	0	-	0	0	-	0	0	-	1	0	-	0	0	-	1	0	-
12–17 years	0	0	-	0	0	-	0	0	-	0	0	-	4	1	25.0	0	0	-	4	1	25.0
Subadult	0	0	-	0	0	-	0	0	-	0	0	-	0	0	-	0	0	-	0	0	-
18–25 years	4	3	75.0	6	2	33.3	3	1	33.3	1	0	-	0	0	-	14	6	42.9	14	6	42.9
26–35 years	10	1	10.0	25	11	44.0	1	1	100.0	2	1	50.0	0	0	-	38	14	36.8	38	14	36.8
36–45 years	9	2	22.2	27	18	66.7	0	0	-	2	2	100.0	0	0	-	38	22	57.9	38	2	57.9
≥46 years	3	3	100.0	9	6	66.7	0	0	-	0	0	-	0	0	-	12	9	75.0	12	9	75.0
Adult	4	0	-	13	6	46.2	1	0	-	40	4	10.0	0	0	-	58	10	17.2	58	10	17.2
Total	30	9	30.0	80	43	53.8	5	2	40.0	45	7	15.6	13	1	7.7	160	61	38.1	173	62	35.8

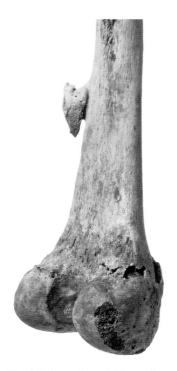

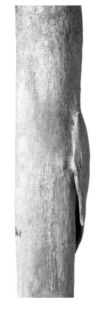

Fig 55 Enthesopathy on left femur of 26–35-year-old male primary inhumation [239] (scale c 1:2)

Fig 56 Ossified haematoma on left femur of ≥46-year-old male portion [21001] (scale c 1:2)

related to an episode that had also resulted in bone fracture. Portion [49203] had a bony spur on the right acromial clavicle, adjacent to a healed fracture and resulting from ossification of the trapezoid ligament. Possible soft-tissue trauma was given for portion [20601] as a differential diagnosis for bony spurring at the insertion for tibialis anterior (responsible for ankle dorsiflexion) relating to a tibial plateau fracture (see also below, 'Neoplastic disease'). One example of myositis ossificans was seen, the left humerus of portion [17404] displaying ossification of brachialis and the medial head of triceps, both responsible for elbow flexion and suggesting a hyperextension injury.

In the disarticulated sample, six examples of soft-tissue injury were noted. All affected adult elements and five were consistent with a diagnosis of myositis ossificans. A left proximal humerus from [129] also had rotator cuff disease, whilst a right proximal fibula from [309] had a possible healed fracture. In the right distal femur of [149], the bony change appeared to be in response to a hyperextension injury to vastus intermedius. An ossified haematoma was present on the left lateral proximal and midshaft of a femur from [457].

In total, an almost equal number of right (16) and left (18) elements had evidence of soft-tissue trauma. The femur was the element most frequently involved, with 14 cases, followed by the ulna with six.

ossified haematoma, the result of trauma, was seen in an elderly male (Fig 56) and ossification of the soft tissues surrounding the manubrium was observed in a 36–45-year-old male, [138], and was associated with rib fractures (Table 38).

Enthesophyte formation was also seen in nine portions. All of those portions for which sex could be established (four) were male. Bony spurs affected the areas of attachment for vastus medialis and adductor magnus in the femur, biceps in the humerus, triceps and brachialis in the ulna, and a left second metatarsal. In two instances the soft-tissue injury was most likely

Joint dislocation

Evidence of joint dislocation or subluxation was present in five individuals (5/173: 2.9%), all of whom were adults (5/160: 3.1%) (Table 39).

Mature adult female [595] (≥46 years) had suffered dislocation of the left elbow joint with a healed fracture of the trochlear notch of the ulna (Fig 57). The articular head of the radius was flattened and there was also a healed fracture of the medial condyle of the humerus. As a result, the elbow may have been fixed in flexion, although secondary osteoarthritis in the

Table 38 Soft-tissue trauma in the primary inhumations

Context no.	Age (years)	Sex	Type	Location	Mechanism
[138]	36–45	male	soft-tissue ossification	manubrium	trauma related to upper rib fractures
[175]	26–35	female	enthesopathy	L patella	ligament strain
[178]	18–25	female	enthesopathy	pubes, adductor longus	habitual activity/groin strain
[212]	adult	male	enthesopathy	R femur, adductor magnus/medial head of gastrocnemius	hip adduction/knee flexion
			enthesopathy	R femur, psoas major, iliacus & gluteus minimus	hip flexion, abduction & medial rotation
[215]	26–35	undetermined	enthesopathy	R clavicle, deltoid	shoulder abduction & flexion
[239]	26–35	male	enthesopathy	L femur, vastus lateralis	knee extension
[305]	26–35	male	enthesopathy	clavicles, costoclavicular ligaments	joint tearing/stretching
[340]	36–45	male	enthesopathy	R ulna, triceps	elbow extension
[368]	adult	male	enthesopathy	ulnae, triceps	elbow extension
[369]	36–45	male	enthesopathy	L femur, vastus intermedius	knee extension
[421]	36–45	male	enthesopathy	patellae, quadriceps tendon/patellar ligament	ligament strain
[423]	36–45	male	enthesopathy	L ulna, triceps	elbow extension
			enthesopathy	R femur, short head of biceps	knee flexion
[451]	26–35	male	myositis ossificans	R femur, vastus intermedialis	knee extension
[609]	adult	undetermined	enthesopathy	L fibula, peronius tertius	ankle dorsiflexion

Table 39 Joint dislocation in primary inhumations

Context no.	Age (years)	Sex	Location	Mechanism
[222]	≥46	male	hand, unsided distal interphalangeal joint	
[349]	36–45	male	R foot, first interphalangeal joint	
[582]	18–25	female	L clavicle, sternoclavicular joint	childhood blow to shoulder/fall on outstretched hand
[588]	36–45	male	L hand, carpometacarpal joints	severe trauma to upper L limb
[595]	≥46	female	L elbow joint	severe trauma with fracture to all three arm bones

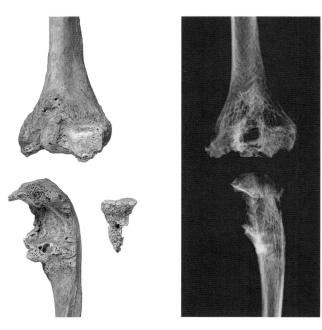

Fig 57 Dislocated left elbow from ≥46-year-old female primary inhumation [595]: left – anterior view (scale c 1:2); right – anteroposterior radiograph (scale c 1:2)

form of eburnation betrays at least minimal movement.

An unusual case of fracture and dorsal dislocation was observed in the carpometacarpal joints of the left hand of 36–45-year-old male [588] (Fig 58). Most joints suffered from secondary osteoarthritis. This form of injury is associated in modern clinical medicine with high-velocity motor vehicle accidents. Such injuries predispose the hand to mechanical disruption and osteoarthritis, as even in modern cases closed

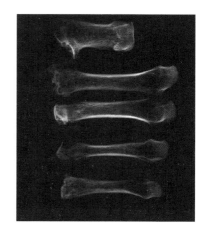

Fig 58 Anteroposterior radiograph of left hand from 36–45-year-old male primary inhumation [588] (scale c 1:2)

reduction (ie, reducing the injury without surgical intervention) can be challenging (Hartwig and Louis 1979, 906–8). Individual [588] also had a healed left elbow fracture, possibly associated with the same traumatic incident.

In addition, gross contour change in the distal radioulnar joint of portion [59003], together with secondary osteophyte formation and eburnation, indicated joint subluxation in the wrist and was possibly associated with an impression fracture in the distal radius. This injury may have been caused by a fall on to an outstretched arm. Severe osteophyte formation and joint contour change in a disarticulated right acromial clavicle from [599] may also have been the result of subluxation.

Fractures

Fractures were visible in 33.5% (58/173) of the primary inhumations – 35.6% of adults (57/160) and 7.7% of subadults (1/13) (Table 40). Males (42/80: 52.5%) were affected more frequently than females (7/30: 23.3) (χ^2 = 7.51, df = 1, p≤ 0.006). Radiographic examination of the disarticulated assemblage was not undertaken, so that in three instances the diagnosis of a healed fracture remains tentative. Twenty-two examples of fractures were noted, most of them well healed. True prevalence rates were affected by the small sample sizes for some elements. Of these, compression fractures affected the spine of nine primary inhumations (9/173: 5.2%) – 6.3% of males (5/80) and 6.7% of females (2/30).

True prevalence rates of bone fracture were compiled for the articulated assemblage (primary inhumations and portions) and include all fracture types (separately discussed below) (Tables 41–2). The number of fractures in each element was insufficient to allow for statistical testing or for measuring any variation in injury rates between the two samples. Fractures involving solely the joint surfaces of the manubrium, patellae, long bones, flat bones and the skull were calculated separately (below, 'Joint fractures').

In the majority of cases the bone fractures were fully healed by the time of death of the individual, though a small number remained unhealed. The primary inhumations contained three burials with healing fractures, where the callus at the site of injury was formed of immature bone, representing 5.2% (3/58) of individuals affected by fractures in the sample. The same number had peri-mortem fractures where there were no visible signs of healing, suggesting that the individual died at or near the time of injury. When calculated by total number of

Table 40 Crude prevalence rate of fractures in the primary inhumations

Age	Female n	Affected	%	Male n	Affected	%	Intermediate n	Affected	%	Undetermined n	Affected	%	Subadults n	Affected	%	Adults n	Affected	%	All individuals n	Affected	%
<4 weeks	0	0	-	0	0	-	0	0	-	0	0	-	5	0	-	0	0	-	5	0	-
1–6 months	0	0	-	0	0	-	0	0	-	0	0	-	0	0	-	0	0	-	0	0	-
7–11 months	0	0	-	0	0	-	0	0	-	0	0	-	0	0	-	0	0	-	0	0	-
1–5 years	0	0	-	0	0	-	0	0	-	0	0	-	3	0	-	0	0	-	3	0	-
6–11 years	0	0	-	0	0	-	0	0	-	0	0	-	1	0	-	0	0	-	1	0	-
12–17 years	0	0	-	0	0	-	0	0	-	0	0	-	4	1	25.0	0	0	-	4	1	25.0
Subadult	0	0	-	0	0	-	0	0	-	0	0	-	0	0	-	0	0	-	0	0	-
18–25 years	4	2	50.0	6	2	33.3	3	1	33.3	1	0	-	0	0	-	14	5	35.7	14	5	35.7
26–35 years	10	0	-	25	10	40.0	1	1	100.0	2	0	-	0	0	-	38	11	28.9	38	11	28.9
36–45 years	9	2	22.2	27	18	66.7	0	0	-	2	2	100.0	0	0	-	38	22	57.9	38	22	57.9
≥46 years	3	3	100.0	9	6	66.7	0	0	-	0	0	-	0	0	-	12	9	75.0	12	9	75.0
Adult	4	0	-	13	6	46.2	1	0	-	40	4	10.0	0	0	-	58	10	17.2	58	10	17.2
Total	30	7	23.3	80	42	52.5	5	2	40.0	45	6	13.3	13	1	7.7	160	57	35.6	173	58	33.5

fractures, the injuries within the body portions appeared to occur nearer the time of death than those from the primary inhumations (Table 43).

Within the assemblage were a number of fracture types rarely observed in archaeological studies. These included a healed but non-united fracture of the waist of the right scaphoid of adult primary inhumation [412] (Fig 59). This type of injury often results from falling on an outstretched hand, which causes the extended wrist to dorsiflex. Secondary osteoarthritis developed and there was some reduction in size when compared to the left bone, but there was no evidence of osteonecrosis.

Primary inhumation [138], a 36–45-year-old probable male, had a healed Duverney fracture of the right ilium (Fig 60). Such fractures normally require severe lateral force, such as provided

Table 41 True prevalence rate of fractures in the articulated assemblage

	n	Affected	%
Primary inhumations			
Male	6090	87	1.4
Female	2262	11	0.5
Subadult	596	1	0.2
All adult	9906	109	1.1
Total	10502	208	2.0
Portions			
Male	1263	19	1.5
Female	402	4	1.0
Subadult	328	0	-
All adult	4059	40	1.0
Total	4387	42	1.0

Table 42 True prevalence rate of fractures by element in the articulated assemblage

		Female n	Affected	%	Male n	Affected	%	Adult n	Affected	%	Subadult n	Affected	%	All individuals n	Affected	%
Primary inhumations																
Frontal	R	19	0	-	53	0	-	77	0	-	6	0	-	83	0	-
	L	19	0	-	54	1	1.9	78	1	1.3	6	0	-	84	1	1.2
	total	38	0	-	107	1	0.9	155	1	0.6	12	0	-	167	1	0.6
Parietal	R	19	0	-	55	1	1.8	79	1	1.3	6	0	-	85	1	1.2
	L	19	0	-	56	0	-	80	0	-	6	0	-	86	0	-
	total	38	0	-	111	1	0.9	159	1	0.6	12	0	-	171	1	0.6
Supraoccipital		20	0	-	53	1	1.9	78	1	1.3	7	0	-	85	1	1.2
Nasal	R	11	0	-	28	6	21.4	41	6	14.6	0	0	-	41	6	14.6
	L	12	0	-	29	4	13.8	43	4	9.3	0	0	-	43	4	9.3
	total	23	0	-	57	10	17.5	84	10	11.9	0	0	-	84	10	11.9
Maxilla	R	18	0	-	49	0	-	72	0	-	2	0	-	74	0	-
	L	19	0	-	50	1	2.0	73	1	1.4	3	0	-	76	1	1.3
	total	37	0	-	99	1	1.0	145	1	0.7	5	0	-	150	1	0.7
Ribs	R	239	2	0.8	647	12	1.9	1058	16	1.5	72	0	-	1130	16	1.4
	L	227	1	0.4	652	6	0.9	1065	8	0.8	89	0	-	1154	8	0.7
	unsided	2	0	-	7	1	14.3	13	2	15.4	11	0	-	24	2	8.3
	total	468	3	0.6	1306	19	1.5	2136	26	1.2	172	0	-	2308	26	1.1

Table 42 (cont)

		Female			Male			Adult			Subadult			All individuals		
		n	Affected	%	n	Affected	%	n	Affected	%	n	Affected	%	n	Affected	%
Thoracic	1	22	0	-	62	1	1.6	20	1	5.0	9	0	-	29	1	3.4
	3	20	0	-	66	2	3.0	21	2	9.5	9	0	-	30	2	6.7
	4	20	0	-	65	3	4.6	20	3	15.0	9	0	-	29	3	10.3
	5	23	0	-	65	2	3.1	20	2	10.0	8	0	-	28	2	7.1
	6	23	0	-	63	2	3.2	20	3	15.0	10	0	-	30	3	10.0
	8	24	0	-	64	2	3.1	18	3	16.7	10	0	-	28	3	10.7
	12	24	0	-	70	0	-	19	1	5.3	9	0	-	28	1	3.6
Lumbar	1	23	1	4.3	71	1	1.4	112	2	1.8	7	0	-	119	2	1.7
	2	23	2	8.7	71	0	-	112	2	1.8	8	0	-	120	2	1.7
Scapula	R	20	0	-	59	0	-	98	0	-	9	0	-	107	0	-
	L	20	0	-	58	1	1.7	99	1	1.0	11	0	-	110	1	0.9
	total	40	0	-	117	1	0.9	197	1	0.5	20	0	-	217	1	0.5
Clavicle	R	21	0	-	58	2	3.4	99	2	2.0	11	0	-	110	2	1.8
	L	22	0	-	63	0	-	106	1	0.9	10	0	-	116	1	0.9
	total	43	0	-	121	2	1.7	205	3	1.5	21	0	-	226	3	1.3
Humerus	R	24	0	-	58	0	-	104	0	-	11	0	-	115	0	-
	L	25	1	4.0	64	2	3.1	111	3	2.7	12	0	-	123	3	2.4
	total	49	1	2.0	122	2	1.6	215	3	1.4	23	0	-	238	3	1.3
Radius	R	23	1	4.3	62	1	1.6	101	2	2.0	7	0	-	108	2	1.9
	L	23	1	4.3	58	0	-	99	1	1.0	10	0	-	109	1	0.9
	total	46	2	4.3	120	1	0.8	200	3	1.5	17	0	-	217	3	1.4
Ulna	R	22	0	-	64	1	1.6	103	1	1.0	8	0	-	111	1	0.9
	L	23	1	4.3	57	0	-	99	1	1.0	11	0	-	110	1	0.9
	total	45	1	2.2	121	1	0.8	202	2	1.0	19	0	-	221	2	0.9
Scaphoid	R	20	0	-	44	0	-	71	1	1.4	2	0	-	73	1	1.4
	L	16	0	-	43	0	-	67	0	-	1	0	-	68	0	-
	total	36	0	-	87	0	-	138	1	0.7	3	0	-	141	1	0.7
Trapezium	R	15	0	-	36	2	5.6	58	2	3.4	1	0	-	59	2	3.4
	L	10	0	-	37	0	-	56	0	-	1	0	-	57	0	-
	total	25	0	-	73	2	2.7	114	2	1.8	2	0	-	116	2	1.7
1st metacarpal	R	17	0	-	52	3	5.8	79	3	3.8	6	0	-	85	3	3.5
	L	23	0	-	46	3	6.5	77	3	3.9	6	0	-	83	3	3.6
	total	40	0	-	98	6	6.1	156	6	3.8	12	0	-	168	6	3.6
3rd metacarpal	R	21	0	-	55	1	1.8	88	1	1.1	5	0	-	93	1	1.1
	L	19	0	-	50	1	2.0	76	1	1.3	4	0	-	80	1	1.3
	total	40	0	-	105	2	1.9	164	2	1.2	9	0	-	173	2	1.2
4th metacarpal	R	21	0	-	51	0	-	85	0	-	5	0	-	90	0	-
	L	24	0	-	48	1	2.1	81	1	1.2	4	0	-	85	1	1.2
	total	45	0	-	99	1	1.0	166	1	0.6	9	0	-	175	1	0.6
5th metacarpal	R	18	0	-	53	1	1.9	83	1	1.2	3	0	-	86	1	1.2
	L	21	0	-	48	2	4.2	79	2	2.5	5	0	-	84	2	2.4
	total	39	0	-	101	3	3.0	162	3	1.9	8	0	-	170	3	1.8
Proximal hand phalanges	R	16	0	-	41	0	-	66	0	-	4	0	-	70	0	-
	L	18	0	-	31	0	-	68	0	-	4	0	-	72	0	-
	unsided	159	0	-	408	1	0.2	638	1	0.2	27	0	-	665	1	0.2
	total	193	0	-	480	1	0.2	772	1	0.1	35	0	-	807	1	0.1
Ilium	R	27	0	-	70	1	1.4	107	1	0.9	10	0	-	117	1	0.9
	L	27	0	-	69	0	-	108	0	-	11	0	-	119	0	-
	total	54	0	-	139	1	0.7	215	1	0.5	21	0	-	236	1	0.4
Femur	R	26	0	-	67	3	4.5	108	3	2.8	10	0	-	118	3	2.5
	L	25	0	-	64	0	-	106	0	-	9	0	-	115	0	-
	total	51	0	-	131	3	2.3	214	3	1.4	19	0	-	233	3	1.3
Tibia	R	25	0	-	55	0	-	105	0	-	11	0	-	116	0	-
	L	22	0	-	58	1	1.7	104	1	1.0	9	0	-	113	1	0.9
	total	47	0	-	113	1	0.9	209	1	0.5	20	0	-	229	1	0.4
Fibula	R	22	0	-	53	4	7.5	99	4	4.0	10	0	-	109	4	3.7
	L	22	0	-	52	3	5.8	98	3	3.1	7	1	14.3	105	4	3.8
	total	44	0	-	105	7	6.7	197	7	3.6	17	1	5.9	214	8	3.7

Table 42 (cont)

		Female			Male			Adult			Subadult			All individuals		
		n	Affected	%	n	Affected	%	n	Affected	%	n	Affected	%	n	Affected	%
Calcaneus	R	22	1	4.5	50	1	2.0	95	2	2.1	2	0	-	97	2	2.1
	L	17	0	-	45	1	2.2	83	1	1.2	4	0	-	87	1	1.1
	total	39	1	2.6	95	2	2.1	178	3	1.7	6	0	-	184	3	1.6
Talus	R	21	0	-	49	0	-	94	0	-	2	0	-	96	0	-
	L	20	0	-	45	1	2.2	86	1	1.2	3	0	-	3	1	33.3
	total	41	0	-	94	1	1.1	180	1	0.6	5	0	-	185	1	0.5
4th metatarsal	R	19	0	-	41	1	2.4	75	1	1.3	4	0	-	79	1	1.3
	L	16	0	-	45	0	-	81	1	1.2	4	0	-	85	1	1.2
	total	35	0	-	86	1	1.2	156	2	1.3	8	0	-	164	2	1.2
5th metatarsal	R	22	0	-	44	1	2.3	87	1	1.1	6	0	-	93	1	1.1
	L	15	0	-	43	0	-	81	0	-	5	0	-	86	0	-
	total	37	0	-	87	1	1.1	168	1	0.6	11	0	-	179	1	0.6
Proximal foot phalanges	R	21	0	-	46	0	-	90	0	-	1	0	-	91	0	-
	L	15	0	-	47	0	-	86	0	-	1	0	-	87	0	-
	unsided	98	0	-	269	1	0.4	489	2	0.4	13	0	-	502	2	0.4
	total	134	0	-	362	1	0.3	665	2	0.3	15	0	-	680	2	0.3
Middle foot phalanges	R	-	-	-	1	0	-	1	0	-	0	0	-	1	0	-
	L	-	-	-	1	0	-	1	0	-	0	0	-	1	0	-
	unsided	15	0	-	74	1	1.4	116	1	0.9	0	0	-	116	1	0.9
	total	15	0	-	76	1	1.3	118	1	0.8	0	0	-	118	1	0.8
Portions																
Nasal	R	2	0	-	8	2	25.0	10	2	20.0	0	0	-	10	2	20.0
	L	2	0	-	8	2	25.0	10	2	20.0	0	0	-	10	2	20.0
	total	4	0	-	16	4	25.0	20	4	20.0	0	0	-	20	4	20.0
Maxilla	R	6	0	-	11	1	9.1	20	1	5.0	1	0	-	21	1	4.8
	L	4	0	-	11	1	9.1	20	1	5.0	2	0	-	22	1	4.5
	total	10	0	-	22	2	9.1	40	2	5.0	3	0	-	43	2	4.7
Ribs	R	62	0	-	146	1	0.7	522	3	0.6	63	0	-	585	3	0.5
	L	62	0	-	164	4	2.4	532	5	0.9	49	0	-	581	5	0.9
	unsided	-	-	-	1	0	-	55	1	1.8	7	0	-	62	1	1.6
	total	124	0	-	311	5	1.6	1109	9	0.8	119	0	-	1228	9	0.7
Thoracic	5	7	0	-	14	1	7.1	53	1	1.9	6	0	-	59	1	1.7
	6	7	0	-	15	1	6.7	57	1	1.8	6	0	-	63	1	1.6
	7	6	0	-	16	1	6.3	57	1	1.8	4	0	-	61	1	1.6
	8	6	0	-	16	1	6.3	53	1	1.9	6	0	-	59	1	1.7
	9	7	0	-	17	1	5.9	57	1	1.8	6	0	-	63	1	1.6
	12	6	1	16.7	17	0	-	58	2	3.4	4	0	-	62	2	3.2
Lumbar	1	6	1	16.7	18	0	-	58	1	1.7	3	0	-	61	1	1.6
	2	6	0	-	19	1	5.3	58	1	1.7	2	0	-	60	1	1.7
	3	9	1	11.1	26	1	3.8	65	2	3.1	3	0	-	68	2	2.9
Clavicle	R	3	0	-	13	0	-	39	1	2.6	3	0	-	42	1	2.4
	L	2	0	-	9	0	-	36	0	-	6	0	-	42	0	-
	total	5	0	-	22	0	-	75	1	1.3	9	0	-	84	1	1.2
Humerus	R	1	0	-	11	0	-	57	1	1.8	7	0	-	64	1	1.6
	L	2	0	-	8	0	-	63	0	-	6	0	-	69	0	-
	total	3	0	-	19	0	-	120	1	0.8	13	0	-	133	1	0.8
Trapezium	R	1	0	-	3	0	-	23	1	4.3	4	0	-	27	1	3.7
	L	1	0	-	3	0	-	21	0	-	2	0	-	23	0	-
	total	2	0	-	6	0	-	44	1	2.3	6	0	-	50	1	2.0
Hamate	R	1	0	-	3	0	-	24	1	4.2	4	0	-	28	1	3.6
	L	1	0	-	3	0	-	21	0	-	2	0	-	23	0	-
	total	2	0	-	6	0	-	45	1	2.2	6	0	-	51	1	2.0
1st metacarpal	R	2	0	-	5	0	-	29	2	6.9	2	0	-	31	2	6.5
	L	1	0	-	4	0	-	22	1	4.5	2	0	-	24	1	4.2
	total	3	0	-	9	0	-	51	3	5.9	4	0	-	55	3	5.5
5th metacarpal	R	1	1	100.0	5	0	-	30	0	-	5	0	-	35	1	2.9
	L	1	0	-	4	0	-	29	0	-	2	0	-	31	0	-
	total	2	1	50.0	9	0	-	59	0	-	7	0	-	66	1	1.5

Table 42 (cont)

		Female			Male			Adult			Subadult			All individuals		
		n	Affected	%	n	Affected	%	n	Affected	%	n	Affected	%	n	Affected	%
Tibia	R	1	0	–	15	0	–	60	0	–	3	0	–	63	0	–
	L	3	0	–	17	0	–	52	1	1.9	3	0	–	55	1	1.8
	total	4	0	–	32	0	–	112	1	0.9	6	0	–	118	1	0.8
Fibula	R	1	0	–	13	0	–	52	0	–	2	0	–	54	0	–
	L	2	0	–	17	1	5.9	50	2	4.0	2	0	–	52	3	5.8
	total	3	0	–	30	1	3.3	102	2	2.0	4	0	–	106	3	2.8
Calcaneus	R	0	0	–	11	0	–	38	1	2.6	1	0	–	39	1	2.6
	L	1	0	–	8	0	–	36	0	–	1	0	–	37	0	–
	total	1	0	–	19	0	–	74	1	1.4	2	0	–	76	1	1.3
Navicular	R	0	–	–	8	0	–	33	0	–	2	0	–	35	0	–
	L	2	0	–	8	0	–	33	1	3.0	1	0	–	34	1	2.9
	total	2	0	–	16	0	–	66	1	1.5	3	0	–	69	1	1.4
4th metatarsal	R	0	0	–	7	0	–	31	0	–	2	0	–	33	0	–
	L	2	0	–	8	0	–	32	1	3.1	2	0	–	34	1	2.9
	total	2	0	–	15	0	–	63	1	1.6	4	0	–	67	1	1.5
5th metatarsal	R	0	0	–	8	0	–	31	0	–	2	0	–	33	0	–
	L	2	0	–	7	0	–	31	1	3.2	2	0	–	33	1	3.0
	total	2	0	–	15	0	–	62	1	1.6	4	0	–	66	1	1.5

Table 43 Healing and peri-mortem fractures as a proportion of total fractures

	Total fractures	Healing fractures	%	Peri-mortem fractures	%
Primary inhumations	208	5	2.4	3	1.4
Portions	42	4	9.5	3	7.1

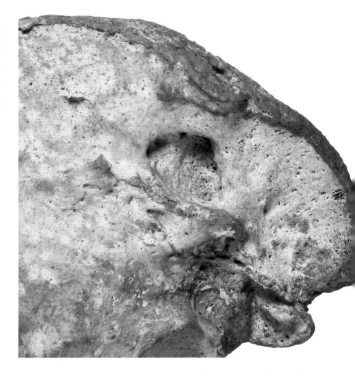

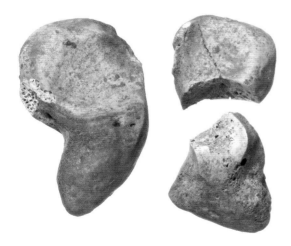

Fig 59 Non-united right scaphoid fracture (with normal left bone) from adult primary inhumation [412] (scale c 2:1)

Fig 60 Dorsal view of fractured right ilium of 36–45-year-old probable male primary inhumation [138] (scale c 4:1)

by a fall from a height or high-impact injuries, although this does not disrupt the pelvic ring (Galloway 1999, 161). A healed sub-circular lesion on the dorsal blade, probably the result of osteomyelitis, suggests the wound may have been open. Considering the present-day mortality rate of such fractures is 50% or higher, owing to blood loss and haemorrhage, this individual was fortunate to survive.

In addition to fractures to the nasal bones and the shaft of the left fifth metacarpal, primary inhumation [133], a 36–45-year-old male, had a severe healed intra-articular impaction fracture of the right calcaneus (Fig 61). The posterior half of the bone, including the majority of the posterior talal articular surface, had been driven down into the trabecular bone of the heel, causing a displaced coronal fracture of the aforementioned articular surface. There was also a vertical intra-articular impression fracture in the facet for the cuboid. A vertical fall on to the foot would cause this type of crushing injury, where the talus drives into the calcaneus. In general, the prognosis is poor, with persistent pain and limping (Resnick 2002, 2897–901; McRae 2003, 483).

A more common form of fracture, though in this case particularly severe, involved adult portion [24305], which had a healed compression fracture of the body of the 12th thoracic

vertebra (Fig 62). The severe nature of the injury caused 40° anterior wedging of the centrum and a large coronal burst fracture in its superior surface. The inferior surface also contained a burst fracture and had slight displacement of a fracture anterior margin (McRae 2003, 370–2).

The true prevalence rate of fractures in the disarticulated assemblage can be seen in Table 44.

Examples of bone fracture which occurred around the time of death (peri-mortem), and those in the very earliest stages of healing, were evident in the primary inhumations, the portions and the disarticulated sample.

The lateral shaft of a left rib of primary inhumation [242], a 36–45-year-old male, had a thick but highly porous deposit of woven bone overlying an oblique, incomplete fracture. A further left rib had an incomplete, long, oblique fracture on the visceral surface of the lateral shaft with the initial growth of reparative woven bone (Fig 63). These indirect fractures may have resulted

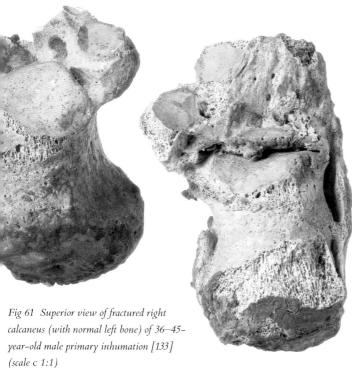

Fig 61 Superior view of fractured right calcaneus (with normal left bone) of 36–45-year-old male primary inhumation [133] (scale c 1:1)

Table 44 *True prevalence rate of fractures in the disarticulated assemblage*

Element	n	Affected	%
L patella	28	1	3.6
R ribs	275	7	2.5
Unsided ribs	98	5	5.1
L ribs	259	4	1.5
R 2nd metatarsal	25	1	4.0
L proximal femur	70	1	1.4
Sternum	48	1	2.1
R mid clavicle	65	1	1.5
L 1st metatarsal	18	1	5.6
L acromial clavicle	65	1	1.5
R acromial clavicle	64	2	3.1
L mid clavicle	67	1	1.5
R acromion	53	2	3.8
L mid radius	48	1	2.1
L distal humerus	68	1	1.5
R proximal fibula	53	1	1.9
R distal fibula	37	1	2.7
L distal tibia	53	1	1.9

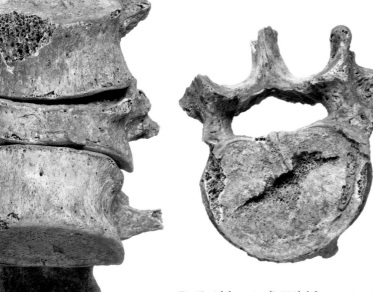

Fig 62 Adult portion [24305]: left – anterior view of 11th thoracic to first lumbar vertebrae with fractured 12th thoracic vertebra; right – superior view of fractured 12th thoracic vertebra (scale c 1:1)

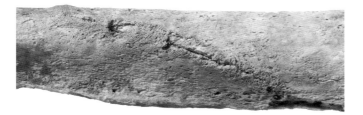

Fig 63 Visceral aspect of healing fracture in the left rib of 36–45-year-old male primary inhumation [242] (scale c 2:1)

from crushing and bending forces, perhaps the result of a fall or anteroposterior compression of the ribcage (Galloway 1999, 107). Their early stage of healing reveals that this individual died just a matter of days or weeks after the incident, perhaps owing to injury to vital organs within the ribcage, blood loss or infection.

Portion [57002], a 26–35-year-old female, suffered peri-mortem fractures in the lower thoracic and the lumbar spines. The 12th thoracic vertebra had a compression fracture in the centre of its superior body surface. Compression was also evident in the first lumbar vertebra, where there was clear superior overlap on the anterior aspect of the body. In the third lumbar vertebra, compression led to retropulsion of the central posterior border of the superior body, an injury that can compromise the neural canal (Maat and Mastwijk 2000, 149; Resnick 2002, 2992) (Fig 64). All these vertebrae were well preserved and provided excellent examples of peri-mortem lesions, having sharp edges with no evidence of remodelling. The vertebral centra suffered mechanical failure following hyperflexion of the spine, perhaps owing to a fall on to the feet or buttocks (Galloway 1999, 95–6; McRae 2003, 351). The fractures would not in themselves have proved fatal but it seems probable that death was related to the same incident.

Male primary inhumation [124], aged ≥46 years, had an unreduced spiral midshaft fracture, with non-displaced butterfly segment, of the right femur. There was clear overlap of the broken ends and shortening of the limb when compared to the left side, suggesting that this was an unstable fracture (Fig 65). The location of the fracture implies that considerable force was involved, as, for example, in a high-impact collision or a fall from a height (Galloway 1999, 180). It is also possible that this was a compound (open) fracture with extensive soft-tissue damage that could cause blood loss, arterial injury, fat embolisation, shock and infection, as well as associated life-threatening injuries to the viscera or cranium (Resnick 2002, 2870–2). Although the fractured ends of the bone had no visible remodelling, small deposits of immature new bone represent the initial stages of healing and suggest that this individual died within approximately three weeks of receiving the injury (Lovell 1997, 145) (Fig 66).

In the disarticulated assemblage, a healed fracture of a right clavicle and another of the left distal tibia had associated secondary infection (above, 'Osteitis and osteomyelitis'), and a healed radial fracture had significant rotational deformity,

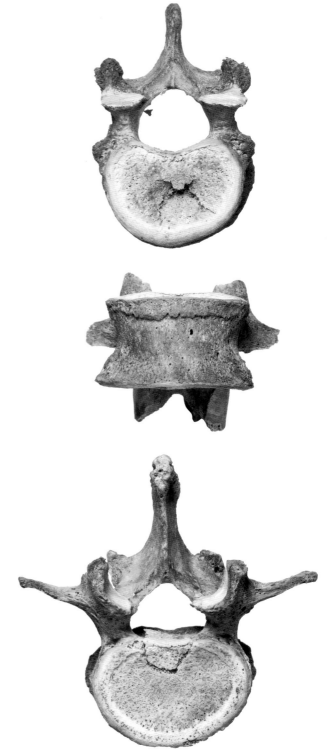

Fig 64 Peri-mortem compression fracture in 12th thoracic (top) and first and third lumbar (middle and bottom) vertebrae of 26–35-year-old female portion [57002] (scale c 1:1)

suggesting an absence of (or ineffective) reduction and splinting. Healed blunt-force injuries were noted on two left frontal bones and one right parietal. Whilst such injuries may have been acquired through accident, assault is also a possibility (the location on the left frontal possibly suggesting a right-handed assailant). A healed avulsion fracture was noted in the styloid

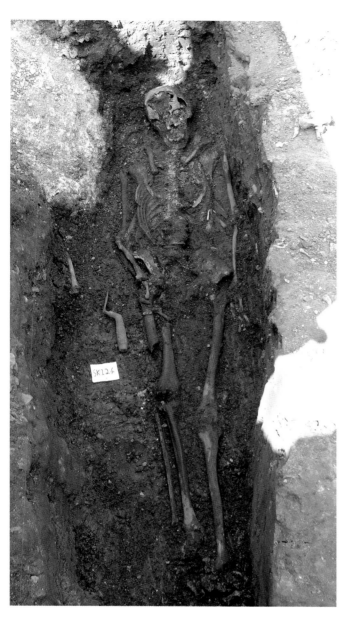

Fig 65 *Male primary inhumation [124], aged ≥46 years, under excavation*

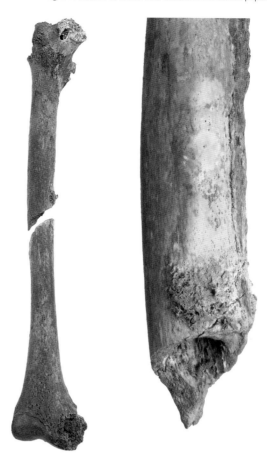

Fig 66 *Unhealed right femoral midshaft fracture from ≥46-year-old male primary inhumation [124]: left – anterior view (scale c 1:4); right – detail of medial view, showing non-displaced butterfly fragment and new bone growth (scale c 1:1)*

process of a right distal ulna. Avulsion injuries also affected a first lumbar vertebra, where the superior endplate had a 'bow-shaped' anterior profile with an excavated area (evidence of disc herniation) immediately behind, and the lateral border of a right cuboid. This last injury had healed but remained un-united. A posterior ring fracture was present in a 12th thoracic vertebra and a possible compression fracture of a fifth lumbar vertebra was indicated by reduction of the height of the anterior body, leading to a wedge-shaped profile.

Two unsided rib fractures were in the process of healing at the time of death whilst the disarticulated sample also contained several examples of peri-mortem injury, including a pertrochanteric fracture of a left femur that was continuous with a contemporaneous three-part spiral fracture of the proximal shaft ([355]), possibly resulting from major trauma (Resnick 2002, 2867–8) (Fig 67). These injuries attest to the likely presence of accident victims (Chapter 5.7).

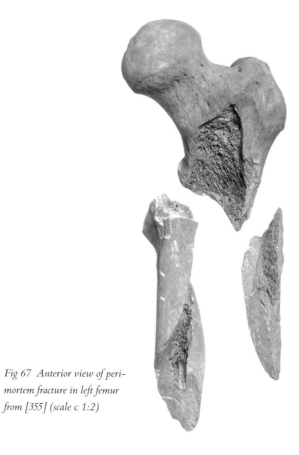

Fig 67 *Anterior view of peri-mortem fracture in left femur from [355] (scale c 1:2)*

JOINT FRACTURES

Fractures involving solely the joint surfaces of the manubrium, patellae, long bones, flat bones and the skull were calculated separately. Details for primary inhumations and portions are listed below (Table 45).

INTERPERSONAL VIOLENCE

A small selection of the fractures noted are suggestive of interpersonal violence. Male [414], aged 26–35 years at death, had suffered a projectile injury to the right, superior, supraoccipital region of the skull (Fig 68). A well-defined circular pit (max Diam 4.4mm) contained a rounded fragment of metal. The fragment lay flush with the ectocranial surface of the occipital bone and a slight rise in the endocranial surface could be felt. This may have been the result of a blow from a sharp object where the end remained in the bone or possibly an embedded piece of shrapnel. The metal fragment prevented the injury from closing.

Blunt-force cranial trauma, consistent with either assault with a blunt weapon or possibly a blow from a falling object, affected 36–45-year-old male [423]. A diamond-shaped depression (32.5 × 14.6mm, × 0.8mm deep) lay immediately to the left of the midline of the frontal bone. The injury was well healed. Blunt-force trauma may also have been the cause of a small depressed area in the cranium of [119], a male aged ≥46 years. A healed sharp-force injury, resulting from assault with a bladed weapon, was seen in the right parietal of 36–45-year-old male [572] (Fig 69).

Six primary inhumations (6/173: 4%), all males (6/80: 8.8%), had fractured nasal bones. These may have been caused by falls or by running into stationary objects, but may also have resulted from punches delivered during episodes of interpersonal violence. Six primary inhumations, again all male, had metacarpal fractures. In four cases these involved Bennett's fracture-dislocations of the first metacarpal bone, usually the result of axial force possibly exerted during the landing of a punch (Dandy and Edwards 1998, 225; McRae 2003, 338). The remaining two cases involved fractured fifth metacarpal shafts, again possibly the result of punching. Two of these individuals had both nasal and metacarpal fractures.

Amongst the portions, two males had nasal fractures. Three

Table 45 True prevalence rate of joint surface fractures

			Female			Male			Adult			Subadult			All individuals	
		n	Affected	%	n	Affected	%	n	Affected	%	n	Affected	%	n	Affected	%
Primary inhumations																
Distal radioulnar	R	22	0	-	59	0	-	94	0	-	2	0	-	96	0	-
	L	23	1	4.3	51	0	-	89	1	1.1	1	0	-	90	1	1.1
	total	45	1	2.2	110	0	-	183	1	0.5	3	0	-	186	1	0.5
Radiocarpal: for scaphoid	R	23	0	-	63	0	-	96	0	-	0	0	-	96	0	-
	L	20	0	-	58	0	-	90	1	1.1	1	0	-	91	1	1.1
	total	43	0	-	121	0	-	186	1	0.5	1	0	-	187	1	0.5
Coxal: acetabulum	R	27	0	-	64	0	-	103	0	-	4	0	-	107	0	-
	L	28	0	-	65	1	1.5	108	1	0.9	2	0	-	110	1	0.9
	total	55	0	-	129	1	0.8	211	1	0.5	6	0	-	217	1	0.5
Femorotibial: lateral	R	26	1	3.8	62	0	-	112	1	0.9	3	0	-	115	1	0.9
	L	23	0	-	63	1	1.6	109	1	0.9	2	0	-	111	1	0.9
	total	49	1	2.0	125	1	0.8	221	2	0.9	5	0	-	226	2	0.9
Proximal tibiofibular	R	18	0	-	38	1	2.6	71	1	1.4	1	0	-	72	1	1.4
	L	12	0	-	39	0	-	63	0	-	2	0	-	65	0	-
	total	30	0	-	77	1	1.3	134	1	0.7	3	0	-	137	1	0.7
Talofibular	R	22	0	-	47	0	-	87	0	-	2	0	-	89	0	-
	L	17	0	-	49	3	6.1	89	3	3.4	2	0	-	91	3	3.3
	total	39	0	-	96	3	3.1	176	3	1.7	4	0	-	180	3	1.7
Portions																
Distal radioulnar	R	22	0	-	59	0	-	94	1	1.1	2	0	-	96	1	1.0
	L	23	0	-	51	0	-	89	0	-	1	0	-	90	0	-
	total	45	0	-	110	0	-	183	1	0.5	3	0	-	186	1	0.5
Radiocarpal: for lunate	R	20	0	-	56	0	-	87	3	3.4	1	0	-	88	3	3.4
	L	21	0	-	50	0	-	83	0	-	1	0	-	84	0	-
	total	41	0	-	106	0	-	170	3	1.8	2	0	-	172	3	1.7
Femoropatellar	R	25	0	-	63	0	-	110	0	-	3	0	-	113	0	-
	L	24	0	-	63	0	-	110	1	0.9	3	0	-	113	1	0.9
	total	49	0	-	126	0	-	220	1	0.5	6	0	-	226	1	0.4
Femorotibial: lateral	R	26	0	-	62	0	-	112	0	-	2	0	-	114	0	-
	L	23	0	-	63	1	1.6	109	2	1.8	2	0	-	111	2	1.8
	total	49	0	-	125	1	0.8	221	2	0.9	4	0	-	225	2	0.9

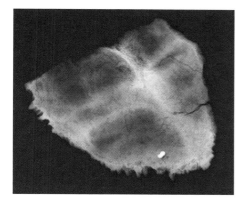

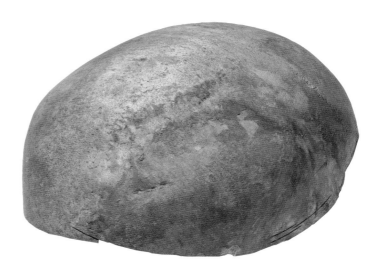

Fig 69 *Healed sharp-force injury to the right parietal of 36–45-year-old male [572] (scale c 1:2)*

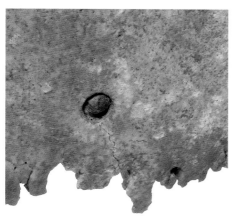

Fig 68 *Right occipital of 26–35-year-old male [414], containing a metal fragment from a projectile injury (view scale c 2:1; radiograph scale c 1:2)*

adults of undetermined sex had suffered first metacarpal fractures (two of which were Bennett's fracture-dislocations), while a fifth metacarpal from a male portion had a neck fracture, commonly referred to as a boxer's fracture because of its aetiology (McRae 2003, 342).

Joint disease

Spinal joint disease

Crude prevalence rates for the primary inhumations are given in Table 46. Osteophytosis and intervertebral disc disease were more prevalent amongst the female inhumations, whilst Schmorl's

nodes affected a greater proportion of males.

One 12–17-year-old subadult had evidence of disc herniation (Schmorl's nodes), affecting one vertebra. This was the only evidence for spinal joint disease in the subadult sample.

True prevalence rates were calculated for the articulated assemblage as a whole by vertebral joint (eg, first to second cervical vertebra). The overall adult pattern of joint disease demonstrated that osteoarthritis was most common in the cervical, upper thoracic and lower lumbar spine, intervertebral disc disease in the lower cervical spine, and Schmorl's nodes in the mid to lower thoracic spine; ostephytosis was least common at the cervico-thoracic border (Fig 70).

Males and females had similar rates of osteoarthitic change (8.0% and 8.6% respectively), intervertebral disc disease (2.3% and 3.3%), osteophytosis (26.7% and 25.3%), and fusion resulting from joint degeneration (0.1% for both sexes). However, male rates of Schmorl's nodes were higher (12.8%) than female (8.8%) (Table 47). When calculated by individual, 45.3% (45/80) of males were affected compared to 33.3% (10/30) of females, a statistically significant difference (χ^2 = 4.58, df = 1, p< 0.04). Whilst this pattern may relate to the different levels of weight-bearing or manual activity performed by the

Table 46 *Crude prevalence rate of spinal joint disease in the primary inhumations*

	n	Schmorl's nodes		Fusion		Osteophytosis		Osteoarthritis		Intervertebral disc disease	
		n	%	n	%	n	%	n	%	n	%
Male	80	45	56.3	3	3.8	52	65.0	35	43.8	15	18.8
Female	30	10	33.3	0	-	22	73.3	12	40.0	8	26.7
Subadult	13	1	7.7	0	-	0	-	0	-	0	-
All adult	160	69	43.1	4	2.5	91	56.9	53	33.1	28	17.5
Total	173	70	40.5	4	2.3	91	52.6	53	30.6	28	16.2

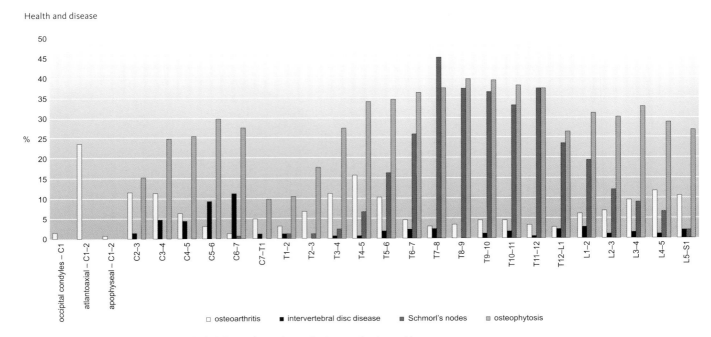

Fig 70 Distribution (true prevalence rate) of adult spinal joint disease for the articulated assemblage

Table 47 True prevalence rate of spinal joint disease in the articulated assemblage

	n	Schmorl's nodes		Fusion		Osteophytosis		Osteoarthritis		Intervertebral disc disease	
		n	%	n	%	n	%	n	%	n	%
Male	2218	285	12.8	3	0.1	592	26.7	177	8.0	50	2.3
Female	791	70	8.8	1	0.1	200	25.3	68	8.6	26	3.3
Subadult	353	1	0.3	0	-	0	-	0	-	0	-
All adult	4330	557	12.9	4	0.1	1143	26.4	303	7.0	92	2.1
Total	4683	558	11.9	4	0.1	1143	24.4	303	6.5	92	2.0

sexes, because of the small female sample size it should be viewed with caution.

True prevalence rates calculated for the primary inhumations and portions separately, and full details by vertebra, may be found in the project archive (Chapter 1.6).

In the disarticulated sample, 616 vertebrae were observable and the true prevalence rates of joint disease (by vertebra) are shown in Table 48. One example of spinal ankylosis was recovered from the disarticulated assemblage and consisted of eighth and ninth thoracic vertebrae joined at the apophyseal facets.

SERONEGATIVE SPONDYLOARTHROPATHY

Possible evidence of ankylosing spondylitis was noted in the disarticulated bone from [457] with characteristic anterior fusion of second to fifth thoracic vertebrae. Psoriatic arthritis is a possible secondary diagnosis.

Extra-spinal joint disease

OSTEOARTHRITIS

Osteoarthritis is the most commonly observed joint disease in humans, affecting the synovial joints of the body (Ortner 2003,

545). The crude prevalence rate of extra-spinal osteoarthritis, with eburnation of the joint surface the diagnostic factor (Rogers and Waldron 1995), increased with advancing age (Fig 71, Table 49). There was no statistically significant difference between males and females. In contrast, at Newcastle Infirmary, 13.6% (26/191) of the articulated adults displayed degenerative joint disease (including osteoarthritis) in the extra-spinal joints, a rate more than twice that seen here (Boulter et al 1998, 126).

Contexts with extra-spinal osteoarthritis considered to be secondary to other classes of disease, such as trauma, were then removed from the overall crude prevalence rates. The results may be seen in Table 50.

True prevalence rate was calculated for each major adult joint where eburnation was recorded as present (Table 51). Insufficient numbers of affected joints prevented comparison of the primary inhumations with ten affected portions, and with samples from other sites. In the smaller joints, the most commonly affected facets were the distal ends of the first metatarsals (right: 3/89: 3.4%; left: 3/98: 3.1%).

The disarticulated assemblage also contained examples of extra-spinal osteoarthritis affecting a right mandibular condyle, left first proximal hand phalanx, right proximal humerus, right

Table 48 True prevalence rate of spinal joint disease in the disarticulated sample

Vertebral joint	n	Schmorl's nodes		Fusion		Osteophytosis		Osteoarthritis		Intervertebral disc disease	
		n	%	n	%	n	%	n	%	n	%
C1	32	0	-	0	-	0	-	0	-	0	-
C2	33	0	-	0	-	0	-	1	3.0	0	-
C3	27	0	-	0	-	1	3.7	1	3.7	0	-
C4	34	0	-	0	-	5	14.7	2	5.9	1	2.9
C5	15	0	-	0	-	2	13.3	2	13.3	1	6.7
C6	14	0	-	0	-	2	14.3	0	-	0	-
C7	17	0	-	0	-	2	11.8	2	11.8	1	5.9
C8	1	0	-	0	-	0	-	0	-	0	-
T1	27	0	-	0	-	4	14.8	2	7.4	0	-
T2	28	1	3.6	0	-	6	21.4	2	7.1	0	-
T3	20	0	-	0	-	5	25.0	0	-	0	-
T4	23	1	4.3	0	-	11	47.8	0	-	0	-
T5	19	0	-	0	-	5	26.3	0	-	0	-
T6	19	0	-	0	-	5	26.3	0	-	0	-
T7	22	3	13.6	0	-	4	18.2	0	-	0	-
T8	12	3	25.0	1	8.3	3	25.0	0	-	0	-
T9	15	1	6.7	1	6.7	3	20.0	0	-	1	6.7
T10	16	3	18.8	0	-	5	31.3	0	-	0	-
T11	13	5	38.5	0	-	3	23.1	0	-	0	-
T12	22	1	4.5	0	-	5	22.7	0	-	0	-
T13	1	0	-	0	-	0	-	0	-	0	-
L1	29	3	10.3	0	-	9	31.0	0	-	0	-
L2	18	1	5.6	0	-	3	16.7	0	-	0	-
L3	30	3	10.0	0	-	8	26.7	0	-	1	3.3
L4	30	3	10.0	0	-	8	26.7	0	-	1	3.3
L5	52	3	5.8	0	-	10	19.2	0	-	3	5.8
L6	0	0	-	0	-	0	-	0	-	0	-
S1	47	1	2.1	0	-	8	17.0	0	-	1	2.1
Total	616	32	5.2	2	0.3	117	19.0	12	1.9	10	1.6

glenoid scapula and left acromion (shoulder), with one right radius and ulna, a right distal humerus (elbow), two distal hand phalanges, one right and one left trapezium (hand and wrist), a right acromion and associated acromial clavicle and two first metatarsals. Joints were not catalogued and so these data

remain separate for the purposes of calculating true prevalence rates.

GOUT

Gout leads to painful crystal formation within articular cartilage as a result of kidney malfunction or an excess of uric acid (Resnick 2002, 1519). Two adult females from the primary inhumations had unilateral para-articular erosive lesions on the heads of the first metatarsals, possibly the result of gouty arthritis. This represents crude prevalence rates of 6.7% (2/30) of females, 1.3% (2/160) of adults and 1.2% (2/173) of all

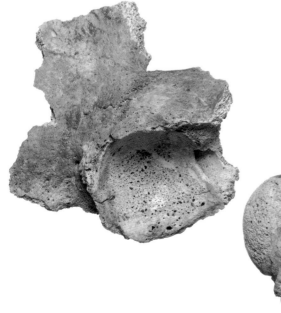

Fig 71 Osteoarthritis in the left hip of 36–45-year-old male primary inhumation [358]: the femoral neck appeared short with para-articular new bone formation, suggesting that an underlying aetiology of a slipped femoral epiphysis was probable, but the absence of the right femur prevented morphological comparisons (scale c 1:2)

Table 49 Crude prevalence rate of extra-spinal osteoarthritis in the primary inhumations

Age		Female			Male			Intermediate			Undetermined			Subadult			Adult			All individuals	
	n	Affected	%	n	Affected	%	n	Affected	%	n	Affected	%	n	Affected	%	n	Affected	%	n	Affected	%
<4 weeks	0	0	-	0	0	-	0	0	-	0	0	-	5	0	-	0	0	-	5	0	-
1–6 months	0	0	-	0	0	-	0	0	-	0	0	-	0	0	-	0	0	-	0	0	-
7–11 months	0	0	-	0	0	-	0	0	-	0	0	-	0	0	-	0	0	-	0	0	-
1–5 years	0	0	-	0	0	-	0	0	-	0	0	-	3	0	-	0	0	-	3	0	-
6–11 years	0	0	-	0	0	-	0	0	-	0	0	-	1	0	-	0	0	-	1	0	-
12–17 years	0	0	-	0	0	-	0	0	-	0	0	-	4	0	-	0	0	-	4	0	-
Subadult	0	0	-	0	0	-	0	0	-	0	0	-	0	0	-	0	0	-	0	0	-
18–25 years	4	0	-	6	0	-	3	0	-	1	0	-	0	0	-	14	0	-	14	0	-
26–35 years	10	1	10.0	25	0	-	1	0	-	2	0	-	0	0	-	38	1	2.6	38	1	2.6
36–45 years	9	1	11.1	27	2	7.4	0	0	-	2	0	-	0	0	-	38	3	7.9	38	3	7.9
≥446 years	3	2	66.7	9	2	22.2	0	0	-	0	0	-	0	0	-	12	4	33.3	12	4	33.3
Adult	4	0	-	13	2	15.4	1	0	-	40	1	2.5	0	0	-	58	3	5.2	58	3	5.2
Total	30	4	13.3	80	6	7.5	5	0	-	45	1	2.2	13	0	-	160	11	6.9	173	11	6.4

Table 50 Crude prevalence rate of primary extra-spinal osteoarthritis in the primary inhumations

Age		Female			Male			Intermediate			Undetermined			Subadult			Adult			All individuals	
	n	Affected	%	n	Affected	%	n	Affected	%	n	Affected	%	n	Affected	%	n	Affected	%	n	Affected	%
<4 weeks	0	0	-	0	0	-	0	0	-	0	0	-	5	0	-	0	0	-	5	0	-
1–6 months	0	0	-	0	0	-	0	0	-	0	0	-	0	0	-	0	0	-	0	0	-
7–11 months	0	0	-	0	0	-	0	0	-	0	0	-	0	0	-	0	0	-	0	0	-
1–5 years	0	0	-	0	0	-	0	0	-	0	0	-	3	0	-	0	0	-	3	0	-
6–11 years	0	0	-	0	0	-	0	0	-	0	0	-	1	0	-	0	0	-	1	0	-
12–17 years	0	0	-	0	0	-	0	0	-	4	0	-	0	0	-	0	0	-	4	0	-
Subadult	0	0	-	0	0	-	0	0	-	0	0	-	0	0	-	0	0	-	0	0	-
18–25 years	4	0	-	6	0	-	3	0	-	1	0	-	0	0	-	14	0	-	14	0	-
26–35 years	10	1	10.0	25	0	-	1	0	-	2	0	-	0	0	-	38	1	2.6	38	1	2.6
36–45 years	9	1	11.1	27	1	3.7	0	0	-	2	0	-	0	0	-	38	2	5.3	38	2	5.3
≥46 years	3	2	66.7	9	0	-	0	0	-	0	0	-	0	0	-	12	2	16.7	12	2	16.7
Adult	4	0	-	13	1	7.7	1	0	-	40	0	-	0	0	-	58	1	1.7	58	1	1.7
Total	30	4	13.3	80	2	2.5	5	0	-	45	0	-	13	0	-	160	6	3.8	173	6	3.5

Table 51 True prevalence rate of extra-spinal osteoarthritis by joint

Joint			Female			Male			All adults	
		n	Affected	%	n	Affected	%	n	Affected	%
Primary inhumations										
Acromioclavicular	R	17	0	-	46	3	6.5	80	2	2.5
	L	15	0	-	50	3	6.0	83	3	3.6
	total	32	0	-	96	6	6.3	163	5	3.1
Humeroradial	R	22	0	-	63	1	1.6	102	1	1.0
	L	22	0	-	55	2	3.6	102	3	2.9
	total	44	0	-	118	3	2.5	204	4	2.0
Proximal radioulnar	R	22	0	-	61	1	1.6	100	1	1.0
	L	22	0	-	54	0	-	96	0	-
	total	44	0	-	115	1	0.9	196	1	0.5
Distal radioulnar	R	22	0	-	59	0	-	94	0	-
	L	23	0	-	51	1	2.0	89	1	1.1
	total	45	0	-	110	1	0.9	183	1	0.5
Coxal	R	27	0	-	64	0	-	103	0	-
	L	28	1	3.6	65	1	1.5	108	2	1.9
	total	55	1	1.8	129	1	0.8	211	2	0.9

Table 51 (cont)

Joint		Female			Male			All adults		
		n	Affected	%	n	Affected	%	n	Affected	%
Portions										
Acromioclavicular	R	2	0	-	9	0	-	33	I	3.0
	L	I	0	-	7	I	14.3	33	2	6.I
	total	3	0	-	16	I	6.3	66	3	4.5
Coxal	R	12	0	-	42	0	-	71	0	-
	L	6	0	-	37	I	2.7	57	I	1.8
	total	18	0	-	79	I	1.3	128	I	0.8
Femoropatellar	R	4	0	-	21	0	-	55	0	-
	L	4	0	-	21	0	-	47	I	2.1
	total	8	0	-	42	0	-	102	I	1.0
Femorotibial: lateral	R	4	0	-	20	0	-	55	0	-
	L	3	0	-	22	I	4.5	46	I	2.2
	total	7	0	-	42	I	2.4	101	I	1.0
Femorotibial: medial	R	4	0	-	21	0	-	28	0	-
	L	3	0	-	22	0	-	46	I	2.2
	total	7	0	-	43	0	-	74	I	1.4

primary inhumations. One portion from probable male [59801] and an adult left first metatarsal from the disarticulated assemblage were also affected, giving an overall true prevalence rate of 1.3% (4/306 first metatarsals) (Chapter 7.8, 'The status of the buried population', for further discussion).

ROTATOR CUFF

Rotator cuff injuries at the shoulder, affecting the muscles and tendons of supraspinatus, infraspinatus, teres minor and subscapularis, may be caused by trauma or advancing age (Resnick 2002, 3075). Bone changes reflecting damage to the rotator cuff were observed in 16 adult primary inhumations (16/173: 9.2%), including one female (1/30: 3.3%) and 14 males (14/80: 17.5%). Three adult portions and eight humeri from the disarticulated assemblage were also affected, giving a total true prevalence rate of 7.4% (36/487 proximal humeri).

JOINT ANKYLOSIS

Joint ankylosis was observed in the sacroiliac joints of one ≥46-year-old male primary inhumation (bilateral), one ≥46-year-old male portion (unilateral) [21001] and one disarticulated male left ilium ([457]). These examples may have been related to an inflammatory arthropathy (ankylosing spondylitis, psoriatic arthritis, Reiter's disease), or diffuse idiopathic skeletal hyperostosis (DISH), or to trauma, joint disease or old age, but insufficient quantities of the skeletons survived to enable diagnosis.

OTHER EXTRA-SPINAL JOINT DISEASE

Primary female inhumation [452], aged 26–35 years, had an atrophic right mandibular facet, with no apparent articular surface remaining. This may have resulted from lack of mastication following the loss of all the mandibular and maxillary teeth.

Primary female inhumation [279], aged 18–25 years, had

a large dorsal bunion on the superolateral aspect of the right first metatarsal head, just proximal to the articular head, with initial signs of similar growth on the left bone. This form of dorsal bunion can lead to hallux limitus or hallux rigidus, and almost certainly to osteoarthritis (Lapidus 1940, 627–37; Schumacher n d).

Congenital and developmental abnormalities

Dental anomalies

Very low rates of Carabelli's cusp were noted, affecting only three male and one subadult primary inhumations and one adult portion. Just one female tooth had an enamel pearl and low numbers of teeth were affected by all other dental anomalies (Tables 52–3). Male [414], aged 26–35 years, had a severe overbite and the dental crowding was so severe in 26–35-year-old female [455] that the sockets of the mandibular central incisors lay behind (lingual to) the lateral incisors. A small selection of unusual anomalies was noted in the primary inhumations (Table 54), all with a true prevalence rate of 0.1% (1/1558). There was no evidence of the transposition of teeth.

Spinal disorders

A number of contexts from the articulated sample displayed minor congenital anomalies in the form of vertebral border shifts (Powers 2008, 64–8 (after Barnes 1994)) (Table 55). The most commonly observed segmentation failure was spina bifida occulta, the incomplete fusion of the posterior neural arches of the sacral segments and or lumbar vertebrae, which affected 3.7% of adult elements (Table 56). This is one of the most frequently reported developmental defects from archaeological samples (Roberts and Manchester 2005, 55), and compares to a crude prevalence rate of 12.5% of the articulated sacra (6/48),

Table 52 True prevalence rate of dental anomalies in the articulated assemblage

	n (teeth)	n (sockets)	Carabelli's cusp		Enamel pearls		Crowding		Protosylid cusp		Peg teeth		Impaction		Rotation	
			n	%	n	%	n	%	n	%	n	%	n	%	n	%
Primary inhumations																
Male	1049	1593	3	0.3	0	-	15	1.4	1	0.1	5	0.5	2	0.2	11	1.0
Female	367	596	0	-	1	0.3	6	1.6	0	-	1	0.3	2	0.5	5	1.4
Subadult	75	116	1	1.3	0	-	0	-	0	-	0	-	2	2.7	2	2.7
All adult	1483	2314	3	0.2	1	0.1	21	1.4	1	0.1	6	0.4	4	0.3	17	1.1
Total	1558	2430	4	0.2	1	0.1	21	1.3	1	0.1	6	0.4	6	0.4	19	1.2
Portions																
Male	99	280	0	-	0	-	0	-	0	-	1	1.0	0	-	0	-
Female	71	172	0	-	0	-	0	-	0	-	0	-	0	-	2	2.8
Subadult	1	29	0	-	0	-	0	-	0	-	0	-	0	-	0	-
All adult	243	572	2	0.8	0	-	0	-	0	-	0	-	1	0.4	5	2.1
Total	244	601	2	0.3	0	-	0	-	0	-	0	-	1	0.4	5	2.0
Primary inhumations & portions																
Male	1148	1873	3	0.3	0	-	15	1.3	1	0.1	6	0.5	2	0.2	11	1.0
Female	438	768	0	-	1	0.2	6	1.4	0	-	1	0.2	2	0.5	7	1.6
Subadult	76	145	1	1.3	0	-	0	-	0	-	0	-	2	2.6	2	2.6
All adult	1726	2886	5	0.3	1	0.1	21	1.2	1	0.1	6	0.3	5	0.3	22	1.3
Total	1802	3031	6	0.2	1	0.1	21	1.2	1	0.1	6	0.3	7	0.4	24	1.3

Table 53 Crude prevalence rate of dental anomalies for the primary inhumations

	n	Carabelli's cusp		Enamel pearls		Crowding		Protosylid cusp		Peg teeth		Impaction		Rotation	
		n	%	n	%	n	%	n	%	n	%	n	%	n	%
Primary inhumations															
Male	80	3	3.8	0	-	11	13.8	1	1.3	5	6.3	2	2.5	9	11.3
Female	30	0	-	1	3.3	4	13.3	0	-	1	3.3	2	6.7	5	16.7
Subadult	13	1	7.7	0	-	0	-	0	-	0	-	2	15.4	1	7.7
All adult	160	3	1.9	1	0.6	15	9.4	1	0.6	6	3.8	4	2.5	15	9.4
Total	173	4	2.3	1	0.6	15	8.7	1	0.6	6	3.5	6	3.5	16	9.2

Table 54 Unusual dental anomalies in the primary inhumations

Context no.	Age/sex	Tooth	Anomaly
[369]	male	R mandibular 1st molar	three roots
[109]	male	maxillary 1st incisors	stunted roots
[407]	male	R maxillary lateral incisor	peg tooth
[131]	female	L mandibular 3rd molar	+5 cusp pattern (Bass 1987, 279)

whilst the same proportion of the disarticulated sacra from Newcastle Infirmary (2/53: 3.8%) also demonstrated spina bifida occulta (Boulter et al 1998, 117–19). In the disarticulated sample an example of a hypoplastic neural arch with a posterior hiatus was noted in a fourth lumbar vertebra (1/246: 0.4%). A second and a third cervical vertebra found disarticulated within [457] formed a single 'block'. Partial (left) sacralisation also affected adult disarticulated context [457].

Female [523], aged 36–45 years, was affected by a series of vertebral defects (Fig 72). The sixth cervical vertebral body and bifurcated neural arch were congenitally fused to the seventh cervical vertebra, forming a block vertebra. She also had a hypoplastic spinous process on the sixth cervical vertebra and a bifurcated neural arch with irregular left superior apophyseal articulation on the seventh cervical vertebra. In the first thoracic vertebra the left costal facet was absent, the neural arch bifurcated and the left superior articular facet faced to anterior (rather than to posterior as normal) in order to articulate with the seventh cervical vertebra. There was hypoplasia of the first thoracic body with vertically restricted posterior margins on midline, while the second thoracic vertebra had a bifurcated neural arch. These changes all represent delays in development (Barnes 1994, 117–23). The fused vertebrae resulted from type II Klippel-Feil syndrome, which is normally asymptomatic and probably the result of autosomal dominant transmission (ibid, 67–9). She also had merged first and second left ribs together with a rib spur, possibly a secondary consequence of the changes in the lower cervical/upper thoracic spine (ibid, 73–4).

Table 55 Vertebral border shifts in the articulated assemblage

Border shift	Female			Male			Adult			Subadult			All individuals		
	n	Affected	%	n	Affected	%	n	Affected	%	n	Affected	%	n	Affected	%
Occipitocervical border	30	0	-	69	0	-	131	0	-	8	0	-	139	0	-
Expression of occipital vertebrae	30	0	-	69	0	-	131	0	-	8	0	-	139	0	-
Precondylar process	30	0	-	69	0	-	131	0	-	8	0	-	139	0	-
Bipartite occipital condyles	30	0	-	69	0	-	131	0	-	8	0	-	139	0	-
Atlas occipitalised	30	0	-	69	0	-	131	0	-	8	0	-	139	0	-
Epitransverse process (R)	30	0	-	69	1	1.4	131	0	-	8	0	-	139	0	-
Cervicothoracic border	30	1	3.3	82	3	3.7	162	4	2.5	16	0	-	178	4	2.2
Expression of cervical rib: bony tubercle	30	1	3.3	82	0	-	162	1	0.6	16	0	-	178	1	0.6
Cervical rib: complete with articular facets	30	0	-	82	1	1.2	162	1	0.6	16	0	-	178	1	0.6
Stunted transverse process C7	30	0	-	82	2	2.4	162	3	1.9	16	0	-	178	3	1.7
2nd rib attaches to mesosternum only	30	0	-	82	0	-	162	0	-	16	0	-	178	0	-
Thoracolumbar border	30	9	30.0	89	22	24.7	178	43	24.2	14	2	14.3	192	45	23.4
Hypoplastic rib 12	30	4	13.3	89	2	2.2	178	9	5.1	14	0	-	192	9	4.7
Aplastic rib 12	30	0	-	89	1	1.1	178	1	0.6	14	0	-	192	1	0.5
Transitional facets on T11	30	6	20.0	89	4	4.5	178	29	16.3	14	2	14.3	192	31	16.1
T13 present	30	0	-	89	0	-	178	0	-	14	0	-	192	0	-
Lumbar rib & facet on L1	30	0	-	89	2	2.2	178	3	1.7	14	0	-	192	3	1.6
Transitional facet on L1	30	2	6.7	89	1	1.1	178	3	1.7	14	0	-	192	3	1.6
Lumbosacral border	37	3	8.1	117	9	7.7	197	19	9.6	12	0	-	209	19	9.1
Ala-like transverse process L5 – non articulating (R)	37	0	-	117	0	-	197	0	-	12	0	-	209	0	-
Ala-like transverse process L5 – articulating (L – partial sacralisation)	37	1	2.7	117	1	0.9	197	2	1.0	12	0	-	209	2	1.0
Ala-like transverse process L5 – articulating (R – partial sacralisation)	37	1	2.7	117	1	0.9	197	3	1.5	12	0	-	209	3	1.4
Complete sacralisation L5	37	0	-	117	2	1.7	197	2	1.0	12	0	-	209	2	1.0
L6 present (no ala-like wings, non articulating)	37	0	-	117	2	1.7	197	4	2.0	12	0	-	209	4	1.9
Ala-like transverse process L6 – articulating (R – partial sacralisation)	37	0	-	117	1	0.9	197	1	0.5	12	0	-	209	1	0.5
Complete sacralisation of L6	37	0	-	117	0	-	197	0	-	12	0	-	209	0	-
Anterior cleft between S1 & S2	37	0	-	117	0	-	197	0	-	12	0	-	209	0	-
S1 & S2 apophyseal joints & anterior cleft	37	0	-	117	0	-	197	1	0.5	12	0	-	209	1	0.5
Incomplete lumbarisation of S1 L	37	0	-	117	0	-	197	0	-	12	0	-	209	0	-
Incomplete lumbarisation of S1 R	37	1	2.7	117	1	0.9	197	5	2.5	12	0	-	209	5	2.4
Complete lumbarisation of S1 (bilateral)	37	0	-	117	1	0.9	197	1	0.5	12	0	-	209	1	0.5
Sacrocaudal border	27	6	22.2	88	19	21.6	135	30	22.2	3	0	-	138	30	21.7
Complete separation of S5	27	0	-	88	1	1.1	135	1	0.7	3	0	-	138	1	0.7
Incomplete sacralisation of 1st caudal vertebra	27	4	14.8	88	13	14.8	135	20	14.8	3	1	33.3	138	21	15.2
Complete sacralisation of 1st caudal vertebra	27	3	11.1	88	6	6.8	135	11	8.1	3	0	-	138	11	8.0

Table 56 True prevalence rate of neural arch non-union in the articulated assemblage

	Female			Male			Adult			Subadult			All individuals		
	n	Affected	%	n	Affected	%	n	Affected	%	n	Affected	%	n	Affected	%
C1	27	1	3.7	63	1	1.6	121	2	1.7	6	0	-	127	2	1.6
L5	35	0	-	108	1	0.9	183	1	0.5	11	0	-	194	1	0.5
L6	0	0	-	3	0	-	5	1	20.0	0	0	-	5	1	20.0
S1	36	2	5.6	113	15	13.3	180	21	11.7	12	0	-	192	21	10.9
S2	35	0	-	101	6	5.9	166	8	4.8	7	0	-	173	8	4.6
S3	32	1	3.1	97	7	7.2	157	10	6.4	6	0	-	163	10	6.1
S4	30	3	10.0	90	30	33.3	144	37	25.7	4	1	25.0	148	38	25.7
S5	27	16	59.3	79	63	79.7	126	90	71.4	3	1	33.3	129	91	70.5
All vertebrae	864	23	2.7	2497	123	4.9	4620	170	3.7	326	2	0.6	4946	172	3.5

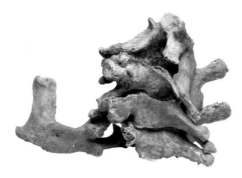

Fig 72 Vertebral anomalies in the spine of 36–45-year-old female primary inhumation [523]: posterior view of sixth cervical to second thoracic vertebrae (scale c 1:2)

Scoliosis was observed in one primary inhumation and an articulated portion. Context [15001], a portion of a 36–45-year-old male, displayed scoliosis at the junction of the lumbar and sacral vertebrae. The first two sacral bodies were laterally wedged to the left, the fifth lumbar vertebral body compensated through wedging on its right side. Primary inhumation [175], a 26–35-year-old female, had severe scoliosis with mid–lower thoracic curvature to the left side and upper lumbar curvature to the right. This was associated with advanced secondary osteoarthritis and fusion of some apophyseal joints. The ribcage was asymmetrical with deformation and thinning of the right 11th and 12th ribs (Fig 73). Idiopathic scoliosis usually manifests between 10 and 12 years of age, possibly owing to inheritance of a dominant trait (Aufderheide and Rodríguez-Martín 1998, 66). Primary inhumation [551], a male aged ≥46 years, had left lateral wedging of the fifth lumbar vertebra. There was no evidence of scoliosis and this may have been a developmental adjustment to asymmetry at the lumbosacral border.

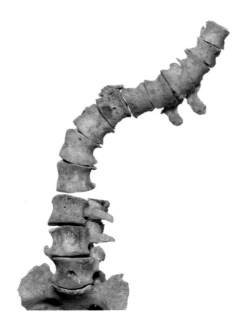

Fig 73 Severe idiopathic scoliosis in 26–35-year-old female [175] (scale c 1:4)

Spondylolysis is the unilateral or bilateral separation of the posterior neural arch of a vertebra, generally caused by repetitive spinal trauma in teenagers. Apart from slight lower back discomfort the condition normally causes no symptoms unless it is associated with vertebral body dislocation (Roberts and Manchester 2005, 106). Six articulated contexts had spondylolysis in the vertebral column, one in the third lumbar vertebra (1/187 of this vertebra; 0.5%), four in the fifth lumbar vertebra (4/194: 2.1%) and one in a sixth lumbar vertebra (1/5: 20%). Four of these originated from the primary inhumation sample (4/173: 2.3%). In four cases there was bilateral separation whilst the other two were unilateral. Two examples of spondylolysis, both affecting the fifth lumbar vertebra, were found within the disarticulated assemblage (2/52: 3.8%), bringing the overall prevalence rate for this vertebra to 2.4% (6/246).

Extra-spinal disorders

Ten primary inhumations (10/173: 5.8%), one articulated portion and three disarticulated elements (3/7571: <0.1%) displayed minor extra-spinal anomalies.

Probable male primary inhumation [340], aged 36–45 years, exhibited a slight protrusion of the posterior cranial vault (bathrocephaly). This developmental anomaly results from excessive enlargement of the lambdoid suture during growth. Adult [443], of intermediate sex, had bony growths on the right third and fourth ribs terminating in articulating facets indicative of partial bridging of the ribs (also known as incomplete merging) (Barnes 1994, 72–4). The right scapula of [385], an 18–25-year-old adult of undetermined sex, had a deviated glenoid fossa (c 45° posterior to normal position). The glenoid neck was unusually small and the fossa irregular, with a shallow horizontal notch running across the centre of the articular surface. The tip of the acromial process was also angled slightly to posterior. Such hypoplasia (dysplasia) of the glenoid neck can lead to joint instability. The cause of the condition is uncertain but it may be due to a failure of cartilage in this region to ossify, possibly as a result of an inherited trait (dominant gene) (Resnick 2002, 4583–6). The arm appeared normal with defined muscle attachments.

The radii of [369], a 36–45-year-old male, also from the primary inhumation sample, had unusually deep depressions in the articular head, and sub-triangular extensions of the articular surfaces on to the anteromedial aspect of the proximal shaft (Fig 74). Both extensions were well defined, smooth and had no evidence of joint disease. The lateral aspect of the proximal shaft of the left ulna was slightly concave. In the right ulna there was an inferior extension to the radioulnar facet, continuing into a substantial concavity in the lateral aspect of the proximal shaft. This condition probably represents some form of fibrous fusion within the spectrum of radioulnar synostosis, an anomaly of longitudinal segmentation that is bilateral in 60% of cases (Resnick 2002, 4589–90).

Two primary inhumations, both male, had sesamoid bones

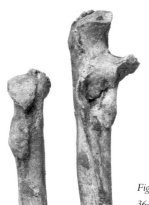

Fig 74 Bilateral radioulnar synostosis in 36–45-year-old male [369] (scale c 1:2)

resulting in crescent-shaped depressions in the superior rims of the acetabula (os acetabulum). In both cases the left os coxa was affected. Although this condition can be associated with dysplasia, there was no evidence of such in these individuals (Martinez et al 2006). However, amongst the disarticulated material was one example of developmental hip dysplasia, again with malformation of the left acetabulum (1/110 disarticulated ilia; 0.9%; 1/472 total ilia; 0.2%).

Adult [40210] from the primary inhumations, of undetermined sex, had a relatively common form of tarsal coalition with cartilaginous or fibrous union of the calcaneus and navicular in the right foot, and elongation of the posterior border of the navicular. This can be asymptomatic or may be associated with painful flat-foot deformity (Resnick 2002, 4593). One male and two adults of undetermined sex were affected by type II os navicularum, where an accessory ossicle is incorporated into the posterior tibial tendon on the medial side of the foot. In all three cases, the ossicle did not survive although its presence was attested by a flattened articular surface on a shortened medial end of the navicular. Although often asymptomatic, the condition can be aggravated by trauma, habitual activity or poorly fitted shoes, leading to inflammation and pain (Wheeless 2011).

Portion [22306], from an 18–25-year-old male, had bilateral bipartite medial cuneiforms, where the superior halves of the bones are separated from their inferior halves. This is a developmental anomaly that may or may not be symptomatic (Elias et al 2008). Two portions of adults of undetermined sex had osseous defects in third cuneometatarsal joints, presenting as sub-circular pits in the articular surfaces of the lateral cuneiforms and third metatarsals. These lesions may represent a form of tarsal coalition with a strong genetic link (Regan et al 1999). Symphalangism affected the feet of two male primary inhumations (2/173: 1.2%).

In the disarticulated material, a group of foot bones from [179] contained an unusually short third metatarsal – 2.2% (1/45) of disarticulated third metatarsals and 1.3% of all third metatarsals (1/80). This condition (brachymetatarsia), which usually presents between 4 and 15 years of age, is often asymptomatic but may lead to foot pain and increased risk of hallux valgus. Brachymetatarsia has a reported 25:1 female bias

and clinical incidence of just 0.02% (Thomas et al 2009, 246). Context [190] contained an adult mandible with a bifurcated left condyle. This is again generally asymptomatic but can lead to joint malfunction (Barnes 1994, 166). The condition was present in 0.5% of left mandibles (1/200).

HALLUX VALGUS

Hallux valgus describes a deformity where the great toe is angulated laterally towards the other toes of the foot. Untreated, this can lead to joint disease and bunion formation. Although it is found in individuals who do not wear shoes, it is commonly associated in modern populations with restrictive footwear (Resnick 2002, 1361; McRae 2003, 181; Mays 2005, 139) (Fig 75).

Of the 30 females in the primary inhumations, four (13.3%) had suffered from the condition. This compared to a male crude prevalence rate in the group of just 5.0% (4/80). This pattern remained when the prevalence rate by element was calculated for the articulated contexts as a whole, with 18.4% (7/38) of female and 7.8% (8/103) of male first metatarsals affected (Table 57). Therefore, although the sample size is small, it appears that females were more susceptible to hallux valgus, possibly as a result of gender-related shoe choice. In total, 6.3% (10/160) of adults and 5.8% (10/173) of all primary inhumations had suffered from hallux valgus.

The true prevalence rate for all articulated contexts was 7.7% (19/248) with 8.2% (19/233) of adult first metatarsals affected. A greater proportion of right than left first metatarsals were affected for each sex, though this pattern was not observable for the adult assemblage as a whole.

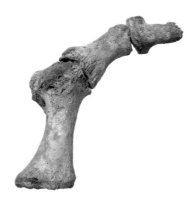

Fig 75 Right great toe from [360], an adult with hallux valgus and a large bunion (scale c 1:2)

Table 57 True prevalence rate of hallux valgus by side in all articulated contexts

Sex	Observable		Affected		%	
	Right	Left	Right	Left	Right	Left
Female	18	20	4	3	22.2	15.0
Male	49	54	4	4	8.2	7.4
All adults	111	122	9	10	8.1	8.2

The disarticulated material contained one right and one left first metatarsal with evidence of hallux valgus, with bunion formation in the remains from [360]. When the disarticulated material is included, the overall true prevalence rate of hallux valgus is 4.4% (21/474 adult first metatarsals).

MUSCULAR DYSTROPHY

Subadult [298], aged 12–17 years, from the primary inhumations, had a small and very gracile skeleton, though overall the elements remained fairly well proportioned (Fig 76). Approximate stature based on right humeral length was 1.54m (5ft 0in). Excess curvature was evident in the acromial shafts of the clavicles, and the site photograph revealed them to be unusually positioned, orientated on the long axis of the body with the acromial ends pointing superiorly (Fig 77). All long-bone shafts, except for the tibiae and fibulae, were slightly thicker on the left side, but insufficient survival prevented analysis of any possible

difference in length. There was a clear discrepancy between the hand bones, with the left metacarpals much longer than the right (eg, second right metacarpal 54.8mm, left 59.2mm).

This degree of gracility can be found in individuals suffering from muscular dystrophy (MD), a condition that leads to progressive myogenic atrophy (muscle wasting). The most common form is Duchenne's MD. Often inherited, it occurs only in males, who usually do not survive beyond 15 years of age. Individual [298] was *c* 17 years old at death and was perhaps affected by a lesser form of the disease, such as facioscapulohumeral MD or Becker's MD, which chiefly affects the upper body (Resnick 2002, 4751).

UNIDENTIFIED CONGENITAL SYNDROME

Probable male [269], aged 26–35 years, from the primary inhumations, had severe bone changes to all the surviving elements of the skeleton (the cranium, upper body and lower

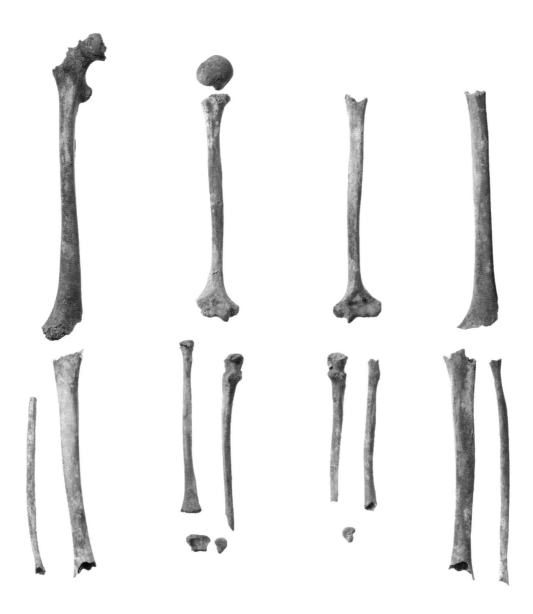

Fig 76 12–17-year-old primary inhumation [298] with possible muscular dystrophy (scale c 1:4)

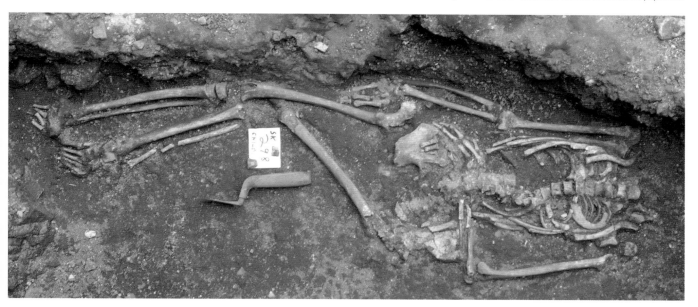

Fig 77 *12–17-year-old primary inhumation [298] under excavation showing the unusual position of the clavicles*

legs and feet were absent owing to truncation).

There was bilateral and symmetrical Erlenmeyer flask deformity, abnormal cortical thinning and a lack of metaphyseal concavity, named after the piece of laboratory equipment that the distal femur subsequently resembles (Faden et al 2009, 1334) (Fig 78), with similar changes to the right radius and ulna (the left bones did not survive), the proximal ends of the first metacarpals, the distal ends of the second to fifth metacarpals,

and the proximal ends of the proximal and middle hand phalanges (Fig 79). Radiographs (Figs 78–9) reveal modelling deformities and cortical thinning. The os coxae were slightly light in weight and had enlarged ischiopubic rami, resulting in reduced obturator foramina size (Fig 80).

All surfaces on the surviving skeleton consisted of mature bone and all joint surfaces appeared healthy. Erlenmeyer flask deformity can be found in cases of Gaucher's disease, Niemann-

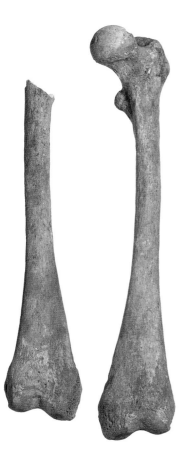

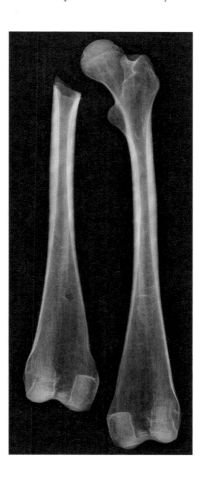

Fig 78 *Femora of 26–35-year-old probable male primary inhumation [269] (view and radiograph scale c 1:4)*

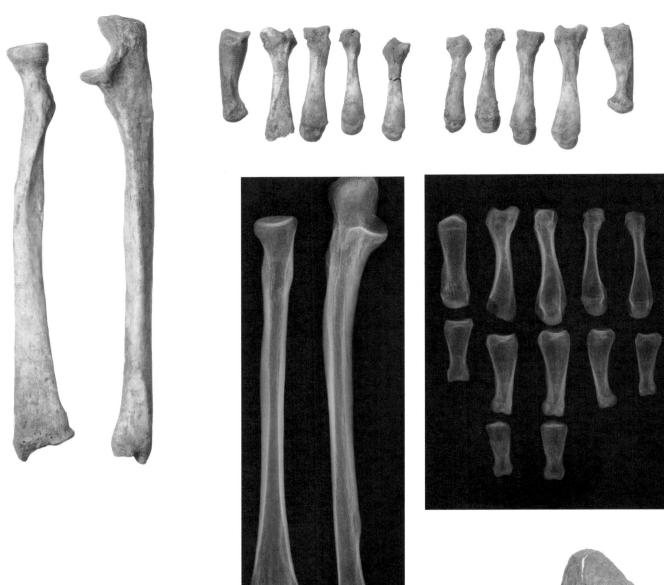

Fig 79 *Right forearm and hands of 26–35-year-old probable male primary inhumation [269] (scale c 1:2)*

Pick disease, fibrous dysplasia, anaemia, osteopetrosis, metaphyseal dysplasia and heavy metal poisoning (Resnick 2002, 2245–6). The lack of further macroscopic or radiographic changes to this skeleton would be unlikely in adult individuals with the majority of these disorders. It is possible that a milder form of Niemann-Pick disease, where lipids accumulate in the cells of the liver, spleen and brain, was responsible – perhaps type B, which is a chronic form involving the nervous system and sphingomyelinase deficiency, or type E, a form with visceral involvement found in adults (ibid). Insufficient skeleton survives for a definitive diagnosis.

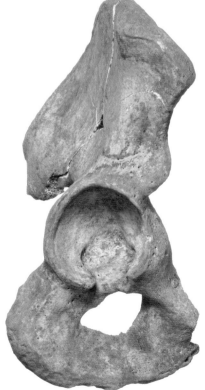

Fig 80 *Right os coxa of 26–35-year-old probable male primary inhumation [269] (scale c 1:2)*

Neoplastic disease

Six primary inhumations bore signs of neoplastic disease (6/173: 3.5%), three males (3/80: 3.8%) and one female (1/30: 3.3%). In addition, adult male [119] had a small, depressed area on the ectocranial surface of the left frontal, between glabella and the left orbit. Shallow depressions in the outer table of the cranium may be the result of soft-tissue lesions, such as epidermoid or sebaceous cysts, and the lesion appeared to be healed but still remodelling. However, as a differential diagnosis of blunt-force trauma could not be excluded, this example was not included in the statisics.

Male [124] (group 21) and female [411] (group 22) both displayed benign (button) osteomata, located on the right frontal and right parietal respectively (2/173 primary inhumations; 1.2%). Button osteoma also affected cranial fragments from two unsexed adults and one female from the disarticulated assemblage, with one, [174], presenting with two lesions, one on each parietal. In total, 0.4% each of the supraoccipital (1/232), left frontal bones (1/245), right frontal (1/239) and left parietal (1/230) and 0.9% of the right parietal bones in the assemblage (2/229) were affected.

In three primary inhumations (3/173: 1.7%) and two portions, bony changes were noted that were consistent with a putative diagnosis of osteochondroma, a relatively common, benign bone tumour (Aufderheide and Rodríguez-Martín 1998, 381). In four cases the proximal tibia was affected, a small bony spur protruding from the lateral or posterior-lateral aspect of the shaft. Radiographs were taken of two of the examples, but unfortunately it was not possible to confirm diagnosis, and soft-tissue trauma associated with a fibula fracture remains a differential diagnosis for portion [20601]. In total, 0.8% (4/498) of proximal tibiae in the skeletal assemblage were affected. Radiographic confirmation

was achieved for a further osteochondroma consisting of a large area (16.5 × 14.8 × 7.9mm) of abnormal bone growth on the palmar aspect of the distal shaft of the right first metacarpal of portion [25706] – a true prevalence rate of 0.4% (1/279). The radiograph shows a metacarpal bone with a likely sessile osteochondroma. It is unlikely to have caused any symptoms in life at this location and this size.

Two examples of malignant neoplastic conditions were also identified, in [543] and portion [34320]. The left mandible of [543] was found in two parts, owing to extensive necrosis between the position of the second molar and the ramus. The remaining bone was finely porous and the lingual aspect revealed resorption of cortical bone. The separated portions of the mandible ended in blunt points (Fig 81). No new bone growth, evidence of expansion or osteomyelitis were present and the localised nature of the lesion discounts a diagnosis of syphilis, leprosy or lupus vulgaris (Ortner 2003, 537). With an absence of reactive bone, it is possible that this lesion represents metastatic spread of an oral carcinoma, but this is rarely seen in the mandible and a plasma cell myeloma is also considered (Resnick 2002, 2194). Given the date of burial, a further differential diagnosis is phosphorous necrosis of the mandible or 'phossy jaw', an industrial disease resulting from chronic exposure to white phosphorus vapour that particularly affected those who worked in the match factories (Porter 1997, 400; Resnick 2002, 3614–16, Roberts and Cox 2003, 300). This example represents a true prevalence rate of 0.5% (1/200 left mandibles).

The remains in portion [34320] displayed mixed osteoblastic osteolytic and osteosclerotic lesions in the sacrum, femoral diaphysis, ischium, thoracic and lumbar vertebrae. A secondary fracture had occurred in the weakened 11th thoracic vertebra. Radiographic examination was inconclusive but secondary

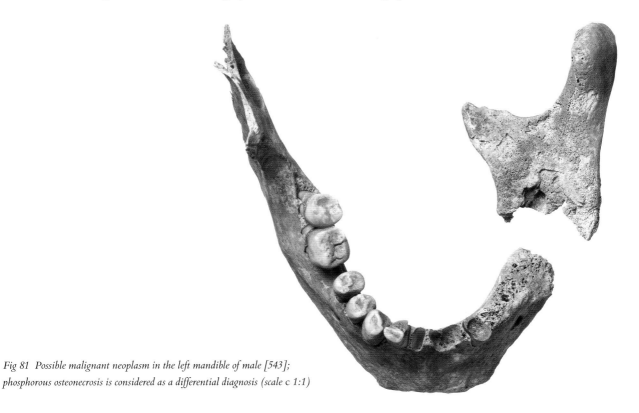

Fig 81 Possible malignant neoplasm in the left mandible of male [543]; phosphorous osteonecrosis is considered as a differential diagnosis (scale c 1:1)

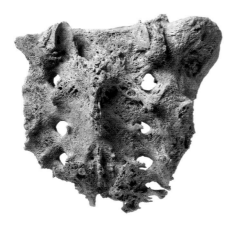

Fig 82 Possible secondary carcinoma in the sacrum and lumbar vertebrae of female portion [34320] (scale c 1:2)

spread from a carcinoma of the breast or lung is plausible (Ortner 2003, 535) (Fig 82).

In comparison, just 1.9% (4/210) of the population at Newcastle Infirmary presented with benign neoplasms and although a possible malignant carcinoma was identified (1/210: 0.5%), a differential diagnosis of brucellosis was given (Boulter et al 1998, 130).

Circulatory disease

Aneurysm

A slightly depressed suboval area in the central part of the third and fourth segments of a disarticulated sternum from [295] suggests that the adult from whom this bone came may have suffered from an aortic aneurysm. Such weakening of the walls of the aorta may be the result of atherosclerosis (a loss of elasticity, commonly in the abdomen) or may occur as a secondary complication in venereal syphilis (usually in the thorax), where invasion by the infectious spirochete destroys the integrity of the arterial wall (Aufderheide and Rodríguez-Martín 1998, 78–9). In this latter condition, pressure from the expanding vessel commonly results in cavitations on the sternum or manubrium and is the most probable diagnosis in this instance.

The diagnosis of aortic aneurysm was a particular specialism of Archibald Billing (Chapter 7.8, 'Waxes, resins and injections'), and this example is thus of particular interest.

Freiberg's disease

Contour change to the superior aspects of the necks of the second metatarsals and subchondral cysts in the left bone of [27201], a portion from a male aged 36–45 years at death, suggests a diagnosis of Freiberg's disease, osteochondrosis of the second metatarsal head. This condition may be caused by trauma resulting from biomechanical imbalance caused by a second metatarsal which is longer than normal; it affects three times as many females as males (Aufderheide and Rodríguez-Martín 1998, 86).

Osteochondritis dissecans

This condition is characterised by the presence of a small area of bone necrosis on a joint surface. It may be a result of chronic or acute trauma, but it has also been described as idiopathic. It most commonly develops in adolescent males. A detached fragment of bone may heal and reattach to the joint surface or a depressed and pitted lesion may remain (Aufderheide and Rodríguez-Martín 1998, 81–2; Ortner 2003, 351).

Twelve primary inhumations were affected (12/173: 6.9%), including six males (6/80: 7.5%) and two females (2/30: 6.7%). The knee, hip, shoulder, elbow and foot were all affected. In six instances fragments had reattached to the joint surface – for example, in the bilateral lesions seen in the radial facet of the humeri of 36–45-year-old male [137]. Four portions also showed evidence of the condition, and osteochondritis dissecans remains a possible differential diagnosis for the changes seen in the left knee of syphilitic male [398] (see above). One adult left patella from the disarticulated assemblage was also affected.

True prevalence rates for the skeletal assemblage as a whole can be seen in Table 58. The locations affected include the glenoid scapula, a joint that is rarely involved (Aufderheide and Rodríguez-Martín 1998, 83).

Table 58 True prevalence rate of osteochondritis dissecans for the entire assemblage

Element	n	Affected n	%
Glenoid scapula	425	1	0.2
Distal humerus	489	4	0.8
Proximal ulna	470	1	0.2
Ilium	472	1	0.2
Distal femur	501	4	0.8
Patella	275	2	0.7
Proximal tibia	491	2	0.4
Foot phalanx	1386	1	0.1
1st metatarsal	306	1	0.3

Pressure necrosis

Cavitations in the ischial tuberosities of 26–35-year-old female [282] suggest pressure necrosis; similar changes were noted in the left tuberosity of a disarticulated adult ischium from [263]. In primary inhumation [282] osteophytes bordered the tuberosity of the left calcaneus (the right was unobservable). These areas are common locations for pressure sores (bedsores or decubitus ulcers). Although they have a multifactoral aetiology, they are frequently associated with older and bedridden patients (Coletta 1999, 545–6; Cunha et al 2000; Resnick 2002, 2406–7).

The presence of two individuals (1/173 primary inhumations; 0.6%) with bony lesions suggestive of bedsores is intriguing. Whilst such injuries remain a problem in the care of bedridden patients today, staff at the London Hospital were aware of the problem and strove for better preventative

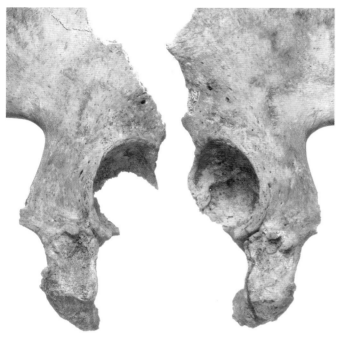

Fig 83 *Pressure necrosis in the ischial tuberosities of 26–35-year-old female [282], suggesting she had suffered from bedsores (scale c 1:2)*

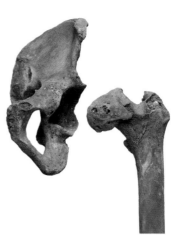

Fig 84 *Perthes' disease in the left hip of 26–35-year-old male portion [40207] (scale c 1:4)*

measures (Chapter 5.8). They were also keen to ensure patients did not stay too long in their care (Chapter 5.5, 5.6). It is equally possible, however, that a patient might have been admitted to the premises already suffering the effects of a long confinement at home.

Perthes' disease (osteochondrosis)

A 'mushroom-shaped' left femoral head, considerable joint contour change and an enlarged left acetabulum in 26–35-year-old male portion [40207] was consistent with Perthes' disease, osteochondrosis of the femoral head (Fig 84) (Aufderheide and Rodríguez-Martín 1998, 84–5). An absence of shortening in the limb and the relatively normal morphology of the acetabulum indicates a late onset (after 10 years of age). The interruption of the blood supply may also have been traumatically induced (Ortner 2003, 346) and the sex of the individual is consistent with the modern clinical male to female ratio of 4:1 in avascular necrosis of the femoral head (Aufderheide and Rodríguez-Martín 1998, 89).

Scheuermann's disease

Anterior kyphosis and extension of the vertebral bodies of the thoracic spine indicate that two male primary inhumations ([137], aged 36–45 years at death, and [119], aged ≥46 years) and adult portion [57001] had suffered from Scheuermann's disease (juvenile kyphosis). This condition appears around puberty and results from damage to the intervertebral discs weakened by minor repetitive trauma in the context of a congenital predisposition (Resnick 2002, 3728). The result is narrowing of the joint spaces and disruption of the anterior endplates, often

accompanied by aching pain and fatigue (Resnick 2002, 3729; Ortner 2003, 464). Schmorl's nodes were present in all instances.

Hypertrophic osteoarthropathy

The remains of 12–17-year-old primary inhumation [391] presented with finely pitted new bone on the visceral surfaces of the ribs, the shafts of both humeri, the lateral aspect of the left ulna, the right clavicle, the inferior aspect of the sternal shaft, the shafts of the femora, tibiae and fibulae, medial bodies of the cuneiforms and the left third to fifth metatarsals. Diffuse layers of immature subperiosteal new bone appeared to have been laid down in a single episode. The largely appendicular, bilateral and symmetrical distribution indicated a diagnosis of secondary hypertrophic osteoarthropathy. The visceral rib changes are likely to relate to the infectious pulmonary disease that precipitated the condition. In some subadults the condition may instead result from congenital intrathoracic lesions (Aufderheide and Rodríguez-Martín 1998, 91).

Symmetrical and diffuse new bone formation on the tubular bones of 26–35-year-old male [105] are also indicative of secondary hypertrophic osteoarthropathy. The mixed nature of the lesions (woven and lamellar bone) and distribution again suggest that this was secondary to pulmonary disease (Matos and Santos 2006, 193–4; Santos and Roberts 2006, 47). Possible indications of the early stages of tuberculosis were noted (see above) and staining on the teeth indicates that this man had also been a smoker.

Unidentified circulatory condition

The hand phalanges, second to fifth metatarsals and unsided proximal foot phalanges of ≥46-year-old male [462] had enlarged nutrient foramina. The cause remains unknown though this has been found in cases of both beta-thalassemia and Gaucher's disease (above, 'Congenital and developmental abnormalities') and may be related to increased arterial supply (Resnick 2002, 2171, 2174).

Nutritional and metabolic disorders

Cribra orbitalia

Cribra orbitalia affected 22.0% (38/173) of the primary inhumations, closely comparable to the rate of 22.4% noted at Newcastle Infirmary (Boulter et al 1998, 94–6). These porous lesions in the orbital roof develop during childhood, remodelling in adulthood. Traditionally they have been presented in palaeopathology as evidence of iron deficiency anaemia. Some authors have recently suggested, however, that they result from megaloblastic anaemia acquired through a combination of maternal vitamin B12 deficiency and gastrointestinal infections at the time of weaning (Walker et al 2009, 119), whilst others have suggested a link with malarial infection (G Western, pers comm).

Males and females were equally affected, with a crude prevalence rate of 32.5% (26/80) and 33.3% (10/30) respectively. Two subadults also had orbital lesions (2/13: 15.4%). This compares well with the roughly contemporary and geographically local assemblage from the Catholic Mission of St Mary and St Michael, Whitechapel, where an adult crude prevalence rate of 26.5% was noted (Henderson et al in prep), and with Greenwich Hospital, where 32.7% (35/107) of the population were affected (Boston et al 2008, 55), but is significantly higher than the rates seen at Newcastle Infirmary, where just 8.9% (5/56) of articulated crania and 1.4% (42/295) of disarticulated crania were affected (Boulter et al 1998, 98). In the case of the two subadult populations, the discrepancy in size is so great (St Mary and St Michael's contained 437 subadults) that direct comparison is not possible.

The true prevalence rates for the primary inhumations and portions can be seen in Table 59. Of the observable orbits from

Table 59 True prevalence rate of cribra orbitalia in the articulated assemblage

		Right		Left		Total	
		n	%	n	%	n	%
Primary inhumations							
Male	grade 1	15	32.6	14	29.2	29	30.9
	grade 2	5	10.9	8	16.7	13	13.8
	grade 3	1	2.2	1	2.1	2	2.1
	observable orbits	46	-	48	-	94	-
	total cribra	21	45.7	23	47.9	44	46.8
Female	grade 1	6	31.6	5	26.3	11	28.9
	grade 2	4	21.1	3	15.8	7	18.4
	grade 3	0	-	0	-	0	-
	observable orbits	19	-	19	-	38	-
	total cribra	10	52.6	8	42.1	18	47.4
Subadult	grade 1	0	-	0	-	0	-
	grade 2	2	66.7	1	33.3	3	50.0
	grade 3	0	-	0	-	0	-
	observable orbits	3	-	3	-	6	-
	total cribra	2	66.7	1	33.3	3	50.0
All primary inhumations	grade 1	21	29.6	19	26.0	40	27.8
	grade 2	12	16.9	13	17.8	25	17.4
	grade 3	1	1.4	1	1.4	2	1.4
	observable orbits	71	-	73	-	144	-
	total cribra	34	47.9	33	45.2	67	46.5
Portions							
Male	grade 1	1	8.3	2	25.0	3	17.6
	grade 2	2	16.7	0	-	2	11.8
	grade 3	0	-	0	-	0	-
	observable orbits	12	-	8	-	17	-
	total cribra	3	25.0	2	25.0	5	29.4
Female	grade 1	2	50.0	2	50.0	4	50.0
	grade 2	0	-	0	-	0	-
	grade 3	0	-	0	-	0	-
	observable orbits	4	-	4	-	8	-
	total cribra	2	50.0	2	50.0	4	50.0
Subadult	grade 1	0	-	0	-	0	-
	grade 2	0	-	0	-	0	-
	grade 3	0	-	0	-	0	-
	observable orbits	1	-	1	-	2	-
	total cribra	0	-	0	-	0	-
All portions	grade 1	5	27.8	4	26.7	9	27.3
	grade 2	2	11.1	0	-	2	6.1
	grade 3	0	-	0	-	0	-
	observable orbits	18	-	15	-	33	-
	total cribra	7	38.9	4	26.7	11	33.3

the articulated assemblage, 46.5% (67/144) had lesions consistent with cribra orbitalia. This compares with a true prevalence rate of 41.3% at the Catholic Mission of St Mary and St Michael (Henderson et al in prep).

Males and females were equally affected, with an overall male true prevalence rate of 44.1% (49/111 orbits) and an overall female true prevalence rate of 47.8% (22/46). Of the subadult orbits, 37.5% (3/8) were affected. The condition was also noted in 21 right (nine male, two female, one subadult) and 20 left (seven male, two female) orbits from the disarticulated assemblage.

Porotic hyperostosis

Healed or healing porotic lesions were present on the external (ectocranial) surface of the crania of 18 male (18/80: 22.5%) primary inhumations and one female (1/30: 3.3%) (19/173: 11.0%). One female and two male portions were affected, as were a number of disarticulated cranial bones – 0.8% (1/123) disarticulated supraocciptals; 0.7% of right (1/135) and left (1/137) frontal bones; 14.5% (18/124) of right parietals; and 16.1% (20/124) of left parietals. The overall true prevalence rates are shown in Table 60.

Thirteen of the 18 primary inhumations (72.2%) with one or both orbits observable had also suffered from cribra orbitalia.

Rickets

Vitamin D is vital for effective bone mineralisation. If an individual is deficient in this, the result will be softened and weakened bones that can no longer support the body weight and become bowed (Mays et al 2006, 1). The remains of 15 primary inhumations had evidence of such vitamin D deficiency (15/173: 8.7%), including eight males (8/80: 10.0%) and four females (4/30: 13.3%). This evidence consisted predominantly of the bowing of the lower limbs, as seen in male [572] (Fig 85), though in three instances the upper limbs were involved, suggesting that the individual had been deficient in vitamin D whilst they were still crawling. Seven portions were also affected (four male and one female) as were 11 collections of long-bone elements from the disarticulated assemblage, representing a minimum of three adults who had suffered the condition during childhood and survived.

There was no evidence of active rachitic changes amongst

the subadults, in marked contrast to the high rates reported for a number of contemporary groups (eg, Miles et al 2008; Henderson et al in prep). This may simply be a function of the extremely small size of the subadult assemblage, and is discussed further in Chapter 7.8 ('The status of the buried population').

Osteoporosis

Lightweight thoracic vertebrae with concave fractures were present in the spine of male primary inhumation [365] and were confirmed radiographically to have an appearance consistent with a diagnosis of osteoporosis (Brickley and Ives 2008, 165). A series of secondary joint changes (Schmorl's nodes and osteophytes) were also present and the third and fourth thoracic vertebrae had sharp-edged, transverse impression fractures in the anterior portion of the superior body, with collapse of the central body. This gives a crude prevalence rate of just 0.6% (1/173) for the primary inhumations.

More enigmatic were changes noted in the spine of female portion [57002]. Again the vertebrae were light, with compression fractures and an irregular trabecular structure, but the appearance of the vertebrae was not typical of osteomalacia and the individual was only 26–35 years old at death, a young age to be suffering from loss of bone density unless there was another underlying medical condition. Nevertheless, osteomalacia remains a strong possibility.

Diffuse idiopathic skeletal hyperostosis (DISH)

Four male (4/80: 5.0%) primary inhumations and one female (1/30: 3.3%) had flowing, 'candle-wax' osteophyte formation

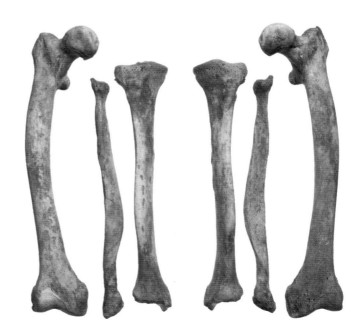

Fig 85 Resolved rachitic changes in 36–45-year-old male [572] with coxa vara, anterior and medial bowing of the femoral shafts, anterior bowing of the tibiae and mediolateral flattening of the fibulae (scale c 1:5)

Table 60 True prevalence rate of porotic hyperostosis for the entire assemblage

Element	n	Affected n	Affected %
R parietal	229	39	17.0
L parietal	230	42	18.3
R frontal	239	20	8.4
L frontal	245	20	8.2
Supraoccipital	232	18	7.8

in the thoracic spine. In two cases, fusion of four or more contiguous vertebrae and extra-spinal enthesophyte formation confirmed the diagnosis of diffuse idiopathic skeletal hyperostosis (DISH) (2/173: 1.2%) (Resnick 2002, 1477).

A sixth thoracic vertebra from the disarticulated material displayed unilateral osteophyte formation characteristic of the changes seen in DISH. However, without contiguous fusion to the adjacent vertebra it was not possible to form a definitive diagnosis.

The causes of DISH remain unknown and though diabetes mellitus and obesity are thought to have a correlation with the condition, the only clearly linked feature is advancing age (Aufderheide and Rodríguez-Martín 1998, 1478, 1496–7).

Miscellaneous disorders

Evidence for a number of pathological bone changes that did not readily fall into the previous categories was also seen.

Endocranial lesions

Conditions that result in the inflammation or haemorrhage of the meningeal vessels may result in the formation of new bone on the endocranial surface of the skull. The underlying aetiology may be traumatic, infectious or metabolic (Lewis 2004, 93).

Amongst the primary inhumations, two adult males, [451] and [529] (2/80: 2.5%), and a subadult, [122], aged 12–17 years (1/13: 7.7%) were affected, giving a crude prevalence rate of 1.7% (3/173). The lesions were healed in the case of [529] whilst 26–35-year-old male [451] had lesions with a 'hair on end' appearance together with newly formed woven bone (Lewis 2004, 90: type 2 and 4). He had also been suffering from a pulmonary infection at the time of his death. In the subadult, a thin layer of finely pitted, grey woven bone was present on the supraoccipital, indicating that the pathological process was active at the time of death. The appearance conformed to Lewis type 2, and may have resulted from haemorrhage (Lewis 2004, 89, 95). Although no concurrent skeletal pathology was noted, discoloration of the crowns of the molar and premolar teeth may have resulted from illness and/or malnourishment during growth.

Three portions (two female and one male) also presented with endocranial lesions. In all instances, bone formation was active at the time of death.

One subadult (parietals and supraoccipital) and three adult cranial fragments (supraoccipital) from the disarticulated assemblage (4/123 supraoccipitals; 3.3%) were affected. One of the adult fragments, [341], presented with fine, grey woven bone in the vascular channels and another, [289], with similar new bone growth on the floor of the transverse sinus. Pronounced vascular impressions were noted in the left parietal and frontal bones of an adult from [457].

True prevalence rates for the entire assemblage are shown in Table 61.

Table 61 *True prevalence rate of endocranial lesions for the entire assemblage*

Element	n	Affected n	%
R parietal	229	2	0.9
L parietal	230	2	0.9
Supraoccipital	232	10	4.3
L squamous temporal	168	1	0.6

Hyperostosis frontalis interna (HFI)

Hyperostosis frontalis interna (HFI) affected the frontal bones of four adults from the disarticulated assemblage, but was not noted in any of the articulated material – 3.3% (8/484) of the frontal elements were affected. This bone formation is a normal aging phenomenon triggered by hormonal changes.

Paget's disease of bone

Irregularity and thickening of the cranial vault with coarse trabeculae and no differentiation between the outer and inner tables, together with thickened and porous sphenoid and perpendicular plate of the ethmoid, indicate that 26–35-year-old male [336] had suffered from Paget's disease of bone (Ortner 2003, 436–7). The diagnosis was confirmed by radiograph, in which the cranial vault had a 'cotton wool' appearance. Male [367], aged 36–45 years at death, had a heavy and thickened left scapula. Radiography showed trabecular thickening and occasional marginal sclerosis, consistent with the condition (Resnick 2002, 1961). Although the scapula is not the most common site for pathological changes to occur, one study found 9.8% of sufferers were affected in this location (Brickley and Ives 2008, 224). The crude prevalence rate of Paget's disease of bone in the primary inhumations was 1.2% (2/173). Amongst the disarticulated material, a fragment of left parietal from [431] displayed a thickened appearance consistent with a possible diagnosis of Paget's disease.

Paget's disease of bone is asymptomatic in 80% of individuals but the remainder suffer bone pain. Having first been described by Sir James Paget in 1876 (Altman 1993), its aetiology remains unknown (Aufderheide and Rodríguez-Martín 1998, 413–14). It would have presented an even greater mystery to the medical profession in the early 19th century, but given it is often asymptomatic those sufferers in this assemblage may not have presented with any indications during life. Seven disarticulated bones with probable Paget's disease were noted at Newcastle Infirmary (Boulter et al 1998, 96–7).

Disuse atrophy

Probable disuse atrophy was noted in an extremely gracile adult right humerus from [344], but as there were no other associated remains it was not possible to determine the cause of any possible paralysis. The humerus had been longitudinally sawn (see Fig 174), though both halves were present, and this enabled the thin but regular cortex to be seen. This element was clearly of some interest to those teaching or learning in the medical school. Interestingly, a radius and ulna with possible disuse atrophy were noted at Newcastle Infirmary (Boulter et al 1998, 104).

Deformities related to restrictive clothing

Three female primary inhumations and a male portion demonstrated changes in bone morphology that appeared most likely to be related to the wearing of restrictive garments.

Bilateral and symmetrical crowding of the metatarsals of 26–35-year-old female [411], who also suffered from hallux valgus, and a rounded and smooth-sided deposit of mature bone on the lateral aspect of the head of the fifth metatarsal of 26–35-year-old male portion [40401] may have resulted from the long-term wearing of shoes that were too narrow, whilst tapered and folded ribs indicate that 26–35-year-old female [216] and 36–45-year-old female [259] had habitually worn corsets or stays. In the latter case, the appearance of the ribcage was complicated by the presence of a series of healed fractures (see above).

The right parietal from an adult probable female from [457] presented with an unusually deep pachyonian depression that had resulted in the perforation of the outer table of the cranial vault. It is unlikely that this had any clinical significance during life.

5

The life of the London Hospital

It may seem a strange principle to enunciate as the very first requirement in a hospital that it should do the sick no harm. It is quite necessary nevertheless to lay down such a principle, because the actual mortality in hospitals, especially those in the crowded cities, is very much higher than any calculation founded on the mortality of the same class of patient treated out of hospital would lead us to expect. (Nightingale 1863, iii)

5.1   The governors and house committee

The London Hospital was run by its governors, and the charity was headed by an appointed president. Before his death in 1834 the president of the hospital was the duke of Gloucester; the governors then approached the duke of Cambridge, uncle of the future Queen Victoria, who accepted the role (Clark-Kennedy 1962, 247–8). The prospect of such illustrious company attracted a large number of subscribers. In return for their subscriptions, the governors gained the right to recommend patients for treatment. A donation of 5 guineas bought the right to recommend patients for one year, and in return for a donation of 30 guineas the donor became a 'life governor'. One guinea bought the right to recommend outpatients only, and payments were monitored – on 3 February 1831 Mr Thomas Saddington was informed that unless he kept up donations of at least 1 guinea a year he would lose his right to recommend patients (RLH, LH/A/5/19, 18). Governors were also limited to recommending one inpatient and up to four outpatients at any one time, although in certain cases exceptions were made, as in September 1838 when four cases recommended by Mr J Mears were admitted after being considered urgent by the physicians and surgeons (RLH, LH/A/5/22, 144). The medical staff were forbidden from becoming governors.

A number of local businesses also paid to enable their workers to use the facilities of the hospital, and in 1825, in recognition of the services given to their workers, the London Dock Company began directly contributing to the hospital funds with a one-off payment of 30 guineas and an annuity of 10 guineas. A letter in 1830 from John Davis, of Rupert Street, Goodman Fields, indicates that it was not just large companies that used the hospital in this way: Davis sent 'a puncheon of milasses [molasses] … in consideration of the able and kind treatment experienced by three or four of my Labourers who have been confined within these walls during the past year' (RLH, LH/A/5/18, 305).

A request from Robert Peel, however, asking if the London Hospital would provide his new police officers (the Metropolitan Police Act was passed in 1829) 'medical and surgical attendance … during illness' was turned down. The committee stated that, unless Peel could supply additional funds, they simply had too much work owing to 'the extension of the Docks and Buildings in the neighbourhood' and the many associated accidents. If funds were provided, the hospital offered Peel the same terms as given to the East India Company and the Corporation of Trinity House and the dock companies (RLH, LH/A/5/18, 295–7).

Governors' powers also extended to the election of the medical officers of the hospital (Lawrence 1996, 55) and, in the case of the London Hospital, to the election of the house governor (Chapter 5.9). At the endowed hospitals, by contrast, many of these responsibilities lay with the treasurer, who was employed by the hospital and worked there full-time. Staff elections could involve hard-fought campaigns, with governors not above using underhand tactics to generate votes for their favoured candidate. In the past, attempts had been made to control some of these – annual subscribers to the charity were not permitted to vote in elections until after a probationary period (initially one week but later a year), in order to prevent candidates from persuading people to become governors solely to vote in their favour (Clark-Kennedy 1962, 176), and those under the age of 21 were not permitted to vote, in order to prevent governors from subscribing their children to increase their household's voting power (ibid, 201–2). In spite of these measures, the election of William John Little to the post of assistant physician in 1839 was fraught with scandal, culminating in the publication of a letter purporting to be from Dr Little, but in fact written by supporters of his opponent, a Dr Fox, announcing that he was withdrawing his candidacy (ibid, 251–3).

The governors of the London Hospital met quarterly, but most did not take an active role in the running of the hospital. This was entrusted to an elected committee of the house (later called the house committee). The house committee met once a week, and submitted a report to the governors at their quarterly general court (Clark-Kennedy 1962, 30). At their weekly meetings they admitted patients and dealt with other issues concerning the running of the hospital. They received and accepted tenders for work and provisions, dealt with grievances from staff and patients and controlled the finances of the hospital.

Two house visitors were appointed from their number to walk the wards of the hospital and ensure that it was being properly run. Their period of duty was for a fortnight, but some took the job more seriously than others. At times the visitors' reports to the house committee comprise no more than a cursory comment, to the irritation of those who were more thorough (RLH, LH/A/16/4). In 1840 the chairman of the house committee drew the attention of the committee members to 'the importance of a more strict attention to their duties' when appointed as house visitors, and subsequently a notice was to be sent to the visitors at the beginning of their fortnight's duty reminding them of this and requesting that they arrange to attend the hospital at the same time (RLH, LH/A/5/22, 358, 375).

Once a year the governors held an anniversary dinner to commemorate the date of the hospital's foundation and encourage donations (Figs 86–7). These dinners were lavish affairs, held, during the earlier years of the charity, in the City. Later a sermon was preached by an eminent member of the clergy in the hospital chapel, followed by a dinner at the London Tavern (Clark-Kennedy 1962, 195). In 1835 the Tavern bill for the dinner came to £106 3s 6d (RLH, LH/A/5/21, 160).

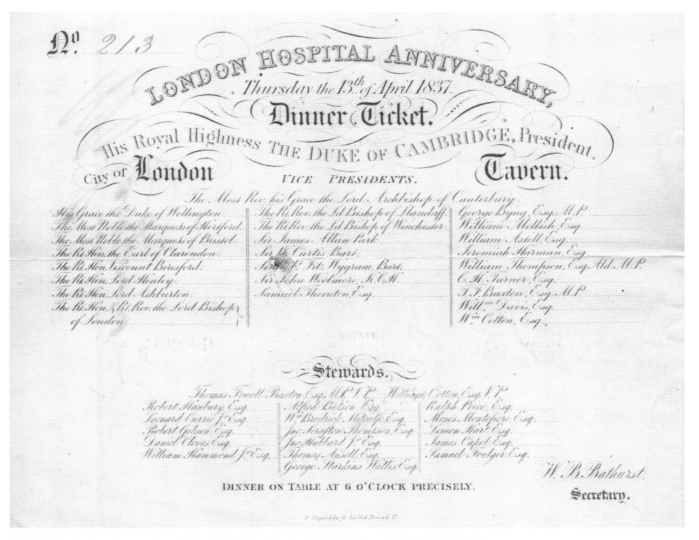

Fig 86 Ticket for the anniversary dinner, 13 April 1837 (Royal London Hospital Archives, RLH, LH/A/23/23, 3)

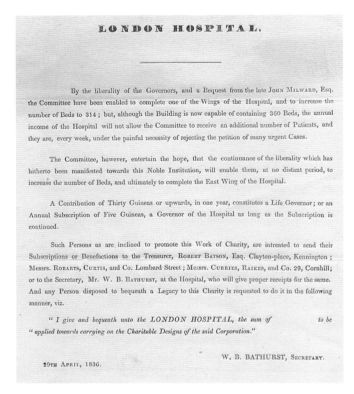

Fig 87 Printed appeal for contributions towards the completion of the extension to the east wing, 29 April 1836 (Royal London Hospital Archives, RLH, LH/A/23/30)

5.2   Plans for expansion

The large number of people applying for treatment and the comparatively small number of beds for patients had long caused problems for the hospital. To an extent the difficulty of accommodating patients could be managed by attempting to limit the length of a patient's stay in the hospital and by excluding certain patients whom the hospital was unlikely to be able to help (below, 5.3 and 5.5), but this did not resolve the problem.

The scale of the overcrowding is emphasised by the case of Adam Bowman, a 'poor man without any friends in this Country' for whom Mr D Willink of the Dutch Church, Austin Friars, wrote to the hospital giving 7s weekly for his continued care. The hospital replied that 'although they would feel very happy to meet his wishes, if practicable, the crowded state of the House and the urgent want of Beds, obliged them to request that Mr Willink would procure the removal of the Patient referred to as he is not altogether suitable for an inmate of a Hospital' (RLH, LH/A/5/19, 78–9).

As the hospital's finances improved, the governors were keen to try to accommodate a greater number of patients. In October 1822 the house committee began to look at the costs involved in increasing the number of patients that the hospital could take in from 250 to 300, and on Christmas Eve they resolved to work towards this goal by increasing the number of inpatients from 250 to 265 (159 surgical and 106 medical), and then to 270 (160 surgical and 110 medical) (RLH, LH/5/A/5/17,

184). These patients were to be accommodated within the existing wards, but at times the wards became very full and in 1823 the president of the charity, the duke of Gloucester, suggested making plans to enlarge the hospital 'in the not too distant future' when he addressed the governors at the annual festival (ibid, 213). By August 1825 it was again reported that 'the Hospital was extremely crowded last week and that more beds were fitted up than the wards could properly contain' (RLH, LH/A/5/18, 46). On 2 May 1829 the women's wards were completely full, leading to the resolution that patients should be transferred to the surgeons' wards (ibid, 263) (Fig 88).

Whilst expansion was on hold, improvement works were undertaken in 1825 with the provision of additional water closets, a bench for the garden and improvement works to the west wing worth over £600, carried out by Thomas Burton (RLH, LH/A/5/18, 15, 31, 36, 42, 51). The work included adding doors to the lobbies to keep out drafts, mop boxes and plate racks for the ward sinks and 'fitting up new Bread Room and Scullery for the house governor' (ibid, 73). Although they did not yet possess sufficient funds to consider further expansion, the house committee was keen to compare the position of the London Hospital with that of the other hospitals in the metropolis, and in 1827 a list of data comparing the relative intake between 1820 and 1826 was compiled (Fig 89). This demonstrates that, despite the vast numbers of patients treated at the London, in terms of patient throughput the hospital still lagged behind St Thomas's and St Bartholomew's.

The hospital's accumulating fund was due to mature in 1831 (or when the contents reached £25,000), and in June 1830 the hospital received a legacy of £10,000 from a Mr Holland, making the means to expand available. In January 1830 the house committee and past officers were called together 'to take into consideration the propriety and expediency of commencing building to increase the accommodation of the Hospital by enlarging one of the wings' (RLH, LH/A/5/18, 306). They resolved that 'the largely increased application for admissions

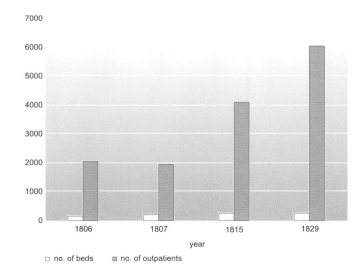

Fig 88 Hospital expansion shown by an increase in the number of beds and outpatients between 1806 and 1829 (RLH, LH/A/5/18, 310)

render an extension of the accommodation for Patients highly desirable' (ibid, 307), and set up a subcommittee to look into the practicalities and costs. The increasing number of applications for treatment that came with the rapid expansion of the neighbourhood meant that the existing 272 beds were insufficient. Additional space would also allow for the segregation of certain patients from the main wards (ibid, 310).

On 25 March 1830, the resolution to build the extension was unanimously passed at a public general meeting at the London Tavern (RLH, LH/A/5/18, 318), and soon the expanding hospital buildings began to encroach on the enclosed ground to the south. The west wing was chosen as the first to be extended. Four new wards were housed within the extension, which was heated by hot air stoves. Plans were submitted by Mr Mason, the hospital surveyor, and work began later in the year (Fig 90). A Mr Colebatch submitted the lowest tender and was chosen to undertake the work. As part of his contract he was due a payment of £2199 in the September, on condition that the building had reached 12 inches above the ground. He did not meet this deadline, and so his first instalment for the work was reduced to £1500. By June 1831 they were having to turn away patients (both surgical and medical) (RLH, LH/A/5/19, 68) but on 4 August the new wards were opened and 44 additional patients were admitted (ibid, 91). The final balance for the work was paid to Mr Colebatch in October 1831: total cost £11,526 2s 2d, including a commission for the surveyor of £600 and fences to the east and west for the patients' garden at £78 –s 9d (ibid, 139). In January 1832, with the permission of the royal family, two wards in the new wing were named as William IV and (after his brother, recently deceased) William Frederick, while two wards in the hospital were renamed as Adelaide and Victoria (ibid, 121, 183–5).

The new wing did not completely resolve the issue of overcrowding. On 22 December 1831 the committee reported that Mellish's ward was too full and 12 beds were moved to Bowley's ward, which was unoccupied (RLH, LH/A/5/19, 162). The following month, January 1832, 'The surgeons recommended eight urgent men and four urgent women, 10 proper men and eight proper women' but had sufficient beds only for two men and four women. The physicians recommended five urgent, 14 very proper and two proper men and three urgent, eight very proper and three proper women, but had a mere two spare beds (ibid, 187); by March 1832 'the Patients beds appeared to be, in some parts of the House, too close together' (ibid, 222). In May 1834 the governors reported to the House of Commons Committee on Medical Education that although there was room in the hospital for 360 beds, the funds of the institution allowed for the admission of only 314 patients (RLH, LH/A/5/20, 286).

The problems of covering the running costs of the hospital continued during the 1830s. In 1838 the house committee recommended to the general court to authorise the sale of £2000 of stock held by the charity, 'considering the progressive pressure on the funds of the Institution arising from the increased number of Patients, and the inadequacy of the permanent Income of the Hospital to meet the consequent Expenditure'. At the same time they ordered all the rum in the hospital to be put into one cask and sold (RLH, LH/A/5/22, 13 February 1838, 63). Another sale was necessary the following year (RLH, LH/A/5/22, 19 November 1839, 282–3). Appealing for greater funds, the governors began from 1840 to include in the annual report the number of recommended patients that had been turned away over the previous year because of lack of space: 514 patients had been refused admission in 1839 and the following year this number rose to 568, dropping to 504 in 1841 (RLH, LH/A/15/19–21). When the 'bed state' of the hospital was recorded in May 1840, 347 patients were found to be on the wards, instead of the official number of 314 (below, 5.9), but because the hospital actually

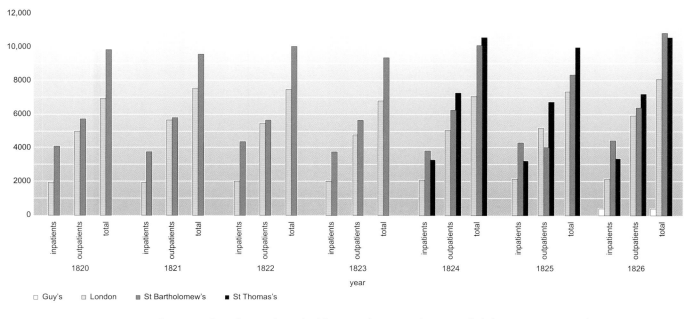

Fig 89 *A contemporary comparison of patient intake at the major hospitals of the metropolis, 1820–6 (RLH, LH/A/5/18, 150, 29 May 1827)*

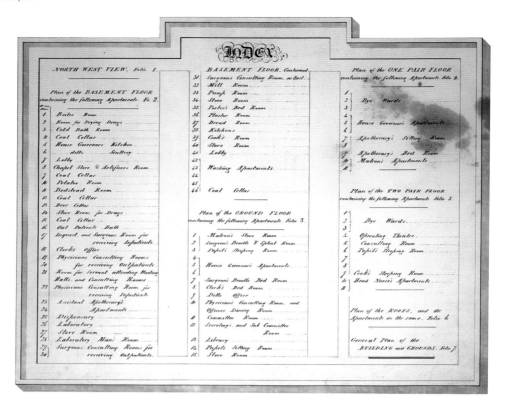

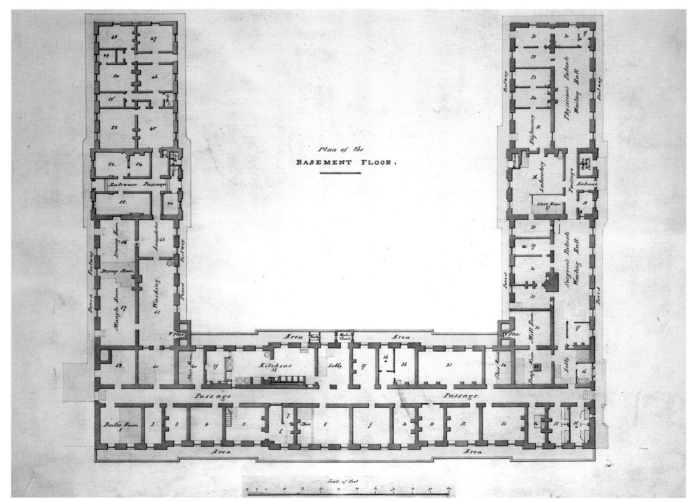

Fig 90 Alfred Richmond Mason's detailed plans of the proposed extension to the hospital, 1832 (Royal London Hospital Archives, RLH, LH/S/2/4) (floor plans have scale bars of 10+100ft; for overall plan see Fig 19)

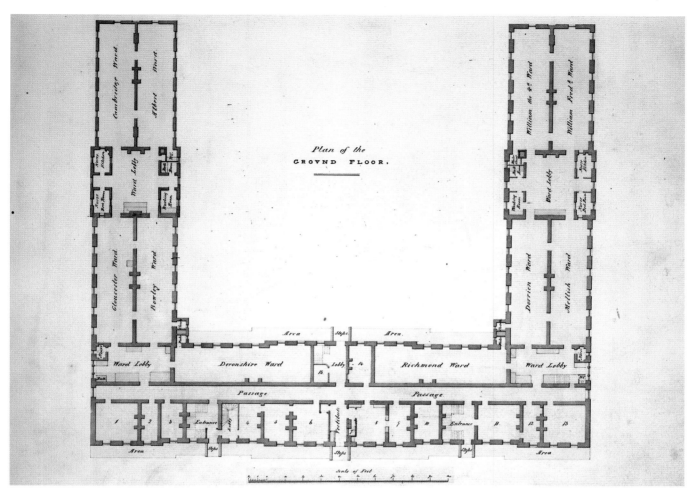

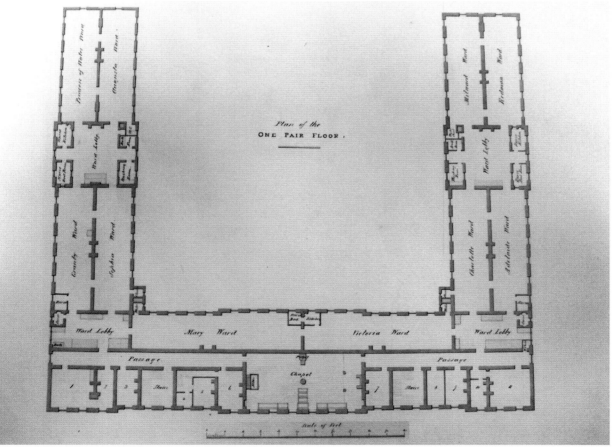

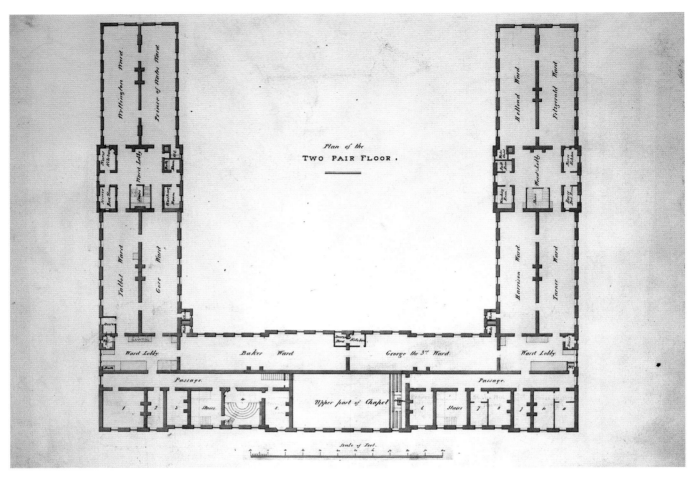

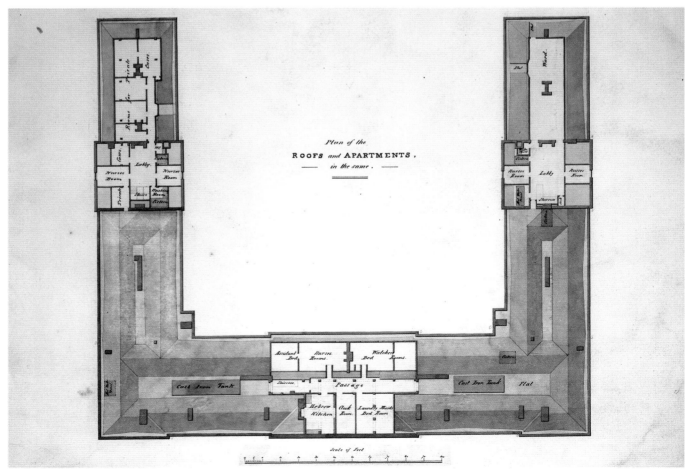

had room for 360 beds this did not necessarily indicate that the building was full. The following month one of the house visitors reported that there were '335 beds on the Wards instead of 314 as stated but not all occupied, nor are the Wards overcrowded' (RLH, LH/A/16/4, 189).

The centenary festival of the hospital in 1840 broke all previous records, raising £10,809, in addition to £1000 raised by the Jewish community for separate accommodation for Jewish patients (Clark-Kennedy 1962, 256). A special meeting of the house committee was summoned for 9 June (RLH, LH/A/5/22, 362, 369). The new wing, at a projected cost of £9000, was intended to include male and female wards for Jewish patients (ibid, 392). Mr Mason, the surveyor, drew up the plans and oversaw the work, for which he was paid a 5% commission (ibid, 420, 434). George and Robert Webb won the contract to construct the new building, with a tender of £8160 (ibid, 435). In October, Mason advised that as the weather was so unfavourable, construction work should not start until the following spring (RLH, LH/A/5/23, 3). Including all extra works they were paid a total of £8726 14s 10d for the construction of the wing, and other expenses such as stoves, baths and the surveyor's commission brought the total to £9452 10s 4d (ibid, 20 September 1842, 291).

The new wing encroached on an area of the enclosed ground to the south of the hospital that had been in use as a burial ground, and the disturbed burials were removed and reinterred (Chapter 3.4, 'Group 22 (relocated burials)'). Mason reported the following November that the wing should be ready by 1 December, although fixtures and fittings were still required (RLH, LH/A/5/23, 153). Following the completion of the wing, the hospital continued to experience difficulties in raising sufficient funds to run the building at full capacity (Clark-Kennedy 1963, 12–13).

5.3 Admissions procedures

In common with the other voluntary hospitals in London – and in contrast to the endowed hospitals – the London Hospital charged no fees to patients, but in order to be admitted to the hospital all but acute cases had to attend one of the weekly meetings of the house committee with a governor's letter of recommendation, although this was no guarantee of admission. The committee interviewed all the applicants and took responsibility for admitting them as inpatients or outpatients, or for refusing treatment, with advice from the principal surgeon and physician on duty that week. On one occasion in July 1837, Dr Gordon failed to attend the meeting and so the committee sought the advice of the apothecary in his stead (RLH, LH/A/5/21, 466). The other voluntary hospitals operated similar systems, and there was not a hospital in London free of both governors' letters and fees until 1828, when Dr William Marsden set up a dispensary on Hatton Garden (which later became the Royal Free Hospital) after he found a girl dying on

the steps of St Andrew's church, Holborn, because she could not get a governor's letter for any hospital in London (Clark-Kennedy 1962, 226).

Emergency cases arising from accidents had always been admitted to the London Hospital at any time, without the need for a governor's letter, but there was a conflict between accommodating the governors' recommended patients and the extra cases admitted by the hospital's medical staff. The issue was an ongoing problem, causing more than a few arguments between the house committee, the house governor and the physicians and surgeons. Matters were brought to a head in November 1822, when the governors asked the secretary to search the hospital records to see if any authority was ever given to the medical officers to recommend patients and when (RLH, LH/A/5/17, 165). During the previous year 260 extra cases had been admitted by the medical staff, a number considered by the committee to be excessive. As a consequence the house committee wrote to all the medical officers to demand that they limit extra cases to those arising from accidents. They were only to be admitted by a surgeon of the hospital, with notice given immediately to the secretary. A ticket with the words 'Extra Case from Accident' marked in red ink was to be attached to the patient's bed, and the surgeon responsible for the case had to fill in a form and present it at the next meeting of the house committee. The admission of these cases was amended in January 1823 to include all cases deemed 'essential for the Preservation of Life' (ibid, 191, 194), although the right of the physicians and surgeons to admit them still had to be defended on occasions (below, 5.9).

In practice, extra cases were often admitted for reasons other than strictly for the preservation of life and defining the urgency of admission created a grey area, as was evidenced by the case of Sarah Murphy, who was admitted as an extra case by the house governor in October 1830. It was stated that she was 'labouring under the effects of a long exposure to a Fever Atmosphere, and although I cannot conscientiously say that her immediate admission is necessary to the actual preservation of life, yet I conceive that the admission as an Extra Case would preserve her from a dangerous and perhaps fatal attack' (RLH, LH/A/5/18, 317). In March 1834 the surgeon Mr Luke sought an amendment to the rules to allow for official admission in other cases requiring immediate admission, such as for the preservation of an eye or a limb (RLH, LH/A/5/20, 253–5).

During the period that the cemetery was in use there was a rise in the total number of patients admitted (Fig 91), facilitated by the expansion of the hospital and an increase in the number of beds. The extra capacity within the hospital was used primarily to admit a greater number of accidents and extra cases, and over time the proportion of inpatients admitted by the governors declined. By 1841 they accounted for only 34.1% of all admitted inpatients, compared with 52% in 1826 (Fig 92).

The admissions policy was on occasion the cause of complaint. In January 1831 a governor wrote of his disgust that Joanna Haines, a poor woman with a leg nearly in a 'state of mortification', had not been seen despite his referral. The committee responded that, the 'crowded state of the House rendering it imperatively necessary to classify cases of applicants for admission into Urgent, Very Proper and Proper Cases', she was later referred as an outpatient instead – 'the Committee have recently been compelled not only to reject Very Proper, but even Urgent Cases, in consequence of the crowded state of the Wards' (RLH, LH/A/5/19, 7).

In February 1826, the committee resolved to allow the apothecary to request that immediate attention be given to patients in the waiting room, if it was in his opinion required (RLH, LH/A/5/18, 70), which indicates that he felt some patients were being overlooked by the medical staff. This is perhaps unsurprising when one considers that by 1827, 90–100 medical patients and 40–50 surgical patients were attending the

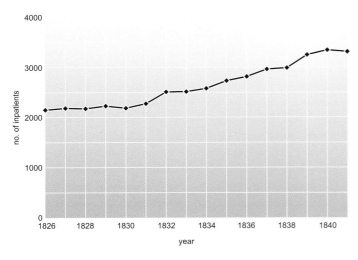

Fig 91 *Numbers of inpatients admitted to the hospital, as recorded in the annual reports (RLH, LH/A/15), with the figure for 1829 provided by the house committee in answer to a question from the House of Commons Medical Committee (RLH, LH/A/5/20, 284–306)*

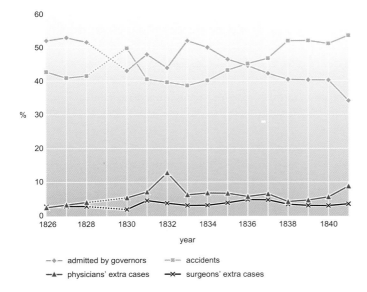

- admitted by governors
- accidents
- physicians' extra cases
- surgeons' extra cases

Fig 92 *Percentages of patients admitted by the governors, as accidents, and by the surgeons and physicians, as extra cases, as recorded in the annual reports (RLH, LH/A/15) (data for 1829 not available)*

hospital each day (ibid, 151). In October 1832 Mr Andrews was chastised for not seeing outpatients when he was supposed to (RLH, LH/A/5/19, 352–4). There were also complaints from the staff that patients were arriving very late in the day, and in October 1829 the committee resolved that inpatients were to be seen at 3pm, outpatients at 12pm and accidents were to be treated as outpatients in the wards to which they were originally admitted (RLH, LH/A/5/18, 205, 288).

5.4 Patients

Like other voluntary hospitals, the London Hospital was intended to serve the working poor. Although detailed registers kept by the hospital of patients have not survived, the 1841 census return from the hospital provides a snapshot of the 312 patients in the hospital on the night of 6 June 1841, listing name, age, sex and occupation, together with place of birth (TNA: PRO, 1841 England census, parish St Mary Whitechapel). The ages of the patients ranged from 8 months to over 80 years, and male patients outnumbered the female, accounting for 64.1% (200/312) of all inpatients (Fig 93). Although 44.9% (140/312) of the patients were born in Middlesex, 10.3% (32/312) came from Ireland, 1% (3/312) from Scotland and 1.9% (6/312) from 'foreign parts'; the remainder (131/312: 42%) were born elsewhere in the United Kingdom. There were some differences according to sex: 55.4% (62/112) of the female patients were born locally as opposed to 39% (78/200) of the male patients, and all of the patients from 'foreign parts' were male (Fig 94).

The information from the census does not allow us to distinguish between those patients who lived locally to the hospital and those who travelled there for treatment. The 14 agricultural labourers listed, none of whom were born locally, may have lived some distance away. In 1826 the house governor reported the case of a man whose leg required amputation, and who had sold his only cow to obtain the money to travel to London for treatment; the house governor, William Valentine, assured him that the Samaritan Society (below, 5.6) would assist him to travel home after the operation (RLH, LH/A/17/5, 3 September 1826). This was a common use of the Samaritan Society's funds. During the year 1839–40 the society provided financial assistance to 192 patients in order that they might travel home after a stay in the hospital, expending a total of £28 17s, and the hospital's annual report of 1841 noted that many of the 'domestic servants, mechanics and labourers' treated at the hospital had come from a distant part of the country for treatment (RLH, LH/A/15/20, 12).

A wide array of occupations is represented in the census return (Table 62), by far the most common being labourer or servant. Excluding agricultural workers, 43 (21.5%) of the men were labourers and 37 (33%) of the women were servants. There are some associations between occupation and place of birth – most strikingly 34.9% (15/43) of the labourers were born in

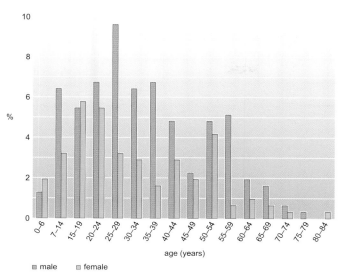

Fig 93 Age and sex of patients, recorded in the 1841 census (TNA: PRO, 1841 England census, parish St Mary Whitechapel)

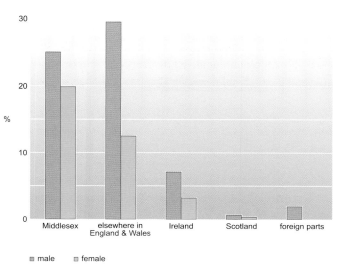

Fig 94 Birthplace of patients, recorded in the 1841 census (TNA: PRO, 1841 England census, parish St Mary Whitechapel)

Ireland, compared with 10.9% for all patients. It is possible that some of the labourers worked in the nearby docks; others who would have done so include five seamen, two sailors, two shipwrights, one ship's cook and an apprentice to sea.

Although the hospital was intended to care for those who could not afford to pay for private treatment, wealthier patients were sometimes admitted as accidents or extra cases. In 1836 Captain H G Pearce donated £5 to the hospital, 'accompanying it with expressions of unbounded gratitude to his Surgeons Mr Hamilton & Mr Scott and for the kindness and attention which he had *received* and *witnessed* in the Hospital' (RLH, LH/A/5/21, 211–12). His hand had been amputated after being shattered as he was trialling improvements to his patent invention. The following year a Mr Affleck donated £10 and thanked the hospital for the care and attention given to his son William Affleck, who had died on Harrison's ward (RLH, LH/A/5/22, 23).

Table 62 Occupations of the 312 inpatients recorded in the 1841 census (TNA: PRO, 1841 England census, parish St Mary Whitechapel)

Occupation	Number	Occupation	Number
Agricultural labourer	14	Lighterman	1
Agricultural labourer's child	1	Lock-maker's wife	1
Apprentice to sea	1	Lunatic-keeper's child	1
Baker	2	Market woman	1
Bargeman	1	Needlewoman	5
Boilermaker	2	Nurse	1
Bootmaker	2	Ostler	1
Bootmaker's wife	1	Painter	1
Brewer's servant	1	Painter's child	1
Brick-maker	1	Painter's wife	1
Bricklayer	3	Paper stainer	1
Bricklayer's wife	1	Parasol-maker	1
Broker	1	Plasterer	1
Brush-maker	1	Policeman	1
Butcher	2	Porter's wife	1
Cabinetmaker	1	Post Office	1
Cabinetmaker's wife	1	Printer's wife	2
Cap-maker	1	Publican's child	1
Carman	3	Railway guard	2
Carman's child	1	Rope-maker	1
Carpenter	5	Rule-maker	1
Carpenter's child	1	Sack-maker's son	1
Carpenter's wife	1	Sailor	2
Coachman	1	Sailor's wife	5
Coal labourer	1	Salesman's son	1
Coal whipper's child	1	Sawyer	2
Comb-maker	1	Sawyer's son	1
Confectioner	1	Schoolmistress	1
Cooper	1	Seaman	5
Coppersmith	1	Sells in sheets	2
Cordwainer	1	Servant (M)	3
Dealer	4	Servant (F)	37
Dealer's son	1	Servant's wife	1
Distiller's labourer	1	Ship cook	1
Dragman	2	Shipwright	2
Dyer	1	Shipwright's wife	1
Engineer	3	Shoemaker	7
Errand boy	1	Shoemaker's child	2
Excavator	1	Shoemaker's wife	2
Farmer's boy	1	Silk [?]ess	1
Farmer's labourer	1	Smith	7
Farrier	1	Smith & farrier	1
Fellowship porter	1	Smith's wife	2
Fireman	1	Stationer	1
Fishmonger	3	Stonemason	3
Floor cloth painter	1	Sugar baker	2
Foreman in docks' wife	1	Tailor	2
Fur dresser	1	Tinplate worker's wife	1
Gardener	5	Tobacco cutter	1
Gardener's child	1	Watchman's wife	1
Glass-maker's wife	1	Waterman	1
Gunsmith	1	Weaver	5
Hairdresser	1	Weaver's wife	3
Iron founder	1	Wheelwright	1
Iron moulder	1	Widow	19
Joiner's child	1	Widow's child	2
Labourer	43	Widow's son, pauper	1
Labourer's child/son	7	Unknown, either illegible or not given	5
Labourer's son, pauper	1		
Labourer's wife	4	Total	312
Land surveyor	1		
Leather ?dresser	1		

5.5   Exclusions

From its inception, the London Hospital excluded some demographic groups and those suffering certain illnesses. Other hospitals had similar rules. At Newcastle Infirmary the incurable and infectious were generally omitted; patients were predominantly local and mostly artisans (Nolan 1998, 36–7). Military personnel buried in Newcastle Infirmary ground may have been from nearby barracks (ibid, 17).

Infectious disease

The governors tried to keep those suffering from infectious diseases out of the hospital as much as possible and passed a 'law' that those with smallpox, 'itch' or any infectious or venereal disease were not to be admitted (Clark-Kennedy 1962, 59).

In 1827 the house governor, William Valentine, accused the medical officers of admitting as extra cases patients suffering from venereal disease and consumption, although at the same time he did suggest that it would be better openly to admit those suffering from venereal disease and keep them on separate wards (RLH, LH/A/17/5, 17 April 1827); it was not until 1858 that a ward was set aside for the admission of women with acute venereal disease (Clark-Kennedy 1963, 35). By 1832, venereal infections were not specifically alluded to in the London Hospital by-laws but measles had been added to the list of excluded infectious diseases. By 1841 the house committee reserved the power to admit those suffering from venereal disease, 'subject to such regulations as they shall, from time to time, establish' (RLH, LH/A/5/23, 22 June 1841, 102).

A watercolour image, labelled 'London Hospital … 1831', of the hand of a probable victim of smallpox (Fig 95), suggests that some patients slipped through despite the restrictions. In April 1841 the house committee received a letter from the Samaritan Society, which stated that 'it is indeed possible that Small Pox may unexpectedly show itself, after the admission of a Patient, whom it is then important to remove as speedily as possible, to prevent the spread of the disorder' (RLH, LH/A/5/23, 75–6). Sometimes this occurred because patients were misdiagnosed on admission. In December 1837 the house committee demanded an explanation from Dr Frampton as to how one of his patients could have been admitted with rheumatism, only to die several days later apparently of typhus fever (RLH, LH/A/5/22, 39). The house committee impressed on Dr Frampton 'the necessity for extreme caution in ascertaining the real circumstances of each applicant, prior to admission, in order to guard against the introduction of improper cases' (ibid, 41). Following this incident and a probable outbreak of typhus fever within the hospital (Chapter 4.1), the physicians and surgeons requested 'a convenient place to examine Accidents and Extra Cases previous to their admission' (ibid, 6 February 1838, 60–1). The surveyor estimated that the cost of the adjustments necessary to provide this space would be £168 5s, and a complex reshuffling of rooms would be required. The improvements were approved by the committee, who obviously felt that such space was necessary.

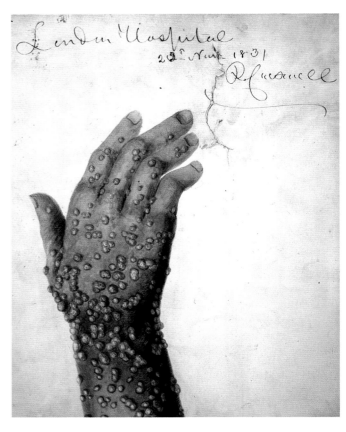

Fig 95   The hand of a patient probably suffering from smallpox, signed and dated: 'London Hospital 23 Nov [?] 1831 R. Carswell' (Wellcome Library, London, L0019716)

The osteological examination of the buried population suggests that those with incurable, infectious and venereal diseases did make their way into the hospital. The crude prevalence rate of tuberculosis in the primary inhumations (1.7%) was similar to that reported for Newcastle Infirmary (Chapter 4.2, 'Tuberculosis'), Bow Baptist church (1.9%) and St Marylebone, Westminster (1.3%; Miles et al 2008, 132), and slightly higher than that at St Mary and St Michael (0.7%) and Sheen's burial ground (0.8%), both in Whitechapel (Henderson et al in prep). The low level of variance between these groups suggests that the buried population at the London Hospital was broadly similar to its contemporaries (see below). However, pathognomonic, bony changes are seen in only a small percentage of those who suffer tuberculosis and the prevalence rate of rib lesions was much lower than that seen at St Mary and St Michael, which may be an indicator of the deliberate exclusion of those with pulmonary disease. A crude prevalence rate of 4.6% for venereal syphilis is significantly higher than the rate seen at St Mary and St Michael (1.9% of adults), Bow Baptist church (0.2%) or St Marylebone (0.3%; Miles et al 2008, 133). Interestingly, the assemblage at the London Hospital showed little evidence of cranial or facial changes and therefore of patients who had very visible soft-tissue lesions. Whilst this may in part be due to the under-representation of cranial elements (Chapter 7.8), it is also possible that it reflects the hospital screening procedure. Nonetheless, the rates remain higher than those seen at Newcastle Infirmary, where just 1.8% of articulated crania and 2.0% of disarticulated (two female and three male) were affected (Boulter et al 1998, 92–3).

Children

At the beginning, children under 7 years of age were admitted officially only in 'cases of compound fractures, or those in which amputation or cutting for the stone may be necessary', though in November 1832 the house committee decided on the inclusion of the clause 'and other cases of equal or greater urgency' to enable a larger number of children to be admitted (RLH, LH/A/5/19, 360, 375). This certainly contributes to the low proportion of subadults in the sample when compared to post-medieval parish burial grounds (Chapter 3.4). Although the results are not statistically significant, there is a higher ratio of subadults to adults in the primary inhumation sample from group 21 when compared to the other groups and it is possible that this reflects the changes in the admissions policy.

In 1837 the house governor suggested that Sophia ward's 'By-Ward' should be appropriated for the very young children in the hospital, but the medical officers did not agree, believing that it would 'systematize and extend the admission of very young children beyond the limits designed by the Committee' (RLH, LH/A/5/21, 384–5). In 1840 the house governor again raised the issue of the admission of children and the establishment of a separate children's ward, after adult patients had complained to the house visitors that they were being annoyed by the children on the general wards. The governors agreed that this should be done and that the rules for the admission of children should be more strictly applied, although this decision affecting patient care was made without consulting the medical officers. When they wrote to complain, the committee said that they had meant to make the suggestion only prospectively (RLH, LH/A/5/22, 385, 399). The 1841 census return includes ten patients (3.21% of the total) under the age of 7 within the hospital, the youngest of whom was aged only 8 months. A further 30 patients (9.62%) were aged between 7 and 14 years. The children appear to have been distributed throughout the hospital, with those aged 7 and over segregated by sex and distributed throughout the main wards.

Subadults, including those under the age of 7 years, were interred in the hospital grounds, albeit in small numbers (Table 12). Presumably the majority of the young patients would have been accompanied on their visit and were thus perhaps less likely to remain unclaimed after death. It is interesting that the largest difference in the age profile between the 1841 census and the primary inhumations is in the older subadult group, with a far smaller proportion of such individuals buried than were present in the hospital on the day of the census (Chapter 7.8, 'Demographic composition of the dissected remains'). Without longitudinal data on patient intake during the period in question, the significance of this pattern cannot be determined, but it is perhaps in part a reflection of the different reasons for admission for those aged under 7 years and the greater risk of death associated with both accident and surgery.

Pregnant women

The early regulations (1810) also excluded pregnant women (RLH, LH/A/1/4, 12–13), although they were clearly admitted on occasion: 'Elizabeth Brazier, an inpatient, having been delivered of a female child in the House on Thursday morning last, Ordered, as its father could not be found, that the said child be sent to the Foundling Hospital immediately' (Clark-Kennedy 1962, 60). The treatment of maternity cases as outpatients was also authorised. In the 18th century Mr Cole, the apothecary, attended every Wednesday afternoon from 3pm to 5pm 'for the Relief of Women with Child and the Distempers incident thereto' (woe betide any woman deciding to get into difficulties in labour on a Thursday!) (ibid, 27).

In 1839, Dr Ramsbotham, who with his son lectured at the college on midwifery and diseases of women and children, suggested that the governors should appoint an obstetric physician to the staff (RLH, LH/A/5/22, 280). Dr Frampton was asked by the committee to enquire as to the practice of the other hospitals in London. He reported back that Guy's, the Middlesex and the University College hospitals all appointed an obstetric physician, although their duties varied: at Guy's the obstetric physician had the care of a ward for women with sexually transmitted diseases; the Middlesex ran an establishment for the delivery of poor married women in their own homes; and at University College the obstetric physician had no particular duties. The medical officers at St George's, St Bartholomew's, St Thomas's, the Charing Cross and the Westminster hospitals all consulted the recognised lecturer on midwifery in their respective schools (ibid, 309–13). The house committee eventually decided that the medical staff could continue to consult Dr Ramsbotham for advice in such cases (as they had already done for the previous 15 years without official sanction) and empowered him to prescribe to patients in such cases, but made it clear that this should not affect the rule that pregnant women should not be admitted to the hospital (ibid, 315, 331).

On the date that the 1841 census was taken, 35.9% of the patients were female, with the proportion dropping to 25.3% for those aged 25–39 (Fig 93). The admissions policy regarding pregnant women may be one of the reasons that fewer women were admitted as inpatients.

'Lunaticks'

'Persons disordered in their senses' were also excluded (1810) (RLH, LH/A/1/4, 12–13). Occasionally a mistake was made: 'Elizabeth Cracroft, an inpatient recommended by Mr David Barclay, being found a Lunatick, the Secretary was ordered to acquaint Mr Barclay thereof and desire him to order her to be removed' (Clark-Kennedy 1962, 60). Epileptics could be treated, but only as outpatients (ibid). However, there is evidence to suggest this was not strictly adhered to (below, 5.11, 'Mental health care').

In the 1790s, the governors of the hospital of Bethlem applied to the London Hospital to use their empty wards to house their female patients during rebuilding work (they would have brought all their own physicians, surgeons and servants), but the governors of the London refused, and the medical staff stated that 'Receiving lunaticks into the House would be a complete subversion of the Principles on which the London Hospital was founded' (Clark-Kennedy 1962, 196). During the period in which the cemetery was in use patients who were considered to be insane were often sent to Messrs Warburton and Talbot's Lunatic Asylum at Bethnal Green. In 1834 the London Hospital was charged 10s a week for the board and upkeep of a deranged patient who had been sent there (RLH, LH/A/5/20, 284).

Incurables

Hospitals considered their purpose to be the rehabilitation of contributing members of society and therefore the London Hospital did not admit those 'in a dieing condition'. Later it was 'Ordered that no Patient deemed incurable by the Physicians or Surgeons … or any Person having an ulcer of long standing, be admitted into the House' (Clark-Kennedy 1962, 60–1). In c 1821, waiting lists for semi-urgent cases were adopted, and continued efforts made to get rid of those with chronic illnesses (ibid, 213).

Those with pulmonary infections were to be excluded only if 'in a state of confirmed consumption' (1832: RLH, LH/A/1/7, 42). William Valentine, the house governor, believed that such patients should be excluded because of a lack of bed space (RLH, LH/A/17/5, 17 April 1827), and consumptives and asthmatics were considered to be more effectively treated as outpatients (Clark-Kennedy 1962, 60–1).

In an effort to make sure that those with no hope of a cure did not remain in the hospital, patients were not supposed to remain in the hospital for longer than two months. In September 1822 the house visitors found that over 50 patients had been in the hospital for more than two months without having their tickets renewed. One patient had been on Talbot ward for 18 months, and another had been in for 14 months (RLH, LH/A/5/17, 50). Following this discovery a resolution was passed not to give any more medicine to patients who had been in the house for longer than two months unless the governor who recommended them gave them a fresh ticket. The house committee also requested an explanation from the surgeons and physicians if their patients exceeded this limit; if satisfactory explanations were given they were often permitted to stay (ibid, 151–3).

On 20 August 1829 the parish was requested to remove from the hospital one John Myler, who had been discharged as 'incurable'. In the third week of September, Myler (or Mylar) was still residing on the wards and the hospital applied to the magistrate to compel the parish to remove him. The reply was received that the hospital must instead apply to the East India Company, with whom he had previously served as a soldier. Despite a reluctance to do so, on the grounds that they had had little success in the past, the hospital wrote to the East India Company. On 12 November the reply was received that, whilst Myler had indeed been a private in the Bombay Artillery, he

had been invalided out and so was no longer the Company's responsibility (RLH, LH/A/5/18, 279, 283, 291). Meanwhile, Myler had been occupying a much-needed bed for a further two months.

The workhouse poor

In the early years of the hospital, a resolution was made by the house committee not to admit anyone who was already in one of the parish workhouses that had their own provision for treating the sick (paid surgeons and apothecaries were employed by the workhouses), unless the person under whose care they had been came with them to explain their case (Clark-Kennedy 1962, 64). Later in the 18th century the house committee decided that paupers should be admitted to the hospital only if their parish officer paid 1 guinea towards their maintenance; by 1788 parishes were charged a fee of 4d a day (Howard 1791, 131; Clark-Kennedy 1962, 170–1).

During the 19th century, the hospital continued to receive payment for the maintenance of paupers, and the amounts received were included within the annual accounts published in the annual reports distributed to governors (Fig 96). The payments were not necessarily consistent, however, and in 1822 the hospital took the decision to discharge a pauper by the name of Peters, who had been a patient for more than seven months, seemingly in the absence of any money from the parish. The parish officers wrote to request that he continue as a patient in the hospital and offered to pay for his upkeep, but the house governor's reply (RLH, LH/A/5/17, 5 February 1822, 84) was that:

the want of the usual security for Peters as a Pauper did not in the slightest degree influence the Committee of this Hospital in their decision relative to his discharge, nor can the offer of payment induce them to continue him as an InPatient, his Physician having reported that nothing more can be done for him; and his continuance therefore in the House only serves to preclude the admission of one more of the numerous applicants, who are every Tuesday rejected for want of room.

In 1835 the coroner's room was appropriated for the house governor to interview prospective recommended patients to find out, before their admission by the governors, whether or not they were paupers (RLH, LH/A/5/21, 79, 89). In 1837 one of the guardians of the Whitechapel Union attended the house committee to complain of the improper conduct of two of the servants of the hospital when they visited the parish workhouse to return a pauper by the name of Mark King, who had been discharged as a patient by the hospital (RLH, LH/A/5/22, 8). The hall porter, Brooks, was also suspended and then dismissed after temporarily losing 24s paid for the maintenance of a pauper (ibid, 13). The 1841 census return includes two paupers, both children – James Turner, the 10-year-old son of a labourer, and John Adams, the 13-year-old son of a widow (TNA: PRO, 1841 England census, parish St Mary Whitechapel).

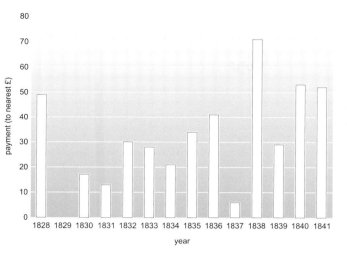

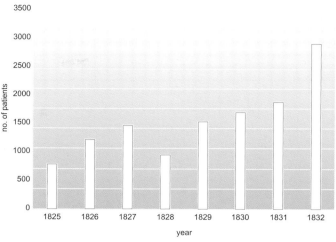

Fig 96 Payments received by the governors for the maintenance of parish paupers, from the figures published in the annual reports (RLH, LH/A/15) (data for 1829 not available)

Fig 97 The number of patients giving thanks between 1825 and 1832, as recorded in the house committee minute books (RLH, LH/A/5/18–19), showing the gradual expansion of the hospital

5.6 Discharging patients

Discharging patients was the responsibility of the physician or surgeon under whom the patient had been admitted. Whether the patient had been cured or merely 'relieved' was marked on their ticket. The patient was then officially discharged at the weekly committee meetings. In line with the spiritual ethos of the hospital (below, 5.11, 'Spiritual care'), the patients were required to return thanks to God, the committee and 'their kind benefactors'. When the hospital chapel was built, all inpatients were required to give thanks the following week at 9am before appearing before the committee at 11am (Clark-Kennedy 1962, 34). If they did not do so they would be refused admission in the future (1810: RLH, LH/A/1/4, 13), and a list of these offenders was kept. Those who did give thanks were given a certificate entitling them to further relief from the hospital should they need it. The clerk would make out the letter of thanks for the patient – presumably many of them could not write – and maintained the logs of 'Certificates for Patients both In. and Out. applying for relief to the Docks and Parishes' (Fig 97).

In December 1831, it was brought to the attention of the committee that William Valentine had been discharging patients without informing their doctors or surgeons (RLH, LH/A/5/19, 165). Given what we know of Valentine's character and duties (below, 5.9, 'The house governor'), it seems likely that, if this were the case, he was taking a pragmatic approach to the issues of a full house.

In addition to being discharged when cured or deemed incurable, patients were, on occasion, discharged for disciplinary reasons. In May 1829 a patient named Coombes tried to defraud the hospital by dictating a letter to another patient, J Corbett (presumably Coombes himself could not write), purporting to be an official missive requesting that the hospital extend to him money and clothes. The deception was discovered and both patients immediately discharged (RLH, LH/A/5/18, 266). Valentine also dismissed two patients for drunk and disorderly conduct (RLH, LH/A/5/19, 273).

Efforts were made to provide some extra assistance to patients and their families through the medium of the Samaritan Society, founded in 1791 by William Blizard, who for several years previously had been delving into his own pockets to help those patients who were in need (Clark-Kennedy 1962, 182). By 1821 William Valentine was chief almoner and honorary secretary of the society, and Blizard was the treasurer; furthermore, the committee included many members of the medical staff. The funds of the society were used to provide help for patients being discharged from the hospital, giving financial support and supplying glasses, artificial limbs and other chirurgical aids, even helping ex-servicemen to obtain their rightful pensions. A considerable proportion of the funds was also used to support convalescing ex-patients at the Margate Sea Bathing Infirmary (ibid, 211–13) (Table 63).

5.7 Casualty

Accidental and 'extraordinary' (acute) cases could be admitted at any time of day or night, without a governor's letter (1832: RLH, LH/A/1/7, 42; Clark-Kennedy 1962, 28). As the committee that agreed admissions met only once a week, the decision to admit acute cases rested with the staff, including the apothecary, who was resident within the hospital. The complaint of Joanna Haines (above, 5.3) indicates that an early form of triage ('Urgent', 'Very Proper' and 'Proper' cases) was used to evaluate accident victims when the number of admissions grew large. This system is believed to have its origins in the Napoleonic Wars, where it was used to assign much-needed resources in the chaos of the battlefield (Iserson and Moskop 2007, 276–7). The system was

Table 63 Accounts of the Samaritan Society 1839–40, published in the annual report, 1840 (RLH, LH/A/15/18)

Patients	Number	£	s	d
			Expense	
Relieved in money	312	76	2	5½
Fares paid or money given to assist home	192	28	17	0
Fares + support of patients at Margate	16	127	13	10
" [ie ditto] in country	1	1	14	6
Lodged + dieted until situations procured, or otherwise disposed of	27	14	8	10
Clothes + mechanics' tools taken out of pawn	9	3	4	4¾
Bread given, where it is probable money would have been misapplied	7	0	12	0
Bibles given	2	0	7	0
Clothing				
Flannel shifts	3	0	12	0
" petticoats	4	0	16	0
" waistcoats	16	2	19	6
" drawers	7	0	15	9
Striped shirts	12	1	10	0
Dowlas shifts	10	1	5	0
Stockings	6 pairs	0	9	0
Shoes	24 "	5	8	3
Guernsey jacket	1	0	3	1
Old clothes supplied to	35			
*Presents of old clothing will be thankfully received				
Mechanical aids				
Wooden legs	3	3	8	0
Artificial arm	1	3	3	0
" palate	1	0	6	0
Trusses, single	35	6	19	6
", double	6	2	4	0
Suspensory bandages	4	0	7	6
Knee caps	10	4	11	6
Lace stockings	4	1	16	0
Eye shades	17	0	17	0
Boot with side iron	1	0	8	0
Instrument for supporting a dislocated shoulder	1	0	18	0
Instrument for leg & club foot	1	1	2	6
Eye glass	1	0	3	6
Catheter	1	0	4	0
Total		293	7	7¼

subsequently adopted more widely by military surgeons and would clearly have provided a practical solution to allocating treatment in a busy hospital.

Those who had suffered accidents and required immediate surgical treatment could therefore be rapidly admitted and this created an inherent tension between the two methods of arrival at the hospital. In 1830 it was recorded (RLH, LH/A/5/18, 309):

that the admission which is at all times freely given by night and by day to cases of accident and extreme urgency is one of the most important benefits conferred by the London Hospital and that the greatly increased number of such cases which during the last years amasses 30 weekly exclusive of a larger number of accidents made Out Patients has of necessity reduced the accommodation for the admission of Patients recommended by Governors.

The volume of such cases is further emphasised by the account that in the week to 23 June 1831 (RLH, LH/A/5/19, 73):

forty nine patients have been brought to the Hospital disabled by accidents, of this number thirty five have been admitted into the House, and fourteen have been treated as Out Patients. During the same period six of those which are denominated Extra Cases have been received into the Hospital: - all independently of Patients admitted by the House Committee.

The accident and emergency function of the hospital became increasingly important over the period in which the cemetery (OA6) was in use (above, 5.3; Fig 92), and contemporary newspaper accounts confirm the accident and emergency function of the London Hospital (eg, *The Times*, 18 July 1804, issue 6078, p 3, col A; 9 April 1806, issue 6706, p 3, col B; 11 August 1806, issue 6813, p 3, col C).

The minute books record a number of instances of the treatment of victims of accident. Although they focus predominantly on the successful treatment of debilitating injury, they also record failures, such as the death of Mr George Friend in July 1831 following an 'extremely serious and dangerous accident' (RLH, LH/A/5/19, 87). The committee had written to his friend James Tomlin, of Crescent, Minories, to 'express the sincere concern which the committee feel at Mr Friend's accident, and their best wishes for his recovery', further stating that 'Mr Friend should continue in the Hospital as long as it may be deemed necessary; during which period all the attentions that can contribute to his convalescence or comfort shall cheerfully be afforded to him' (ibid, 87–8). Despite the ministrations of the hospital, Mr Friend died during the night of Sunday 31 July (ibid, 91).

One of the more dramatic cases successfully treated and outlined was that of John Taylor, aged 19, Prussian by birth and apprenticed to a merchant vessel, the brig *Jane* (under Captain Good), out of Scarborough. Taylor was injured whilst assisting in the lowering of the mast (RLH, LH/A/5/19, 103–6):

This mast is 35 feet in length and about 2 feet in circumference at the bottom; it has at this part an iron bolt 5 inches long and nearly 2 inches round by which it is fitted to the boom … having been lowered to within the distance of about 6 feet Taylor raised his arms to lay hold of it … at this moment a rope by which the mast was suspended slipped or broke … knocking him down on his back and the bolted part was driven through his body and by it he was pinned to the deck of the vessel, the bolt entering the deck above one inch … [it] entered his body between the fourth and fifth ribs about an inch and a half from the centre of the breast bone, passed obliquely downwards and came out between the eleventh and twelfth ribs four inches from the spine. The bolt had a nut to prevent its being forced into the mast and which pressing on his breast chipped out a triangular piece of cartilage leaving the point of the heart with very insecure protection. The ribs were broken, the side of the chest flattened, the jaw-bone badly fractured and the scalp much lacerated. I do not have doubt the bolt passed through the lung, wounding the bag of the heart, and pushing the diaphragm before it. Notwithstanding the fearful mischief described, the man has recovered.

Andrews, the surgeon who operated on Taylor, subsequently attested to his good character and requested that, as the young man would not now be able to carry out manual work, the hospital should set up a small fund to help him. Mr Andrews and William Blizard each contributed a sovereign, though it is not clear if the trust was formed (RLH, LH/A/5/19, 106).

A number of peri-mortem injuries were seen in the buried population: 36–45-year-old male [242], 26–35-year-old female [57002] and perhaps most notably ≥46-year-old male [124] all had injuries that were unhealed at the time of death (Chapter 4.2, 'Trauma'). Such fine examples of healing and peri-mortem injury are rarely observed in archaeological material and they enable more direct comparison with clinical medicine than generally possible: in modern hospitals, imaging of bone fractures takes place soon after the traumatic incident has occurred, before healing starts, but in palaeopathology we

usually see the result of months and years of healing, which can hinder comparison with modern clinical examples of fracture. In comparison, six peri-mortem injuries were reported in the Worcester Royal Infirmary assemblage, all comminuted spiral fractures (Western 2010, 28). The traumatic events that caused these injuries were almost certainly what led on to the person's admission to the hospital. They also ultimately resulted, directly or indirectly, in their deaths: the osteological evidence suggests that male [124] had remained in the wards, receiving care but not successful reduction of his injury, for approximately three weeks before his death.

5.8 Inside the house

On the wards

On 15 September 1788 the hospital was visited by John Howard, prison and hospital reformer, who described the building, which was then occupied by 120 patients on seven of the 18 wards (the remainder having been shut up for two or three years) thus (Howard 1791, 131):

The wards in general are twenty feet wide, and twelve high, and each contains about eighteen beds, which have no testers. Over the doors were square apertures. The passages, which are eight feet wide, are dark. There are no cisterns for water: the vaults are often offensive. […] In a dirty room in the cellar there is a cold and a hot bath, which seem to be seldom used. – The wards were not dirty, but the house has not been white-washed for some years; nor has it, within or without, the appearance of neatness.

By 1840 there were 24 named wards in use in the hospital, arranged over three floors – six wards in the front block of the hospital, six in the east wing and twelve in the extended west wing. The lobbies and 'bye-wards' were also sometimes used to accommodate patients. The wards were divided into male and female wards, and also between medical and surgical cases. In 1840 each ward contained accommodation for between nine and 16 patients. In May 1840 the wards were recorded, with the regular number of beds together with the number of patients actually in each ward (Table 64)

Each ward contained rows of iron bedsteads (an advance from wooden beds, which could become infested with bedbugs (Higgs 2009, 66) and patients generally slept on mattresses filled with straw, which were refilled regularly (RLH, LH/A/5/18, 118), though this was not without attendant problems: 'The Matron having reported that the Beds are overrun with Vermin – Ordered that she make application for any remedy she may be advised' (ibid, 168). On 11 January 1825, the house committee minute books record 'Messrs Dixon and Co to supply 100 blankets' (ibid, 7). In line with general practice, fracture cases were usually placed on a horsehair mattress with a firm base

(Higgs 2009, 66), and 12 horsehair mattresses were purchased in 1836 for the surgical patients. The following year the medical officers requested an additional 12 horsehair mattresses for the surgeons' wards, as well as three more 'fracture beds' for Mr Luke 'on account of the increased admission of accidents' (RLH, LH/A/5/21, 272, 456). In December 1838 the house committee sanctioned the ordering of six coconut fibre mattresses, invented by Captain Wildey as a cheaper substitute for those made of horsehair (RLH, LH/A/5/22, 176). During the expansion of the wards, bedsteads with 'lift up heads' were to be supplied by Mr Shatter at £3 15s for six (ibid, 311). In January 1833 the hospital possessed a number of hydrostatic beds (a recent invention), which, although not in a fit state for use and in need of being made watertight, were evidently effective, for in November that year the house governor requested that three more be ordered for the use of the patients (RLH, LH/A/5/20, 19, 179). These beds were designed to relieve pressure and were specifically invented with the prevention of bedsores in mind (see Fig 83). They consisted of a mattress laid on a sheet of mackintosh or rubberised cloth which in turn sat on a trough of water, enabling the patient to float, supported. Its inventor Dr Arnott considered it superior

even to the pocket-sprung mattress and gave free permission to all to reproduce it with the aim of alleviating suffering (Ryan 1832).

The wards contained wooden lockers for the patients' belongings, numbered to correspond with each bed. In 1825 the house visitors complained that 'the Patients Lockers are continually being brought down into the Carpenters Shop for Repair without doors' (RLH, LH/A/16/4, 71). In spite of the lockers, thefts were a common occurrence. In 1835 William Finn, a boy on Talbot's by-ward, stole a loaf of bread from another patient (ibid, 148). The house governor reported to the house committee in 1827 that instances of theft from the patients on the wards were rife, both by other patients and by visitors, 'many of whom doubtless get into the Hospital for the purpose of stealing whatever they may lay their hands on'. Most recently a watch and some money had been taken. The house governor asked the committee if they would bring charges against anyone caught stealing, but he had reservations about taking such a course of action, fearing that 'by following such a precedent, the governors will have their hands full of prosecutions' (RLH, LH/A/17/5, 13 February 1827).

Each ward had access to water closets, which were not always in perfect working order and were a common cause for comment from the house visitors, who complained of 'offensive smells' emanating from them. They often became blocked and in 1823 they had to be repaired. Not all patients were sufficiently mobile to walk to the water closets, so bedpans were also provided on the wards. Some of the house visitors were concerned, however, that a number of the patients might not be making use of the closets for other reasons, and in 1820 recommended the purchase of a number of loose flannel gowns for patients to use when visiting the closets, worrying that 'many Patients have not apparel sufficient to cover their nakedness' (RLH, LH/A/16/4, 43). In 1828, eight 'night chairs' (commodes) were purchased for the wards (RLH, LH/A/5/18, 224).

Sanitary and hygiene vessels feature strongly in the group of commissioned blue transfer-printed whiteware pottery, recovered during excavation, bearing the image of the London Hospital (below, 5.10). These items would have been in use in the hospital during the second and third quarters of the 19th century. The most frequent and well-preserved pots are the six sputum mugs in refined whiteware with underglaze blue transfer-printed stipple and line decoration (TPW2). These particular one-handled vessels were employed to collect the patient's phlegm, with the water in the mug distilling the contents, which were concealed by a removable funnel (<P1>–<P2>, Fig 98). It is a form that has its origins in tin-glazed ware (Britton 1987, cat no. 60, 118) and Clark-Kennedy (1963, 154) records that as early as the 1750s the London Hospital had pots 'provided in each ward to prevent them [the patients] from spitting against the walls'. Among the other hygiene and sanitary wares discarded here are a plain refined white earthenware (REFW) bedpan (<P3>, Fig 99) with a long tubular handle opening into the interior. This allowed the contents to be emptied with the minimum of unpleasantness and it is of a shape that was improved by the introduction of

Table 64 The beds in the hospital, as recorded on 11 May 1840; principal wards, each with a head nurse in charge, are in italics

Ward	Regular no. of beds, exclusive of extra ones, which vary from time to time	Patients actually in the house
Ground floor		
Mellish	9	12
Dorien	10	13
Richmond	10	10
William IV	10	10
William Frederick	10	10
Gloucester	10	14
Bowley	10	14
Devonshire	10	17
First floor		
Charlotte	12	13
Adelaide	11	12
Milward	12	13
Redman	12	14
Mary	15	19
Victoria	16	18
Sophia	14	14
Granby	13	13
By-Ward	10	12
Second floor		
Harrison	12	12
Turner	13	13
Holland	13	9
Fitzgerald	14	14
George	15	15
Baker	16	18
Talbot	13	13
Gore	14	15
By-Ward	10	10
Total	314	347

the 'Slipper' bedpan from the 1830s onwards (Jackson 2005, 22). The slipper baths, for the comfortable washing of female patients, are mentioned in the 1824 inventory for many of the London Hospital's wards (RLH, LH/A/18/3, fo 32). The collections of the Royal London Museum also feature hygiene and sanitary wares, with a sputum mug (RLHINV/430) that has the number 4 underglaze blue-painted on its base), a chamber pot (RLHINV/119) and a soap dish (RLHINV/108) represented.

The wards sometimes contained more patients than they were intended to accommodate. In 1834 the house visitors reported to the committee that there were two patients in the hospital lying on the floor for want of bedsteads (RLH, LH/A/16/4, 134–5), and in 1837 they reported that there were 55 patients on Gloucester ward – 25 more than the usual number (this is likely to refer to Gloucester together with the adjacent wards, which came under the control of one head nurse). Although every year the hospital was forced to turn away hundreds of deserving cases recommended by the governors, occupancy varied, and sometimes the house visitors noted vacant beds. In January 1832 they noted that there were 18 vacant beds in the women's wards, and in the following month there were found to be 15 empty beds in the accident

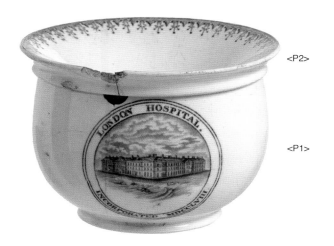

Fig 98 Sputum mug <P1> with funnel <P2> positioned on top, in refined whiteware with underglaze blue transfer-printed (stipple and line) decoration, from [279] (scale c 1:2)

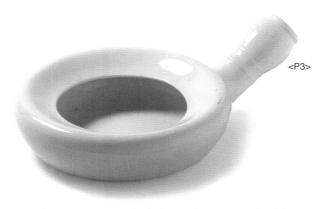

Fig 99 Bedpan <P3> in plain refined white earthenware, from [279] (scale c 1:8)

wards (RLH, LH/A/16/4, 108, 110–11).

The wards were also furnished with chairs and a table, at which the patients who were well enough to leave their beds ate their meals. In 1824 the house visitors recorded that 'George's Bye Ward is in great want of seats, the Patients sitting on the iron coal scuttle' (RLH, LH/A/16/4, 55–6).

The large windows on the wards were fitted with wooden shutters, which were noted 'to be in a bad state of repair by the house visitors in 1836 (RLH, LH/A/16/4, 166). During the day strong sun could cause discomfort to the patients, and the house visitors repeatedly suggested that roller blinds should be fitted (ibid, 148, 166). Photographs from later in the century show this to have taken place (Fig 100).

The lobbies between the wards contained sinks, which could become as offensive as the water closets if they were not kept sufficiently clean. In 1822 it was discovered that the nurses had been dumping dirty poultices in the sinks to hide them before the physicians and surgeons did their rounds (below, 5.10; RLH, LH/A/5/17, 70). The fact that sinks were shared between more than one ward also led to some of the nurses passing the blame for them not being kept clean (ibid, 342).

The detailed documentation regarding the admission and care of patients implies that the wards were highly regulated. Strict segregation of men and women was required (1810: RLH, LH/A/1/4, 15). When children were admitted, general hospitals usually placed older boys on the male wards and girls and younger boys on the female wards (Higgs 2009, 24). The 1841 census, which appears to have been taken ward by ward, seems to indicate that a similar practice was observed at the London Hospital, with boys and girls over the age of 7 placed on the adult wards, but those under that age (both boys and girls) placed together in groups of two, perhaps in the lobbies between the main female wards, which were also used for patients in a state of convalescence (TNA: PRO, 1841 England census, parish St Mary Whitechapel; RLH, LH/A/5/22, 392). The wards were also split between medical and surgical cases, although this division was more flexible. In 1823 the house committee took the decision to admit eight physicians' patients on to the surgical wards, where there was room available (RLH, LH/A/5/17, 202). Suggestions were often made to appropriate wards for other particular cases. Headington suggested that wards be set aside for patients suffering from 'ill conditioned sores' that would be offensive to other patients, and also for depressed and suicidal patients who might be too sensitive to suffer the joking and jeering of their fellow patients on the general wards: 'the mind of the poor Man is as finely framed as that of his Superior and his susceptibility is often more acutely raised from the supposed hopelessness of his condition'. His suggestion does not appear to have been adopted, although in 1822 a room in the attic was set aside for 'temporary lunatics', after the physicians and surgeons argued that a specific ward for convalescing patients was not necessary (RLH, LH/A/5/17, 177).

Normal visiting hours were from 4pm to 8pm in summer and from 3pm to the 'close of day' in winter, every day apart from Sunday (1810: RLH, LH/A/1/4, 30). Exceptions were made for the relations of seriously ill patients and for Jews, who would be

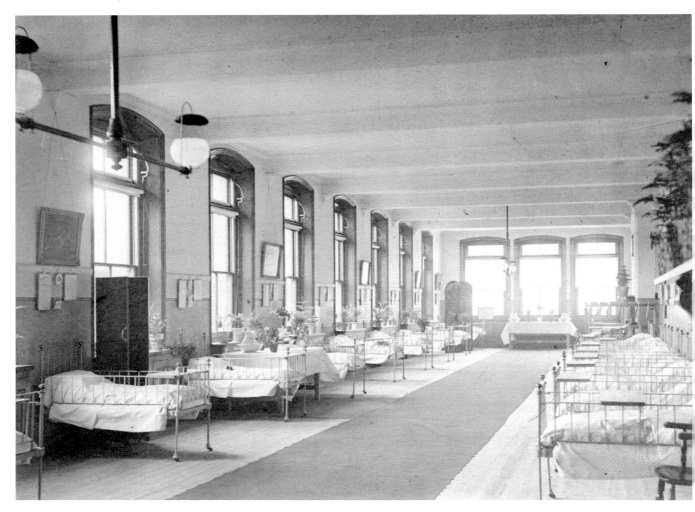

Fig 100 A ward in the newly constructed Grocers' wing, photographed in 1876 (Royal London Hospital Archives, RLH, LH/A/26/32)

unable to visit on the Sabbath (Saturday) – just one of many examples of the hospital being sensitive to the requirements of different religious groups (ibid, 31). Patients were to be in bed by 9pm in summer and 10pm in winter (ibid, 15).

The hospital was whitewashed annually in time for the anniversary celebrations each April (RLH, LH/A/5/18, 6) and the handrails of the banisters to the wards were painted black (ibid, 21). On the suggestion of the medical officers, however, the limewashing of the wards was sometimes delayed until the summer months to minimise disruption for the patients (RLH, LH/A/5/21, 15 March 1836, 223). The response to cholera indicates that limewash was not just cosmetic but was considered to be a disinfectant (Hempel 2006, 40) A deep clean of the hospital was carried out at the same time. In 1837 Priscilla Watson was engaged 'to scour and clean all the Lobbies, passages, staircases and lobbies [sic] in the new wing, waiting Halls, Surgeons, Physicians Rooms the assistant nurses Bedrooms and attick stories likewise all the officers sitting and Bedrooms the Kitchen and men servants bedrooms and all the wainscoating belonging to the above places' in addition to the nurses' sitting and bedrooms, for the sum of £24 (RLH, LH/A/23/31).

The house committee minute books testify to the time and

money required to maintain the buildings in a fit state for the patients. At the end of 1825 the hospital complained to the water company that the supply had been 'very deficient' that past year. Correspondence from William Valentine shows that the fault actually lay in the storage tanks, where valves to the lead pipework were faulty, and the decision was taken to inspect them regularly after this (RLH, LH/A/5/18, 27 December 1825, 61–2). Tenders show that work on the drains and cesspools and repairs to the stairs were needed in 1828 (ibid, 22 January 1828, 190).

Housekeeping appears to have presented a particular problem within the wards. In 1826 an inspection resulted in a complaint about the state of the 'lobbies and closets' and the governors resolved to fine all the nurses 1 guinea. The matron, Mrs Le Blond, blamed the mess on the porters, whom the committee decided to fine instead. At this point the payment of future gratuities was made dependent on compliance with the required standards of cleanliness (RLH, LH/A/5/18, 67). There were still problems at the end of 1830, when Mr Cotton reported the 'swing doors fastened open, three of them by nails driven into the floor, the fourth by a bone thrust under it, thus defeating the object the committee had in view when fitting them with the patent springs' (ibid, 401). The 'steam-table' in the kitchen had been repaired and Tothill, the engineer, had been fixing the vapour bath (ibid, 403). 'I mention all these circumstances to show how much may be wrong, and yet unobserved on an ordinary inspection' (ibid, 404). Cotton recommended a regular timetable of cleaning and reporting faults.

The hospital seems to have attempted to ensure the comfort of both patients and staff. In 1820 warm-air stoves, stoves, fittings for the dispensary, 50 cast or wrought iron bedsteads, 50 lockers for patients, a cast iron vessel for hot water, coal boxes, baths and possibly a movable bath (as used at St George's Hospital) were to be purchased for the new wing (RLH, LH/A/5/16, 381–2), whilst in the spring of 1825 the governors were investigating the heating and ventilation on the wards. They ordered that 'a new stove be procured for the lobby next top the Committee room and also one in the kitchen in Sophia's Ward' (RLH, LH/A/5/18, 23). Although heating had been partially introduced to the wards, discussion on the warming and ventilation of Gloucester ward took place on 19 April 1825 (ibid, 25–6):

> the temperature of the external air was about 42 [6°C], that of the generality of the wards 51–54 [10–12°C] and that of the two under the influence of the new system was from 62–63 [c 17°C] … in the large and long wards cold unpleasant drafts of air pervaded the whole and ventilation was very partial and imperfect and the extremities of the wards particularly cold by their great distance from a fire – small and ineffectual for the comfort of those even within its region.

Being exposed to low temperatures, fluctuations of temperature and drafts can hardly have aided the recovery of the patients.

The governors resolved to complete the heating to a specification that had been provided in an 1823 tender and to place a stove in the chapel. They also decided to replace the water closets at the west end of the hospital, in line with the more effective ones already in place at the east end and on 26 April they further asked the surveyor to draw up plans for a water closet for the matron (RLH, LH/A/5/18, 27). In order to carry out these improvement works, they decided to reduce patient numbers gradually to not less than 260 (ibid, 28). In 1825, the cost of the stoves for the wards was £110 and for the chapel £140 (ibid, 33). The 'warming and ventilation works' were approved on 9 August of that year (ibid, 43).

These works appear to have provided a partial solution. In December 1830 it was recorded that 'During the late cold weather, the temperature has been kept up above 50° [10°C] … Without them [the hot air stoves] the temperature of the wards would, as in other bedrooms, have been below freezing point' (RLH, LH/A/5/18, 407). This also implies that there were still areas of the house without any form of heating. However, rather than lighting fires at night when they had not been needed during the day, the staff shut the windows. 'How offensive they [the wards] must be after having been closed up for seven or eight hours' (ibid, 407). A report by Mr Cotton at this time stated 'the flues were never swept until the fire would

no longer burn' (ibid, 402). By 1831, there were seven fires in the summer and 20 in the winter which had to be attended to (RLH, LH/A/5/19, 156). In the same year, the committee decided to fit Sylvester stoves for the wards (ibid, 384). These appear to have been a patented coal-fired convection heater, and incidentally formed a standard part of Royal Navy equipment for cold climates from the 1820s to 1860s (Battersby 2008, 4). In June, Mr Sylvester wrote explaining the delay in installing the stoves, which had still not appeared (RLH, LH/A/5/19, 64). However, this did not deter the committee, who ordered that 'Mr Sylvester … be directed to furnish immediately an additional Roaster for the Kitchen and a new drying stove for the laundry' (ibid, 77). Unfortunately all did not go smoothly and on 9 February 1832 the committee complained that there had been no hot water to the west wing for several weeks as a result of Mr Sylvester's faulty water tank (ibid, 191). Yet, despite the ongoing challenge of heating the wards, in 1832 the committee decided to forego the expense of purchasing earthenware footwarmers for the patients (ibid, 244).

Whilst clearly aware of the costs of running the house (sometimes apparently at the expense of common sense or patient care), the governors seem to have remained keen to maintain the position of the London Hospital at the forefront of technological advances, as demonstrated by correspondence in 1825 concerning the change from oil gas to coal gas lighting (RLH, LH/A/5/18, 47).

Bending the rules

An audit of the house carried out in November 1832 after a complaint received by the governors suggests that rules on segregation and visiting hours were not always strictly enforced – in addition to a number of apparently unauthorised staff (below, 5.9), relatives of patients were found to be staying overnight. A child called Elger who had been admitted with burns was accompanied for one night by his mother and for three nights by his sister (an incident that provides an intriguing insight into family life as presumably his mother had to work or look after the household on the nights his sister was in attendance). The grandmother of a 14-year-old boy named Pinker, also admitted with burns, had stayed for three nights. It was not just children who had overnight visitors: the mother and the wife of William Hayes had stayed for one night and William Hunt was accompanied by his wife for three nights. When questioned further, the nurses confirmed that the relatives of the sick and dying were regularly allowed to stay overnight, in a victory for compassion over policy (RLH, LH/A/5/19, 390–1).

By the 1830s there were complaints that a number of unauthorised people were present in the hospital with the permission of the matron but without that of the committee, 'a practice which is calculated to introduce abuses' (RLH, LH/A/5/19, 1832, 220). The complaint was raised by one of the more active of the governors, a Mr Tickell (below, 5.9, 'The house governor'). He had carried out an audit and found that a man called John Farrant was staying in the gate porter's lodge (against the explicit orders of the house governor, William Valentine) and several relatives of nurses or servants were coming and going freely (RLH, LH/A/5/19, 393–4):

> a man supposed to be named Gardner professedly a brother of one of the assistant nurses in Mary's Ward, has for a very long period past and until the present time, had constant access to the Ward (which is a female ward) at all times, morning, noon and night, without let or hindrance. This man has lost his nose by the foul disorder [venereal syphilis].

Nurse Redman had her child with her, the head nurse had her nieces and a servant living with her, Nurse Jewell had an unauthorised assistant and her daughter, and Nurse Gloucester had an occasional assistant. Valentine countered that he had removed Gardner from the premises the first time he saw him and that all other apparently unauthorised people had been employed to carry out odd jobs, many of them with the sanction of the committee (RLH, LH/A/5/19, 394–405).

Structural fittings and furniture

Ian Betts and Beth Richardson

A small number of items that may have been installed within the hospital were recovered during the excavation and watching brief.

Deposits across the site produced several fragments of tin-glazed ('delft') wall tile (Fig 101), and it is possible that some of these were installed in the original hospital building. Tin-glazed wall tiles could be used in a variety of locations, but in London were principally used around fireplace surrounds, which is probably the original location of the London Hospital examples.

Two fragments of tin-glazed wall tile, recovered from the deposits dumped to raise and consolidate the enclosed ground behind the hospital, depict a central landscape scene in blue-on-white set within an octagonal powdered purple border, with blue carnation-head corner motifs (<T1>). It is clear from the minutes of the house committee that the majority of this material originated further afield and was brought to the site for the purpose of raising the ground (RLH, LH/A/5/16, 1 July 1817, 150; Chapter 3.1), although items directly associated with the hospital, such as a bone enema syringe, were also present within the machined deposits. Similar tiles are illustrated in Horne (1989, 22–4, nos 33–54). Both Horne's and the London Hospital examples are of London manufacture and may be dated to around 1740–60. Tin-glazed wall tiles are also known to have been installed at St Bartholomew's Hospital in West Smithfield, which has a large collection of tin-glazed tiles believed to have come from the south wing, completed in 1739 and demolished in 1935 (Betts and Weinstein 2010, 64).

Another fragmentary 18th-century tin-glazed wall tile was associated with a grave, although probably from the hospital. It is decorated in blue-on-white and shows part of a seascape with a boat and figures within a circular border (<T2>). The tile could be English or Dutch.

Four tin-glazed wall tiles were collected from the machined deposits across the site. All appear to be from different fireplaces. They comprise a blue-on-white biblical tile, a purple-on-white landscape tile, a purple-on-white military tile and a rare rectangular blue-on-white edging tile. The blue-on-white biblical tile (<T3>) shows Jesus and the Woman of Samaria (John 4: 4–9). This is a Dutch biblical design of probable 18th-century date. Huijg (1978, 145) shows a Dutch tile with the same biblical scene. The decorated purple-on-white tile (<T4>) has a central landscape scene, set within a circular border, showing a man wearing a brimmed

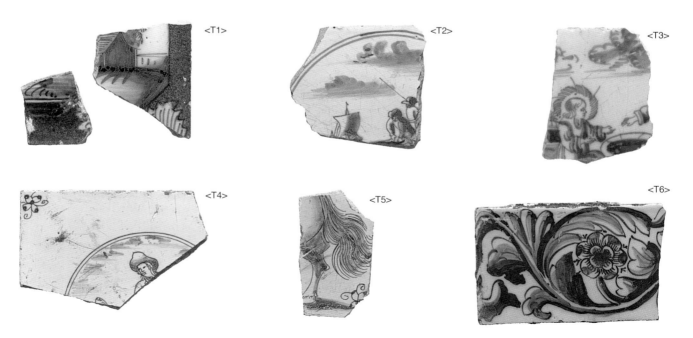

Fig 101 Decorated tin-glazed ('delft') wall tiles <T1>–<T6>, believed to have been used in the London Hospital, recovered from Open Areas 5, 6 and 8 (scale 1:2)

hat; the tile has spider-head corners, indicating that it is a Dutch import. It is painted in a similar style to a Dutch tile illustrated in Pluis (1997, 378, A.03.03.04), dated to c 1660–c 1800, and further tiles dated to c 1750–c 1840 are illustrated in Schaap (1984, 113, no. 138). Interestingly, all these also show a figure wearing a brimmed hat in a landscape scene. The other purple-on-white tile shows the back legs and tail of a horse with a similar spider-head corner (<T5>). This is almost certainly part of a Dutch tile showing a mounted soldier. Two complete tiles from London with mounted figures and very similar spider-head corners are illustrated in Betts and Weinstein (2010, 157, nos 331–2). They are dated to the period c 1700–50, although production could have continued for a few years longer. The dating would again suggest that if the tile is from the hospital it was installed when the hospital was newly built. The blue-on-white rectangular-shaped edging tile (<T6>) measures 63mm in breadth by 7mm in thickness. It has the same running floral design as a complete tile illustrated by Horne (1989, 70, no. 398). This is a London-made tile dating to c 1750–70. Rectangular tin-glazed tiles were used as decorative borders with square tiles in fireplace surrounds. Two tile fireplaces with square and rectangular tiles survive in the London area, one at 12 Kensington Square, the other at Rainham Hall (Betts and Weinstein 2010, 59, 80–1, fig 58).

Other finds included an hourglass-shaped iron pulley (<S11>, Fig 102), which might have had a specific hospital use. Two small, thick copper-alloy discs, dished on the underside and flattened on the top side, their undersides abraded, may have been used as buffers for the feet of small tables, chairs or other items of furniture (<40>, <41>, [650]) (Geoff Egan, pers comm).

Items used by staff or patients

Nigel Jeffries, Jacqui Pearce and Beth Richardson

The machined deposits (OA8) overlying the c 1825 to 1841/2 cemetery produced a small number of items probably belonging to either staff or patients in the hospital. Pottery recovered from the rubble sealing the group 22 burials includes a refined white earthenware (REFW) eight-sided jug with a lion-head spout and applied sprig decoration depicting three different images (<P4>, Fig 103). The first is a cupid holding his bow and arrow on one side; the second, a classical figure of a boy with a rope or vine draped over his shoulder, is applied to the opposite panel; the third type of sprig decoration, positioned towards the top portion of the vessel above these figures, presents a spray of shamrocks flanked by a thistle to the left and a rose to the right, and depicts a common representation of the Union of

Britain and Ireland in 1801.

The most visually striking of all the ceramics is the pot lid in refined whiteware with underglaze three-colour transfer-printed decoration (TPW5; <P5>, Fig 104, left) depicting an invalid male fishing from a large tub in his room with his right leg dressed with a gout sock. Made by the Staffordshire firm of F & R Pratt of Fenton during the 1860s, the image is a reproduction of Theodore Lane's 1828 painting *Enthusiast ('The gouty angler')* (Fig 104, right). The lid itself would have sealed food pastes.

The rubbish also included a complete, heavy green-coloured glass champagne bottle with a distinctive string rim (<G1>, Fig 105), probably made in France, and the handle of a black basalt stoneware teapot.

The deposits overlying the cemetery also produced two brushes (Fig 106), both made from bone, with green staining from the copper wire used to secure the bristles. One (<S13>) is

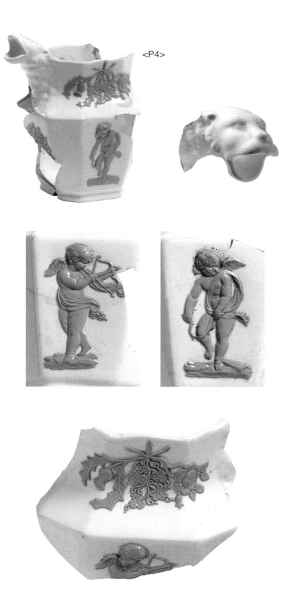

Fig 103 *Refined white earthenware eight-sided jug <P4> (H 170mm) with applied sprig decoration (scale c 1:4); detailed views of the cupid, boy, shamrock and lion-head spout (scale c 1:2)*

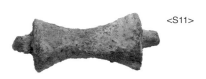

Fig 102 *Hourglass-shaped iron pulley <S11> (scale 1:2)*

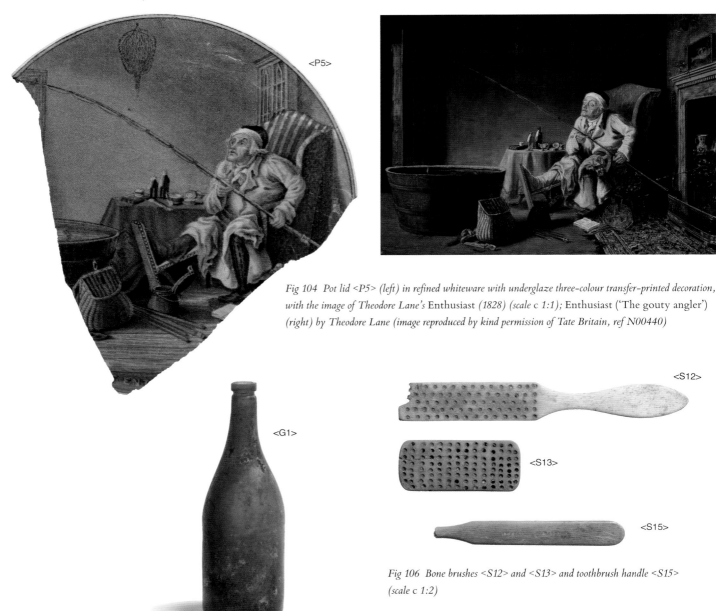

Fig 104 Pot lid <P5> (left) in refined whiteware with underglaze three-colour transfer-printed decoration, with the image of Theodore Lane's Enthusiast (1828) (scale c 1:1); Enthusiast ('The gouty angler') (right) by Theodore Lane (image reproduced by kind permission of Tate Britain, ref N00440)

Fig 105 Green-coloured glass champagne bottle <G1> (scale c 1:4)

Fig 106 Bone brushes <S12> and <S13> and toothbrush handle <S15> (scale c 1:2)

a rectangular nail- or small scrubbing brush; the other (<S12>), with a rectangular head and a waisted, leaf-shaped handle, may be a small hairbrush. If from the hospital these are probably personal items belonging to staff or patients rather than brushes supplied to the hospital, which seem to be mainly for cleaning and decorating, as for example the scrubbing brushes, long scrubbing brushes, brooms and painting brushes supplied by Mr Peter Adams in 1804 (RLH, LH/F/8/11). Other finds associated with the burials include a piece from the base of a bone fan-stick (<S14>, not illustrated), which could have been a casual loss or may have belonged to someone at the hospital; folding fans made of materials such as bone and printed paper were in common use by the late 18th and 19th centuries.

A variety of handles, including some from cutlery or tools, were recovered from the machined deposits in the northern part of area B (below, 5.10, 'Cutlery'). A bone toothbrush handle is

stamped SEATON DALSTON (<S15>, Fig 106). Bone and ivory toothbrushes were in everyday use by the early 19th century; the inscription is probably the name of a Dalston chemist's shop or pharmacy.

A large group of 43 clay tobacco pipes, differing significantly in character, was recovered from the machined deposits across the site (OA8). The pipe bowls span a very wide date range, from some of the very earliest types of pipe made in London – a type AO3, made c 1580–1610, and a type AO5, made c 1610–40, and stamped with a wheel on the heel (<CP1>, Fig 107) – to a single type AO28, current c 1820–60. The wide date range represented suggests more-or-less continuous dumping over a lengthy period, with a high degree of disturbance, but some of the later pipes may have been used within the hospital. Clay pipe bowls made c 1780–1820 (AO27) and so contemporary with the hospital came from the pit (S1, OA5, Chapter 3.1) (<CP2>, Fig 107) and the cemetery (OA6, Chapter 3.4). Many of the pipes are in poor condition and few of the bowls have survived intact, most probably as a result of post-depositional

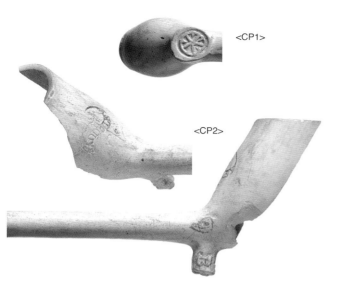

<CP1>

<CP2>

Fig 107 Clay pipe bowls <CP1> (c 1610–40, wheel stamp on heel) and <CP2> (c 1780–1820, BB in relief on heel and 'BADDELEY' stamped on back of bowl (scale c 1:1)

damage. Most have been smoked, some heavily or frequently, and there is no particular emphasis on better-quality pipes.

A second group of 71 bowls, all from [850] (also in OA8), was more closely focused in date range, with four pipe bowls of type AO20 (c 1680–1710) and six of type AO27 (c 1780–1820) but all the rest made c 1730–80 (13 examples of type 11 and 39 of type 12 in Oswald's general typology of 1975, together with nine type AO26 bowls). The main period of deposition, therefore, was in the middle decades of the 18th century, coinciding with the construction of the hospital. It is possible that most of the pipes from this area were used and thrown away by workmen and subsequently disturbed by burials in the official hospital cemetery. Fifty-five pipe bowls are marked by their makers and three of these are also decorated, two with simple vertical ribs and one with the arms of Hanover. It is noteworthy that 26 bowls are marked with the same initials, AG, moulded in relief on the sides of the heel. Most have the initials only, but eight have a crown above each letter and three have stars. Five bowls are of type AO26, with the letter A in line with the long spur and all probably made in the same mould. The other pipes are all Oswald types 11 or 12. It is probable that all were made in the same workshop, and this was most likely located within a relatively short distance of the hospital site. Unfortunately, it has not been possible to identify the pipemaker responsible for their manufacture. Other pipes represented by more than one example are marked RM, probably Richard Manby recorded in Whitechapel in 1746, and ER, possibly Edward Randall, recorded 1719 (Oswald 1975, 141, 143). One pipe was marked with a heel stamp and has the initials WT in relief (<153>). This is an unusually late example of this type of mark, found on a pipe bowl of Oswald type 12 (c 1730–80). It may stand for William Tappin, one of a well-known family of pipemakers, recorded in Blackfriars in 1750–70 (Oswald 1975, 147).

5.9 Staffing the house

The house governor

In 1818, the Revd William Valentine (Fig 108) was elected to the newly established post of house governor, a post that combined the duties previously carried out by the chaplain and the superintendent. The role of chaplain was originally of relatively modest status, whilst that of superintendent was introduced to cover duties that had previously fallen to the apothecary. Commensurate with the new responsibilities, the title of the office was changed to 'house governor'. This gave the position of chaplain greater status and authority within the hospital (Fig 109). The house governor became the highest executive officer and remained so until the roles were separated once more in 1841. The salary Valentine earned as house governor reflected his status: when he retired in 1841 he was receiving £370 per annum, and in addition both he and his family were provided with accommodation in the hospital (RLH, LH/A/5/22, 389–90).

Valentine was one of three candidates chosen for election by the 25 men of the house committee; the others were the Revd Charles James Blenkarne and the Revd Alfred Parrin. James Blenkarne already had established connections within the medical profession and at the time of standing for the post was chaplain to Guy's Hospital, a post he had taken up in 1815 (*The Gentleman's Magazine*, March 1836).

According to later census returns, Valentine was born in Upottery, Devon, in 1787 (TNA: PRO, 1851 England census, parish Stepney). Educated at Trinity College, Cambridge, he

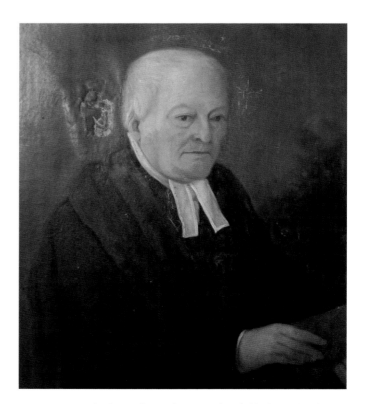

Fig 108 Portait of a cleric at the London Hospital, probably the Revd William Valentine (Royal London Hospital Archives, RLHINV/438)

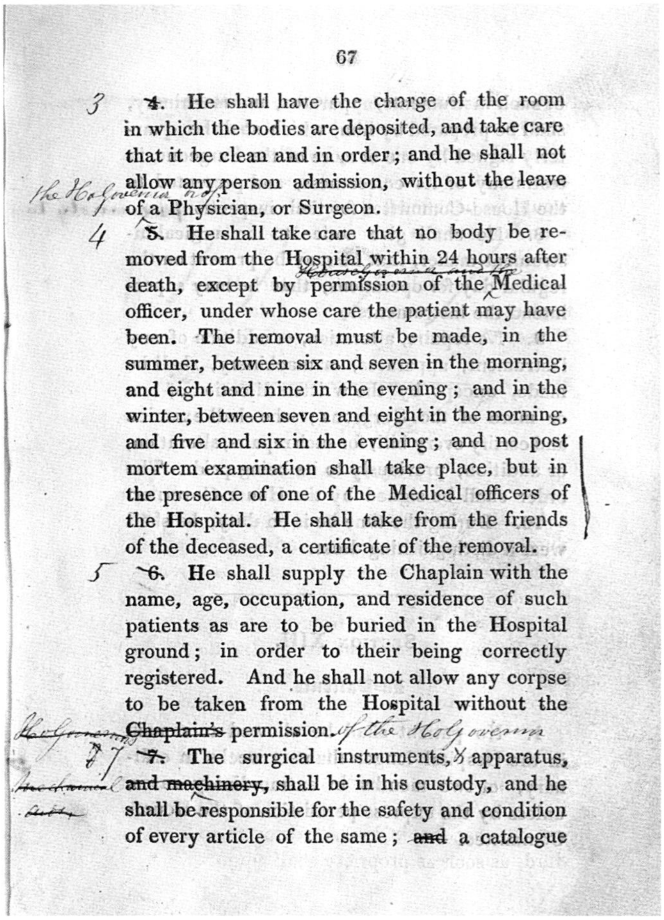

67

3   4. He shall have the charge of the room in which the bodies are deposited, and take care that it be clean and in order; and he shall not *the Ho Governm nof* allow any person admission, without the leave of a Physician, or Surgeon.

4   5. He shall take care that no body be removed from the Hospital within 24 hours after death, except by *permission* of the Medical officer, under whose care the patient may have been. The removal must be made, in the summer, between six and seven in the morning, and eight and nine in the evening; and in the winter, between seven and eight in the morning, and five and six in the evening; and no post mortem examination shall take place, but in the presence of one of the Medical officers of the Hospital. He shall take from the friends of the deceased, a certificate of the removal.

5   6. He shall supply the Chaplain with the name, age, occupation, and residence of such patients as are to be buried in the Hospital ground; in order to their being correctly registered. And he shall not allow any corpse to be taken from the Hospital without the Chaplain's permission. *of the Ho Governm*

7   7. The surgical instruments, *&* apparatus, ~~and machinery~~, shall be in his custody, and he shall be responsible for the safety and condition of every article of the same; ~~and~~ a catalogue

Fig 109 Extract relating to the position of chaplain from the 1832 by-laws (Royal London Hospital Archives, RLH, LH/A/1/7, 67)

began his clerical career in Devon (Crockford 1865, 639). His motivation for moving to London is not known but he began his employment at the hospital as a single man; he later married and by 1841 was living at the hospital with his wife Sarah and their six children (TNA: PRO, 1841 England census, parish St Mary Whitechapel).

Whilst Valentine appears to have been the junior of the three candidates, his ambition to secure the position is demonstrated by an advertisement placed immediately beneath the election announcement in *The Times* (23 October 1818, issue 10495, p 2, col A):

To His Royal Highness the Duke of Glocester [sic], the nobility, ladies and gentlemen, Governors of the London Hospital. Being one of the Gentlemen approved by the House Committee as a candidate for the united offices of Chaplain and House-Governor to the London Hospital, I beg permission respectfully to solicit your vote and interest at the election, fixed for 19th of November next.

Should I have the satisfaction of succeeding to the appointment, it ever will be the first object of my endeavours to perform the duties of this very responsible office with a zeal and faithfulness proportionate to the trust and confidence

thus reposed in me. In confirmation of my possessing the qualifications necessary for so important an office, I beg leave to refer you to the following recommendations.

Beneath this, he published a letter of 'warm recommendation' from nine men who praised him on his 'character, conduct, religious principles and other qualifications' and further stated that since they had not known Valentine before he was put forward for election, their recommendation was made with all the more confidence, clearly trying to distance themselves from the nepotism that was rife within the hospital establishment, and indeed in the medical profession as a whole. Of the nine men who recommended Valentine, seven were members of the house committee. Blenkarne had placed a shorter piece in *The Times* a month earlier (25 September 1818, issue 10471, p 2, col A).

Valentine seems to have been often placed in a difficult position by his role, required to please the sometimes opposing interests of the governors, the medical staff and the patients, and to balance managerial, political and spiritual roles. As the person responsible for enforcing strict adherence to the by-laws and standing orders of the hospital, it was Valentine who was caught in the middle when the governors of the hospital wished to impose their decisions on the medical staff. He was responsible for ensuring that patients in the hospital did not stay longer than necessary, and that only cases permitted by the rules were admitted. In 1823 he questioned the admission of extra cases by the physicians and surgeons, in the belief that according to the by-laws the only cases admitted without recommendation from one of the governors should be those arising from accidents. After receiving a communication from the house committee to this effect, Richard Headington wrote to it to explain that in many other cases admission was absolutely necessary for the preservation of life, and he did not see how he could possibly reduce the number of patients that he admitted (RLH, LH/A/5/17, 197).

In 1827 Valentine called for better descriptions of cases admitted as extra cases by the physicians and surgeons, stating, 'I think it a great hardship on Governors to have their cases rejected by the Committee for want of room, + the Medical Officers permitted to admit whether there be room or not' (RLH, LH/A/17/5, 10 April 1827). In 1838 he questioned the surgeon James Luke as to whether a boy with only a 'simple' fracture of the tibia (as stated on his ticket) should be admitted to the hospital. Luke's reply was indignant (RLH, LH/A/23/32):

As I do not consider you a competent judge in determining accurately the propriety of retaining or discharging a Patient but on the contrary that duty having been left with me by the Governors of the Hospital [...] I have already said that I shall be happy to assign reasons for my advice to the Committee of Governors but I am not called on to assign them to you, whose duty it is to retain Patients when it is directed.

At times Valentine acted as a regulating force, calling into question existing practices (Chapter 7); at others he championed practical needs against opposition from the apparently detached committee. In April 1831, the drug committee resolved that they should buy a vapour bath (probably a steam bath that could also be used with herbal or chemical treatments such as mercury or sulphur (Hancock 1830)) for the patients (RLH, LH/A/5/19, 50). Unfortunately, this well-intentioned decision merely reveals the ignorance of the committee, as when enquiries were made it transpired that there was a vapour bath already in use (ibid, 97). Valentine often provided the checks and balances that would have helped ensure that the best of care was afforded to the patients. He wrote, for example, to question the qualifications of the apothecary in June 1825 (RLH, LH/A/5/18, 32). In October 1832 he complained that the committee were not informing him when they held special meetings (RLH, LH/A/5/19, 342).

Valentine also acted as an official representative of the hospital. Together with James Scott Smith he was instructed to petition parliament in regard to regulations for slaughtering horses, to preserve the purity of the air around the hospital (RLH, LH/A/5/18, 33), and he performed clerical duties elsewhere. He was given leave to work two Sundays at the Institution of the White Chapel Society in 1828 and in March 1829 he preached the Sunday Charity sermon at Stepney church (ibid, 227; RLH, LH/A/5/19, 257).

Perhaps because he was the hospital's chaplain as well as its house governor, Valentine was not insensitive to the distressing situations in which many of the hospital's patients found themselves. He acted as almoner of the Samaritan Society (above, 5.6), distributing that charity's funds to patients of the hospital and providing them with assistance when needed. In 1826 he reported to the house committee the case of a boy who was initially refused admission as an extra case because of a lack of space, but who was brought back the next day by a woman who begged the hospital to take him in, as his mother had gone into labour and they were a family of six with only one 'wretched room' and a straw bed between all of them. Valentine sent some of the old cast-off rugs and blankets from the hospital to the family and was eventually able to admit the boy as someone had just died on one of the wards (RLH, LH/A/17/5, 5 December 1826).

In January 1828 one of the committee, a Mr Tickell, asked that they ascertain 'what the duties of the House Governor in his spiritual character of Chaplain to the London Hospital [are] or whether any alteration or improvement therin is necessary' (RLH, LH/A/5/18, 189–90). Tickell (who, it should be noted, went out of his way to praise the conduct of the 'Romish Priesthood') did not wish to drop his complaint, writing in February that 'the Reverend William Valentine … has been regardless of or inattentive to his spiritual duties … as he has not at all times been ready to visit and pray by or administer the sacrament to The Patients in the wards and also that he has delayed or neglected to attend when applied to or sent to … he has neglected to read the morning service on all other days excepting Sunday … has not daily visited the wards and all parts of the House … has not examined all the provisions and other necessaries brought into the Hospital' (ibid, 198). The vote on whether to take further action split the committee 8 to

2 (ibid, 200), and in March a special meeting was called at which they resolved fully to investigate the complaint (9 to 2 in favour). The committee members who objected (including Tickell) did so as they felt this would deter others from complaining about staff in future (ibid, 202).

The result was recorded in the minute books on 29 January 1828 (RLH, LH/A/5/18, 191):

A report of three of the Members of the Committee [all clergy] to whom it was referred last week the consideration of the duties of the House Governor in his spiritual character of Chaplain was read as follows.

The undersigned Members of the Committee to whom it has been remitted to ascertain and to report what are the duties of the House Governor in his spiritual character of Chaplain to the London Hospital and whether any alteration or improvement therein is necessary having taken the subject into consideration as prescribed by the Resolution of the 22nd January. Report as follows. That in page 12 of the printed bye Laws of the Governor of the year 1820 section 7 under the title 'Chaplain' the duties of the House Governor in his spiritual character of Chaplain to the London Hospital appear to be defined with sufficient clearness and precision and that in their opinion no alteration or improvement therein is necessary – except such incidental addition as neither need not admit of particular enumeration but which every intelligent and conscientious clergyman appointed to that office will supply from his own sense of duty as occasions arise.

Valentine replied (RLH, LH/A/5/18, 192):

I beg here only to say that it is at all times highly agreeable to me to have my duties pointed out and explained by any Governor and that no explanation on that subject could have been more satisfactory to my feeling than that which has come to me under the hands of three Gentlemen so highly respectable and intelligent as those by whom the subject has just been considered and to which it is my wish as it is my duty at all times as far as possible to conform.

In 1826 a complaint was made by a Mr Andrews regarding a patient called John Evans, whom Valentine had sent to St Bartholomew's Hospital to see Mr Lawrence, a surgeon. The man had sold his only cow to travel to London for the treatment of his leg, which in Mr Andrews' opinion required amputation. He did not wish Mr Andrews to operate on him, claiming that he would rather die at home, but in an effort to get him to submit to the operation Valentine reassured him that, if he went to St Bartholomew's instead, the London Hospital Samaritan Society would still assist him with travelling home afterwards. The governors decided that this was not done with any ill will towards Andrews (RLH, LH/A/5/18, 103, 105; LH/A/17/5, 3 September 1826). In July 1830 the committee intriguingly 'Resolved that the House Governors remarks on Mr Bootes reports in the House Visitors Book be erased' (RLH, LH/A/5/18,

346). In March 1832 Valentine was accused of failing to attend a dying nurse, and he had a further confrontation with Mr Andrews over a patient in 1832 (RLH, LH/A/5/19, 217, 273).

Valentine travelled west each summer, writing in August 1827 to the committee 'requesting he might prolong his stay a few weeks/not exceeding a month/ longer which was granted' (RLH, LH/A/5/18, 169) and applying for one month's leave in August 1830 (ibid, 359) and a further break in June 1831, when the Revd Mr James and the secretary were to stand in for him (RLH, LH/A/5/19, 72). Valentine also left the hospital for two extended periods in the 1820s to attend to his parents. In March 1826 he was granted leave of absence to see his dying mother in Devon (RLH, LH/A/5/18, 78), then in March 1828 he travelled back to Devon 'to attend his Father … who was dangerously ill' (ibid, 206).

Despite the apparent formality of the committee, there is repeated evidence that they did not have sufficient control over the workings of the house, nor a proper understanding of the processes required for its effective running. Nevertheless, the conflict led to an examination of Valentine's fitness to practise and the committee realised that they had never taken up Valentine's references. Valentine provided one signed by the rector of Uplyme, Devon, and by his father (RLH, LH/A/5/19, 413).

Valentine played a key role in the hiring and firing of staff. When a man called Brown who had been employed as a cleaner, and then as sub-beadle in the anatomical theatre, tried to extort money for drink from a woman so she could visit her husband (it is not clear if the husband was living or dead), he was dismissed by Valentine (RLH, LH/A/5/19, 413). Valentine also contributed to the discussion of whether staff should receive their annual gratuities, stating in 1828 that 'I have expressed my opinion as to their comparative merits by placing opposite their respective names the sum I should have given them' (RLH, LH/A/5/18, 194).

During Valentine's tenure the duties of the house governor increased in line with the growth of the hospital (above, 5.2), but the role and the London air seem to have preyed on his health. In the summer of 1829 he applied for three weeks' leave to enable him to get country air as he had been 'much indisposed from several colds and inflammation of the Larynx' (RLH, LH/A/5/18, 276). The following two summers he applied for a month's leave (above) and in September 1832 fell sick, missing Sunday services on his doctor's orders. The Revd Mr James of Stepney covered for him in the evening (ibid, 319).

In 1836, one of the house visitors again complained that the roles of chaplain and house governor were incompatible, and could not be 'efficiently discharged by one person'. The issue was regularly raised, perhaps eventually with some foundation. During Valentine's tenure the number of patients in the hospital had increased from 240 to an official figure of 314 (above, 5.2), and proposals to extend the east wing would see this number increase even further. In 1840 the house committee prepared a report for the quarterly court of governors recommending the separation of the roles of chaplain and house governor on the completion of the new wing. As well as the proposed increase in patients, the report reasoned that the characters required of

the chaplain and the house governor were not compatible (RLH, LH/A/5/22, 410–16):

The education, the associations, the pursuits of the Clergy, seem directly and irreconcilably opposed to minute attention to the thousand details which ought daily and hourly to be the subject of the vigilant check of an efficient House Governor, while the enforcement of regularity and discipline throughout the establishment is liable to place in hazard that attachment and respect which it is desirable that the Spiritual head of the Institution should ever be regarded.

They did however consider Valentine's 'long services; his irreproachable character; and the conscientious spirit in which he has, during a period of twenty two years, discharged his laborious duties', and recommended that he be given the option either to stay on as chaplain retaining his present salary, or to be retired on a pension of £300 per annum. In November 1840 Valentine took the difficult decision to resign his post (RLH, LH/A/5/23, 17):

London Hospital
Nov 17th 1840

Gentlemen,
The interview I had with you this morning and other circumstances lead me to believe that in the change proposed to be made with respect to the Offices of Chaplain and House Governor it is your wish to act with unfettered hands; and that it is your opinion the carrying out effectively all the proposed changes depends on my accepting the retiring pension.

You have also intimated your apprehension that my election of retaining the Chaplaincy would prove inconsistent with a prudent foresight and regard to my health, and consequently the welfare of my Family.

Under these circumstances but with deep and painful reluctance I am induced through you to signify to the General Court my election of the retiring pension.

Faithfully + respectfully,
Wm Valentine

Valentine's tenure lasted throughout the period to which the excavated burials date. By 1842 he was the incumbent at the new church of St John Stepney Green (*Old Bailey Proc*, June 1842, Thomas Daniels (t18420613-1895)). Marriage announcements in *The Times* show that by 1848 Valentine was the incumbent of St Thomas, Stepney (*The Times*, 2 October 1848, issue 19983, p 7, col B), where he continued to serve the local population until he died in December 1873, aged 87 (*The Times*, 13 December 1873, issue 27872, p 1, col A).

The surgeons and physicians

Between 1825 and 1842 there were 12 members of medical staff at any one time, comprising three principal surgeons and three principal physicians; from 1827 each of the principals was provided with an assistant (Fig 110, Table 65). The principal physicians and surgeons were responsible for treating the inpatients, and their assistants for tending to the outpatients. As with the appointment of the house governor, the governors advertised for medical staff by announcing a vacancy and election in the newspapers (Lawrence 1996, 59). The provisions of full membership (fellowship) of the Royal College of

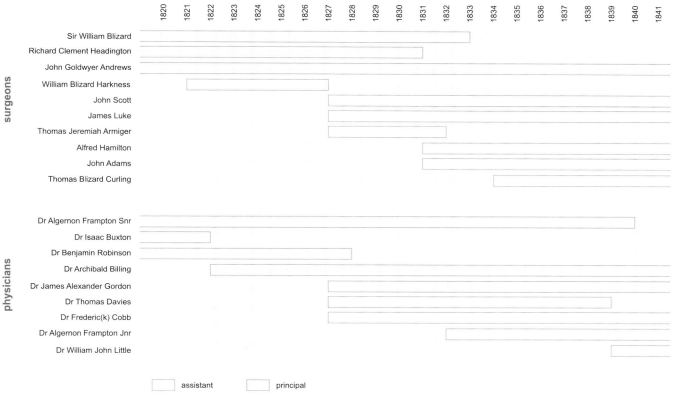

Fig 110 Medical officers of the London Hospital c 1825–42 (for sources see Table 65)

Table 65 References for the dates contained in Fig 110, including the year medical officers were elected, the year of any promotion (from assistant to principal), and the year in which they ceased to be either an assistant or principal officer (ie, the year in which they resigned, died or became a consulting officer)

	Start date	Promotion date	End date	Reference
Surgeons				
John Adams	1831	1850	1868	RCS *Plarr*; *The Times*, 24 September 1831, issue 14652, p 3, col A
John Goldwyer Andrews	1816	-	1849	RCS *Plarr*
Thomas Jeremiah Armiger	1827	-	1832	Clark-Kennedy 1962, 229–30; RLH, LH/A/20/33
William Blizard	1780	-	1833	Clark-Kennedy 1962, 164; RLH, LH/A/5/20, 167
Thomas Blizard Curling	1834	1849	1869	*The Lancet*, 4 September 1869, Medical annotations, 94(2401), 348; RLH, LH/A/5/20, 210; RCS *Plarr*
Alfred Hamilton	1831	1845	1849	*The Lancet*, 24 February 1849, Medical news, 53(1330), 219; RCS *Plarr*; *The Times*, 8 April 1831, issue 14508, p 1, col A
William Blizard Harkness	1821	-	1827	Clark-Kennedy 1962, 230; RLH, LH/A/5/17, 31 July 1821
Richard Clement Headington	1797	1799	1831	Evans and Blandy 1992; *The Times*, 22 February 1831, issue 14469, p 4, col F
James Luke	1827	1833	1861	Clark-Kennedy 1962, 229–30; RCS *Plarr*
John Scott	1827	1831	1845	Clark-Kennedy 1962, 229–30; *Medical Times* 14, 135–6; *The Times*, 19 March 1831, issue 14491, p 3, col A; ibid, 20 November 1845, issue 19086, p 1, col A
Physicians				
Archibald Billing	1822	-	1845	RLH, LH/A/5/17, 127; *Munk's Roll 3*, 203–4
Isaac Buxton	1807	-	1822	RLH, LH/A/5/17, 4 June 1822; *Munk's Roll 3*, 24
Frederic(k) Cobb	1827	1841	1854	Clark-Kennedy 1962, 229–30; *Munk's Roll 3*, 265
Thomas Davies	1827	-	1839	Clark-Kennedy 1962, 229–30; RLH, LH/A/5/22, 227; *Munk's Roll 3*, 289
Algernon Frampton Snr	1800	-	1841	*Munk's Roll 2*, 464
Algernon Frampton Jnr	1832	1844	1851	*Munk's Roll 4*, 11; *The Times*, 3 August 1832, issue 14921, p 1, col A
James Alexander Gordon	1827	1828	1844	Clark-Kennedy 1962, 229–30; *Munk's Roll 3*, 233
William John Little	1839	1845	1863	Clark-Kennedy 1962, 253; *Munk's Roll 4*, 249
Benjamin Robinson	1818	-	1828	*Munk's Roll 3*, 173

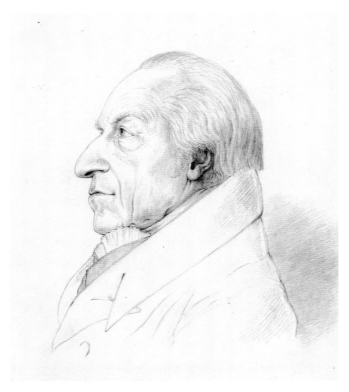

Fig 111 Sir William Blizard; drawn by William Home Clift, c 1818–33 (© The Trustees of the British Museum, Department of Prints and Drawings, 1893,0803.13)

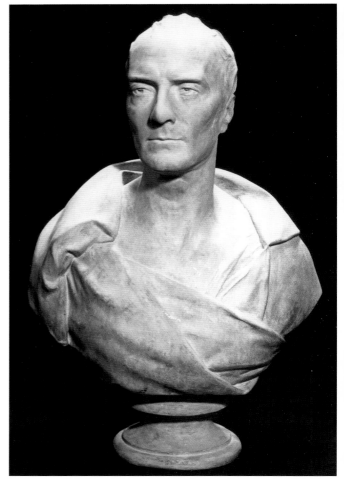

Fig 112 Richard Clement Headington; plaster bust by Thomas Smith, 1831 (Royal London Hospital Archives, RLHINV/147)

Physicians defined an elite group who could not dispense drugs, perform surgery or practise midwifery (ibid, 77). In the early 19th century most medical practitioners were drawn from the artisan or merchant classes (Higgs 2009, 112).

For better or worse, hospital surgeons generally held their posts for longer than did physicians; Sir William Blizard (Fig 111) remained on the London Hospital staff for 54 years, resigning in 1833 when he was 90 years old (Lawrence 1996, 58). Although not as well known today as his contemporary Sir Astley Cooper, Blizard was probably the most illustrious of the medical staff during this period. The son of an auctioneer from Barn Elms in Surrey (Ellis 1986, 5), he studied under John Hunter, founded the London Hospital Medical College with James Maddocks and was knighted in 1803. In addition to his skill as a surgeon he was noted for his religious convictions and for his philanthropy, founding the Samaritan Society in 1791 to provide additional relief to patients (above, 5.6). Although he resigned in 1833, he had performed his last operation (an amputation of the thigh) six years previously at the age of 84.

Richard Clement Headington (Fig 112), who died in 1831, was another active member of the staff and the medical college. Although he wrote little, he was president of the Royal College of Surgeons in 1830, and served on the committee appointed to consider surgical education together with another surgeon from the London, John Goldwyer Andrews. Both Blizard and Headington were subjected to stinging attacks in *The Lancet*; they opposed the appointment of medical coroners, and *The Lancet*'s editor, Thomas Wakley, was suspicious of Headington's motives

for reforming the training of surgeons (Evans and Blandy 1992).

James Luke (Fig 113) started his career at the London in 1821 as demonstrator of anatomy in the medical college (RCS *Plarr*, sub Luke). He became lecturer on anatomy in 1823 and was elected assistant surgeon in 1827. At the time, he was satirised for his (with hindsight well-founded) scrupulous attention to the cleanliness of his instruments. John Scott (Fig 114), who was initially elected assistant surgeon in 1827 and succeeded Headington in the post of principal surgeon in 1831, was less well regarded by his contemporaries. His obituary in the *Medical Times* stated that 'as an operator he was bold but not cool, and rapid without being dexterous' and further that he had 'no sympathy with humanity' (*Medical Times and Gazette* 1846, vol 14, 135–6). Thomas Blizard Curling (Fig 115), a nephew of William Blizard, studied at the London and was appointed to the staff in 1834 (RCS *Plarr*, sub Curling). Well known for his punctuality, he published standard works on diseases of the rectum and testes, was particularly interested in surgical pathology and lectured on morbid anatomy.

Of the physicians, Archibald Billing (Fig 116), an Irishman, pioneered the practice of teaching at patients' bedsides with regular clinical lectures (*Munk's Roll 3*, 203–4). He was also particularly interested in the workings of the heart (Chapter 7.8).

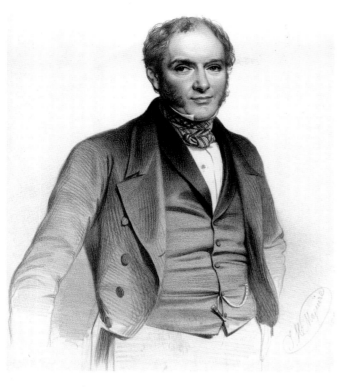

Fig 113 *James Luke, surgeon; lithograph by J H Maguire, 1853 (Royal London Hospital Archives, RLHINV/781)*

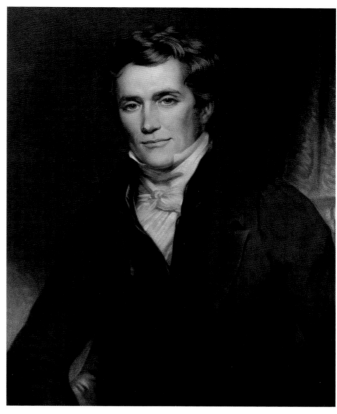

Fig 114 *John Scott, surgeon; engraving by S W Reynolds after a portrait by H Howards RA, c 1835 (Royal London Hospital Archives, RLHINV/798)*

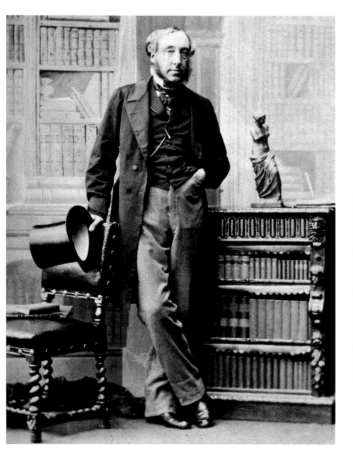

Fig 115 *Thomas Blizard Curling, surgeon; photographed by C Silvy (Wellcome Library, London, V0026236)*

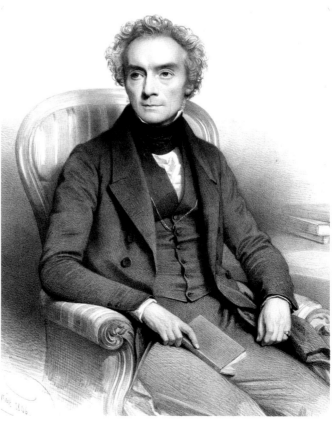

Fig 116 *Dr Archibald Billing, physician; lithograph by Charles Baugniet, 1846 (Royal London Hospital Archives, RLHINV/783)*

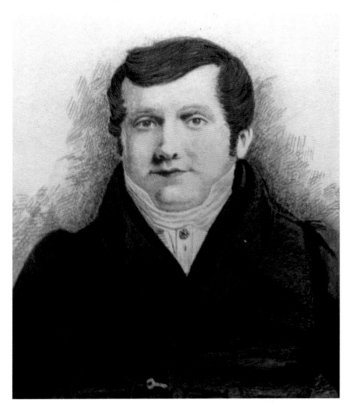

Fig 117 Dr Thomas Davies, physician; lithograph by I Perkhoff, c 1860 (Royal London Hospital Archives, RLHINV/794)

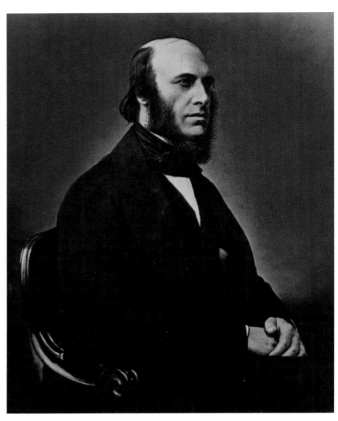

Fig 118 Dr William John Little, physician; photograph c 1863 (Royal London Hospital Archives, RLH/INV/793)

Thomas Davies (Fig 117), after studying in Paris, was among the first to use Laennec's stethoscope for diagnosis in London. Father and son Algernon Frampton senior and Algernon Frampton junior both held posts at the London (*Munk's Roll 2*, 464; *4*, 11). Frederic(k) Cobb, after initially working as demonstrator of anatomy in the medical college at the London, studied medicine at Edinburgh but returned to take up the position of assistant physician at the London in 1827 (*Munk's Roll 3*, 265). William John Little (Fig 118), who suffered from poliomyelitis as a child and had a partially paralysed leg, started the Orthopaedic Institution, which later became the Royal Orthopaedic Hospital (Clark-Kennedy 1962, 252).

The governors of the London Hospital required daily ward visits (excluding Sundays) from at least one physician and one surgeon. In 1827 the house committee noted the visiting days and hours of all the medical staff. Each surgeon and physician visited the hospital twice a week and their visits generally lasted between one and a half and four hours, with the physicians being present for slightly longer than the surgeons (RLH, LH/A/5/18, 153). Once again this separates the character of the London from the other institutions of the metropolis as this workload was far in excess of that required by other medical institutions and may, it is suggested, have dissuaded many Fellows of the Royal College of Physicians from applying for positions at the London (Lawrence 1996, 69).

The medical staff were also permitted to admit their own cases to the hospital, so long as they were deemed 'necessary for the preservation of life'. In 1826 the physicians admitted 55 extra cases and the surgeons 61, but during the 1830s these numbers increased and the physicians generally admitted a greater number of extra cases than the surgeons. Although most of the accidents admitted to the hospital are likely to have been surgical patients these were recorded separately.

The medical officers and the house committee and governors often had different ideas about how the hospital should be run. Mr Headington clashed with the committee in 1822 (RLH, LH/A/5/17, 87–8), complaining that:

I do not think that we meet exactly upon equal terms. The Officers of the Establishment are necessarily much under their control and the Committee having a Giant's strength do sometimes like a Giant use it. It has been my unfortunate lot on several occasions to have been treated by those Gentlemen with I think much want of common courtesy and civility.

It was true that, officially, the medical officers had very little say in the running of the hospital, even in decisions involving patient care, although occasionally their opinion in various matters was sought from the house committee. In November 1835, following a series of contentious decisions made by the house committee, all 12 of the physicians, surgeons and their assistants signed a memorial to the house committee (RLH, LH/A/17/10):

The undersigned Medical Officers of the London hospital

have been unwilling to notice the various inconveniences to which they have of late been subjected by the House Committee, because they hoped that more mature consideration would have led that Body to feel that the cordial co-operation of the Committee and Medical Officers is indispensable to the usefulness and reputation of a public Hospital.

So long as the acts of the Committee were confined to mere dis-courtesy, the Medical Officers were silent; but as they believe that the late proceedings of the Committee will prove injurious to the Charity and detrimental to science, they feel it due to the profession of which they have the honour to be members, to make this their deliberate and unanimous remonstrance. They farther feel it due to the Governors to declare, that there never was a period when the Medical duties were more zealously performed or when, as they regret to add, the Medical Officers have received so little countenance from the House Committee in the discharge of them.

In the first place, the friendly intercourse in the Committee-room between the members of the House-Committee and the Medical Officers, which has existed since the foundation of the Hospital, established, encouraged and fostered, by the best friends and benefactors of the Charity, has been discourteously interrupted, and regulations affecting the welfare of the patients are continually made without in any way referring to those who alone can advise the Committee as to their necessity or expediency.

The memorial went on to set out several grievances that reflected the lack of respect and countenance that the medical officers felt they received from the house committee. Mr Andrews and Dr Gordon had both recently been absent from the hospital, naming their respective assistants to deputise for them in their absence. The committee had decided that this cover was not sufficient and called them to account, in spite of the fact that the assistant physicians and surgeons were required to have equivalent qualifications to the principals, and in contravention of an existing by-law and a resolution of the house committee. In addition to this, one of the hall porters had been noting down the exact times that the medical officers arrived at and left the hospital on the days on which they were required to attend, in the eyes of the staff weakening the 'respect due from the servants of the Hospital to Medical Officers'; the surgery beadle had been ordered not to inform the surgeons of the death of any of their patients, and the committee had refused to authorise the employment of a much needed clinical clerk for the surgeons.

Although there was complaint from some of the members of the house committee regarding the tone of the letter, the conclusion of a special committee established to consider the memorandum was to recognise that communication could be improved between the staff and the house committee. The committee resolved that the medical officers should be informed of 'any proposed Regulations which relate to the

management or Medical treatment of the Patients, or have immediate reference to the duties of the Physicians, Surgeons, or Assists; that thus an opportunity may be afforded for receiving the suggestions of the Medical Officers, previously to such regulations being adopted' (RLH, LH/A/5/21, 171). The medical officers subsequently nominated Dr Frampton (junior) to be their line of communication with the house committee. The medical staff held their own regular meetings and transmitted suggestions and points arising from these to the house committee through Dr Frampton. Once this system was in place, relations between the governors and the house committee appeared to improve, and the house committee was more responsive to the requests of the medical officers, although they did not always acquiesce.

The dressing pupils

Much of the surgical care that the patients received within the hospital was administered by 'dressing pupils', under the supervision of the surgeons and assistant surgeons. They paid the surgeons directly for the privilege of treating the patients, and the hospital benefited from their unpaid labour: in 1834 the fees payable were 30 guineas for 12 months, or 20 guineas for 6 months (RLH, LH/A/5/20, 296). Although they were not appointed by the hospital, the surgeon under whom they were studying was required to introduce them to the house committee before they could be admitted.

The dressing pupils were responsible for carrying out the practical dressing of wounds and injuries and other tasks such as bleeding the patients under the supervision of the surgeons. During most of the 1820s they slept at the hospital. In 1822 the location of their sleeping rooms in the hospital was moved (RLH, LH/A/5/17, 30 July 1822, 131). The pupils were not above playing practical jokes, and in September 1822 two of their number enraged one of the governors, who had been forced 'under the painful necessity of walking bare headed through part of Whitechapel exposed to public ridicule' after they stole his hat and hid it up a chimney whilst he was on a visit to the hospital (ibid, 138). In 1827 the house governor estimated that the number of pupils attending the hospital was between 20 and 30, and during 1827–8 he complained numerous times to the house committee about the misbehaviour of the pupils in the hospital. Allegations were made that some of the pupils were abusing their privileges, being drunk, and on one occasion breaking into a cupboard to leave it in a disorderly state (RLH, LH/A/17/5; /6). In January 1828 there was a dispute between the pupils and Valentine over their conduct, when he reported to the committee that he had seen two of the pupils 'singing, hollowing and leaping' in one of the passages: 'one of them laid hold of a little girl about ten years of age + also an assistant nurse was obstructed by some of them in a not very becoming manner'. When Valentine enquired who they were, he found that one, a Mr Watkins, was known always to hang around the female wards, although he had no patients to attend there, and had also been giving the porter 'half and half'. He was wealthy and thought that as a result he could act as he pleased, stating to Valentine that 'he is able to buy me + my whole family' (RLH, LH/A/17/3). Valentine was of the opinion that letting the pupils reside in the hospital 'serves no purpose, but that of putting money into the Surgeons pockets at the expense of the safety of the Patients, + the constant disorder + [?disrespect] of the charity' (RLH, LH/A/17/6, 20 October 1828). The house governor proposed that only one pupil, the house pupil, should be appointed and allowed to reside at the hospital overnight, and that he should have responsibility for supervising the behaviour of the others.

A house pupil (later two pupils, a senior and a junior house pupil) was subsequently appointed on a weekly basis to reside in the hospital and attend to the patients at night, including any accidents that were brought in. This did not entirely put an end to their tendency to get themselves into trouble with the house committee. There were further complaints of pupils attending drinking parties, inviting a female into the pupils' room, where 'she was employed to perform some service', inviting a performer from the Pavilion Theatre into the hospital, and smoking in and defacing the pupils' room (RLH, LH/A/5/20; /21). This was the kind of conduct satirised in later cartoons (Fig 119). In an attempt to impress upon them the seriousness of their task, the house committee requested in 1835 that the surgeons personally introduce the house pupils at the beginning of their weekly term of office and sign a book of recommendation. They also prepared a charge to be read out to them each week (RLH, LH/ A/5/21, 20 August 1835, 72):

Mr   and Mr
You are, agreeably to the 'Standing Orders' recommended by Mr   one of the Surgeons of this hospital as Gentlemen competent to discharge respective duties of *Senior* and *Junior* House-Pupils, for the ensuing week. The Committee consider this recommendation as an assurance, that you are qualified for the fulfilment of the several important duties thus confided to your care. – they accordingly admit you to the exercise of these duties: trusting, that, by devoting your best attention to the comfort and relief of the Patients, – and shewing due respect to every Authority and Regulation, constituted for the preservation of good order within the Establishment, – you will evince a becoming regard to the Interests and Reputation of the Hospital, and to your own Character, as destined to an honourable profession.
On your thus realizing these expectations of the committee, you will secure to yourselves their approbation, with that of the Governors of the Hospital; but if otherwise, the Committee have determined, that the privilege of Residence, shall, in future, be withheld.

The labour of the house pupils was essential to the efficient running of the hospital, and they paid for the privilege of working there, but they received little thanks or respect from the governors, and the tone of this charge does not appear to have gone down particularly well. The language of the charge was amended after the medical officers of the hospital sent a strongly worded letter to the house committee about how they

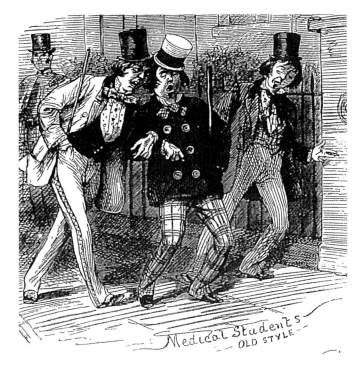

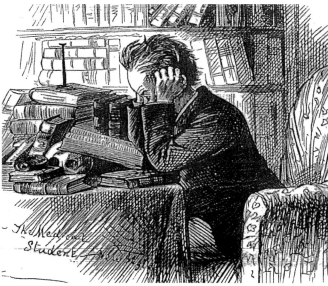

Fig 119 'Notes at a London Hospital': upper – 'Medical Students Old Style'; lower – 'The Medical Student New Style' (Ralston 1879)

treated the medical staff of the hospital generally (RLH, LH/A/ 5/21, 30 December 1835, 170–4). Discontent still simmered under the surface though, and occasionally bubbled up into the sight of the house committee. In August 1840 one pupil was suspended for removing the fastenings on the windows in the pupils' room, 'considering it an insult to the Pupils that they should be prevented opening the windows' (RLH, LH/A/5/22, 403).

Although the role carried with it a large amount of responsibility for patient care, the pupils were sometimes relatively inexperienced; in January 1833 it was noted that the weekly house pupil had been a pupil for only four months

(RLH, LH/A/5/20, 18). Many of the accusations of neglect in treatment at the hospital were levelled at the pupils. Some surgeons and physicians were at pains to emphasise that the students must understand that people who were ill might be difficult but that irrespective of this the students should be understanding and not engage in 'cruel babbling' (Gordon 1833, 10, 16).

When John Weldy was admitted with a fractured thigh in 1836, there being 'no resident or house Surgeon there as in most other Hospitals, he was therefore consigned to the inexperience of a pupil' (below, 5.11, 'Accusations of malpractice'). The pupil did not set his leg correctly, but it was not seen by the supervising surgeon until some days later, and when the mistake was pointed out no steps were taken to correct it (RLH, LH/A/5/21, 24 May 1836, 256–8). The leg was so loosely bandaged that Mr Weldy complained 'that he could feel the bones shift, whenever he coughed or moved however slightly, and that when he used the bed pan he was obliged to keep his hand under his thigh to keep the bones from shifting'. After investigating the incident, the house committee decided that the complaints were unfounded, but the subsequent actions of the committee may suggest otherwise. On 9 August the same year they took steps to regulate the dressing pupils. The number of dressing pupils that could be introduced by each surgeon was limited to six, excluding the three dressing pupils to the outpatients who subsequently became dressing pupils to the inpatients. Every dressing pupil appointed was required to have attended two courses of lectures on anatomy and one in surgery, in one of the medical schools recognised by the Royal College of Surgeons (ibid, 294). In addition, the committee recommended that a house should be provided in the neighbourhood for one of the assistant surgeons to live in, and where he could be called upon if necessary (ibid).

Accusations were also made by the house governor that the pupils sometimes neglected their duties to the patients. In January 1830 he reported to the house committee that they had been asking the nurses and assistant nurses to dress the patients, 'especially when it may be disagreeable or mortified'. A nurse and an assistant nurse were unable to work because they had bad hands from dressing a mortified wound (RLH, LH/A/17/6, 7 January 1830). After the house governor reported that nurses had been dressing burns instead of the pupils, one of the surgeons, Mr Luke, defended them vigorously against such allegations in a letter addressed to the house committee: 'at no time since my first acquaintance with the Hospital, have the duties of the Pupils been more assiduously + attentively performed than they are at the present period; nor do I believe that the Patients of any Hospital in the Metropolis are better or more efficiently dressed than those of the London Hospital' (RLH, LH/A/5/20, 27 March 1834, 253–5).

The ward staff

Nursing underwent radical reforms later in the 19th century, after Florence Nightingale opened her training school for nurses at St Thomas's Hospital in 1860 (Higgs 2009, 128). It was not until 1873 that the governors of the London Hospital were persuaded by the then matron to open their own training school along Nightingale lines (Clark-Kennedy 1963, 57), although as early as 1840 the well-known pioneer of penal reform, Elizabeth Fry, had also made efforts to reform nursing. In 1840 the house committee of the London accepted the request of Elizabeth Fry and Elizabeth Gurney to admit two or three women to the hospital in order to be trained by the matron Mrs Nelson, 'under a distinct understanding that it shall in no manner be permitted to interfere with the discipline of the Hospital' (RLH, LH/A/5/22, 404). These were some of the first women to be trained as nurses by the pioneering Institution of Nursing Sisters (initially called the Protestant Sisters of Charity), which was founded in that year and situated in a home on Raven Row, adjacent to the hospital. At first the partnership appears to have been a successful one, but in 1842 the nursing sisters working in the hospital complained about the cleanliness there, and eventually they were withdrawn (Huntsman et al 2002, 374).

The ward staff of the London Hospital in the second quarter of the 19th century, although untrained, were appointed according to strict regulations. In common with most London nurses, they wore their own clothes to work. In 1830 Valentine reported that whilst the trusts that funded St Bartholomew's Hospital enabled them to buy blue Marino gowns with white robes for the sisters and gowns of 'drab stuff' for the nurses, no other hospitals had uniforms (RLH, LH/A/5/18, 387; LH/A/5/19, 28–9).

In December 1828 the committee reported that they were having problems finding assistant nurses who could read and write and resolved that this regulation could be waived when necessary, so long as those who could not read did not administer medicines (RLH, LH/A/5/18, 242). Nurses were not supposed to dress patients' wounds, although there were allegations that in some instances they did so (see above). Matrons were not trained nurses until the 1870s, but were rather housekeepers and managers of the wards (Higgs 2009, 124).

Although the names of many of the nursing staff are recorded in the hospital records, we know little about these women or their backgrounds. In 1829 the standard salary for the nurses was £16 6s, and for the assistant nurses £12 12s, although hard-working women could earn increases to their wages and gratuities and take their remuneration above £20. The list of nurses awarded gratuities that year includes the length of time that the women had been in the service of the hospital. Of the 17 women listed, three had been working at the hospital for longer than 10 years, and a further five for between five and ten years (RLH, LH/A/5/18, 256). In some instances it is clear that more than one member of the same family were members of staff – nurse Susannah Jewell, for example, of Sophia ward (above, 5.8, 'Bending the rules'; below, 'Caring for the staff') had a daughter who was also a nurse at the hospital (RLH, LH/A/5/19, 243). In October 1836, London Hospital nurse Hannah Shelton, aged 31, was jailed for nine months for stealing a pair of shoes valued at 3s and a table cloth valued at 1s from a friend with whom she was lodging (*Old Bailey Proc*,

October 1836, Hannah Shelton (t18361024-3407)). Isabella Anderson, the nurse of Mellish ward, was described in 1822 as 'a most industrious steady and attentive woman, of an excellent temper; very respectful and exceedingly kind and accommodating to the Patients particularly when irritable from pain or fretfulness of disposition. [She] is decidedly the most deserving Nurse in the House' (RLH, LH/A/5/17, 93). She was given an increase to her salary of £1 1s and a gratuity of £3 3s and was still in the hospital in 1841, when she was listed on the census return as a patient, aged 50–54 (although it is possible there is a mistake in the census, as she does not appear to be on a female ward, though she is included here with the patients). The 1841 census lists 37 nurses working in the hospital, ranging in age from 20 to 49, with just over half of these aged between 35 and 44 (TNA: PRO, 1841 England census, parish St Mary Whitechapel).

As with any large employer, there is some evidence of problematic behaviour amongst the staff. Nurse Margaret O'Bryan was discharged on 15 November 1832 for 'irregularity of conduct' after seven years and four months of service (RLH, LH/A/5/19, 372). In August 1832 a nurse was suspended for neglecting an order from Sir William Blizard. She was not, however, dismissed as Valentine vouched for her hard work (ibid, 302). Finding suitable women to work on the wards and in the house was a concern of the governors, and in 1834 the hospital paid an annual subscription of 1 guinea to the National Guardian Institution as an experiment, in the hope that they would recommend women of good character for employment (RLH, LH/A/5/20, 327–8).

Valentine's input was also vital in the decision over whether annual bonuses should be awarded. In May 1832 the gratuities were withheld from the nurses of Mary, Talbot and Gloucester wards as they had been 'insufficiently attentive to the order of the house governor', and from those of Harrison ward while a complaint was investigated (RLH, LH/A/5/19, 251).

Later in the 19th century old-style, untrained nurses were caricatured as slovenly drunks who failed to care properly for their patients (Fig 120), but in spite of their lack of training some of the nurses were highly skilled and admired by those who knew them. Frederick Treves, who became a student at the London in 1867, described in glowing terms one of the untrained nurses that he had known (Clark-Kennedy 1963, 56):

Without exception she is the most remarkable woman in the Hospital; in appearance a short, fat, comfortable person of middle age with a ruddy face and a decided look of assurance. She was completely without education. Yet her experience of casualties of every kind, and death, was vast and indeed unique. Further, she was entirely self taught (for there were no trained nurses in those days), and of the school of Mrs Gamp, but a woman of courage and infinite resource, an expert in the treatment of the obstreperous and quick to deal with anyone who gave her 'lip.' She was possessed of much humour, was coarse in her language, abrupt yet not unkindly in her manner, indifferent towards and skilled in handling the drunk. She had, like most nurses of her time, a leaning

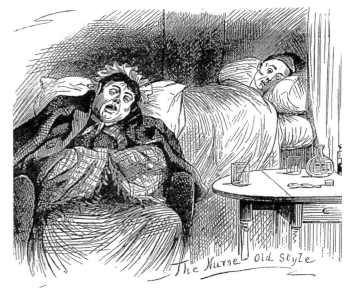

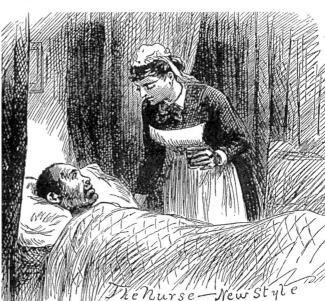

Fig 120 'Notes at a London Hospital': upper – 'The Nurse – Old Style'; lower – 'The Nurse – New Style' (Ralston 1879)

towards gin. But she was efficient even in her cups. She had will power and undertook on her own responsibility the treatment of minor casualties. The dressers regarded her with respect, and from her they learnt the elements of minor surgery and first aid. The house surgeons admired and were a little frightened of her. Her diagnosis of an injury was usually correct, so sound was her observation and so wide her experience.

The apothecary

The role of apothecary was vital to patient care, for a huge number of drugs were required and had to be prepared in the house (see below). Further, in the absence of the physicians it was the apothecary who made judgements on those patients who needed rapid treatment (above, 5.3). Yet this was considered a lowly position on the medical scale.

It was not until 1815 that all practising apothecaries were required to hold a licence from the Society of Apothecaries, for which an apprenticeship and an examination were required. Further details stipulated that the apprenticeship must last five years, that the applicant must have a good standard of Latin and moral conduct and that they should have attended (in addition to chemistry, metria medica and medical theory and practice courses) two courses of anatomy (Lawrence 1996, 104–5). They also needed to complete a placement within a hospital with a cumulative duration of six months (Higgs 2009, 114).

At the London Hospital, the position of apothecary evolved with the growth of the institution, as did that of house governor. Initially, it was seen as a first, and temporary, post for young men. At the start of 1825 the apothecary, Joseph Ward, asked for a pay rise and a permanent contract as his duties had grown with an 'increase in the number of patients' (RLH, LH/A/5/18, 13). The governors at first refused outright, but reconsidered his letter some weeks later. A satisfactory resolution was clearly not reached since Ward resigned in May that year (ibid, 29). Despite his humble position, the apothecary was expected to be available at all hours. Speaking pipes and bells were installed between the dispensary and the lobbies, presumably so that patients could be called to collect medicines (RLH, LH/A/5/19, 27), and the apothecary made the decision to admit extra cases when the surgeons were not available (some responsibility might also have rested with the surgeons' pupils). He accompanied the physicians on their rounds and was responsible for their cases when they were absent from the hospital. The regulations of his office required that he was resident in the house, and not allowed 'to lie abroad' or go out without leave (Clark-Kennedy 1962, 100, 210).

The surgeons' beadle

Until he was relieved of the duty in 1837, the surgeons' beadle (also known as the surgery beadle) rang the 'accident bell' at night to alert staff that they were needed and attended on the assistant physicians with the outpatients during the day (RLH, LH/A/5/21, 443). He notified the surgeons when one of their patients died, and after 1824 he was responsible for taking the burial warrant from the coroner after an inquest and delivering it either to the relatives or to Valentine (RLH, LH/A/5/17, 300). His responsibilities as they related to recently deceased patients put him into a position that was open to exploitation (Chapter 7.2).

The post of surgeons' beadle was held in 1823 by William Hurst (or Hirst) (Millard 1825). He was still in the employ of the hospital ten years later, when he requested a leave of absence in May 1833 (RLH, LH/A/5/20, 82). He did not return to work before his death the following year, and a replacement was appointed in October (ibid, 153–4). An important aspect of the role was looking after the surgical instruments and keeping them clean and in good order and the successful candidate, Edward Harper, had previously worked as a cutler (ibid, 153).

Harper held his post until January 1835, but his successors were almost constantly the subject of complaints from the surgeons for their failure to maintain the instruments. Harper's replacement did not last beyond his three-month probationary period, the surgeons complaining of his 'general inefficiency' and the state of the instruments under his care. In June 1835 the assistant surgeons reported to the house committee (RLH, LH/A/5/21, 34–5) that:

we have inspected the surgical instruments, + find them to be exceedingly deficient, + in a very bad condition. We have arranged a List of those now under the care of the Surgeons Beadle, all of which require to be carefully cleaned, & put in order. We also submit to you a List of such as are necessarily required. If agreeable to the Com[ee], the Asst Surgeons will undertake to examine the Instruments once a quarter, + will report thereon.

Later the same year the surgeons' beadle was dismissed and replaced with a man who had originally applied for a job as door porter (RLH, LH/A/5/21, 109–10, 115). Although he had some experience in a similar role at Westminster Hospital, the newly appointed beadle appeared to be no better at keeping the instruments than his predecessors, and in December 1835 Mr Hamilton suggested to the house committee that a cutler should be engaged by the hospital to attend once a week to sharpen and keep them in good order. This was approved by the committee, and Mr Johnston of Lisle Street was paid 12 guineas to attend once a week for a year, with an additional charge to put them into good repair in the first place (ibid, 135–6, 141–2). Several men in succession held the post of surgeons' beadle during the later 1830s. Even though the upkeep of the instruments had been placed under the care of a specialist contractor, the surgeons continued to complain to the house committee that the surgeons' beadle was failing to keep the items properly catalogued, and in an attempt to ensure his efficiency in this respect a regulation was introduced whereby his quarterly wages were to be withheld until the catalogue of instruments had been certified by the surgeons. This check was not always implemented, and in September 1837 and again in April 1840 Mr Hamilton complained to the house committee that the beadle had been paid without one of the surgeons having certified the catalogue (ibid, 487; RLH, LH/A/5/22, 349). Hamilton also complained on one occasion of 'several silver catheters' and other instruments being missing from the charge of the surgeons' beadle, who was reprimanded for his transgression. In future Hamilton agreed to look over the instruments 'at uncertain times' to ensure that they were always accounted for (ibid, 405).

The beadle worked closely with the surgeons, as is indicated by the decision in January 1825 to wait, on receiving an application for a gratuity from surgeons' beadle William Hurst, pending reports on his conduct from the surgeons (RLH, LH/A/5/18, 8). The close interaction between the pupils and the beadle sometimes led to conflict – a letter of complaint from a pupil is recorded in the minute books for 12 February 1828 (ibid, 193), whilst in March 1832 the subcommittee received a letter addressed to Alfred Hamilton Esq, an assistant surgeon, from Wilmot, attendant in the anatomical theatre, 'containing charges against two of the persons employed in the Hospital (viz Hirst [Hurst] the Surgery Beadle, and Broadbent, an assistant to the Clerk)' (RLH, LH/A/5/19, 216).

Caring for the staff

Working with the sick in a pre-antibiotic era was not without risks. By the start of 1832, the hospital was so crowded that the assistant nurses had to share beds (RLH, LH/A/5/19, 193) and the long hours and hard physical work required to ensure the effective running of the hospital preyed on the health of those who worked there.

The committee appears in general to have shown compassion towards employees whose health was damaged whilst undertaking their duties. In 1824, the governors reported that Ann Maddy, a nurse in Gloucester ward, was in a bad state of health and wished to retire to the country. It was resolved that she should receive a 'gratuity of £5 5s in anticipation of the gratuity she would have been allowed at the usual period' (RLH, LH/A/5/18, 4). Not all staff were so fortunate, however. The gratuity being paid to the former chapel clerk, Robert Weaver, was discontinued as the committee felt that to maintain payments would constitute a pension (ibid, 7). In August 1830 the widow of a late secretary, John Jones, applied for financial help, and the committee asked to inspect John Jones's papers before deciding whether to assist. When William Hurst, the surgeons' beadle, left his post because of ill health and died the following year, an application from his wife for money towards his funeral was refused by the governors on the grounds that he did not die whilst in the service of the hospital (RLH, LH/A/5/20, 312). Despite this evidence, the committee does seem to have felt some ongoing social obligation towards the staff. On 4 August 1831 they discussed whether to award a life pension to Susannah Jewell of Sophia ward, who was 'incapacitated by age and infirmities' at the age of 64 years. A week later she was granted a pension of 20 guineas (RLH, LH/A/5/19, 90, 93).

It was not just upon retirement that the committee were required to consider the health of the staff. In May 1825 the matron, Mrs Le Blond, asked for leave of absence because of ill health and was granted four to five weeks (RLH, LH/A/5/18, 29).

On 7 June 1832, after receiving a complaint from the patients that the principal nurse on Harrison ward was neglectful and 'continually intoxicated', the committee resolved that she should be dismissed (RLH, LH/A/5/19, 261). Her dismissal was postponed, however, until she had recovered from an 'illness having resulted from her attendance on a succession of very bad cases' (ibid, 263). Perhaps it was the strain of this work that had encouraged her drunkenness?

Mr Cotton's report of 1830 (above, 5.8) noted that the hot-water vessel had not been cleaned and contained '3 or 4 inches of mud'. Tothill, the long-suffering engineer, removed this and

became ill (RLH, LH/A/5/18, 403). On 17 November 1831 the committee reported that Tothill was incapacitated by illness resulting from his work. Whether this was the same illness is unclear, but on 1 December that year he died. His widow was given 5 guineas towards funeral expenses, and asked the committee if they could recommend one of her children to an orphan asylum (RLH, LH/A/5/19, 142, 147, 160, 162). Whether they did so is not recorded, but in May 1832 the committee made her a payment of 2 guineas because she was 'in great distress, had several children dependent on her, and was far advanced in pregnancy' (ibid, 258). The intervention of the committee could have been all that lay between Tothill's family and destitution. Later that same year, a 'letter was read addressed to the Committee by Sampson Hanbury, J Buxton and Robert Hanbury Esquires, recommending that a gratuity should be given to the orphan children of the late nurse of Charlotte Ward who died in the Hospital a few weeks ago' (ibid, 213). This unnamed nurse had died in the wake of the cholera outbreak (Chapter 4.1) and the committee felt it necessary 'due to Dr Billing, to state their decided opinion that the later Nurse of Charlotte's Ward, did not die of fever' (ibid, 215–16). In April 1831 the surgeons' beadle was unwell and the committee resolved that the house governor should pay him an advance of 5 guineas on his wages so that he could take country air (ibid, 49).

William Valentine was not immune to the stresses of hospital work and the dangers to health posed by the urban atmosphere (above, 'The house governor'). In addition to the ever-present danger of illness, it appears that occupationally related conditions also affected the staff. Mr Blomfield, the assistant apothecary, lost the use of his hand in March 1832 and it seems likely that this was as a result of what we would now refer to as a repetitive strain injury (RLH, LH/A/5/19, 218). Whilst St Bartholomew's Hospital had a steam-driven drug mill (RLH, LH/A/5/18, 405), in 1822 the medical staff informed the house committee that a drug mill at the London would be 'neither necessary nor expedient', and a subsequent request by the laboratory man for an increase in his wages and additional help to 'pulverize hard substances' was refused (RLH, LH/A/5/17, 106, 108). It appears that a mill was eventually purchased, as a new one was ordered in September 1823 (ibid, 267).

5.10 Food and drink

Diet and provisioning

The by-laws of 1810 provide clear insight into the diet of the patients. In summer breakfast was served at 9am and in winter at 10am. Dinner was served at 1.30pm and supper at 6pm (RLH, LH/A/1/4, 27), and a variety of diets were prescribed to inpatients, depending on their circumstances (Table 66). This list compares unfavourably to the provisions available to pensioners at the Greenwich Naval Hospital, where 1lb of bread, 4 pints of beer, 4oz cheese, 1lb of meat (5 days a week, with pease pudding and extra cheese the other two days) was the usual daily ration (Boston et al 2008, 18). The physicians and surgeons marked their patients' tickets with the kind of diet that they were to be placed on as soon as they were admitted (RLH, LH/A/5/17, 69–70). Food for the patients and servants of the hospital was cooked in the hospital kitchen, and that for the patients transported to the wards. The cook seems to have exerted a firm control over her domain, and was described by the gate porter in 1826 as 'more like a Tyger than a woman' (RLH, LH/A/17/5, 27 June 1826). In 1830 the house governor worried about provoking her anger by suggesting to the house committee that the remains of the meat boiled down for beef tea and broths, which the cook had been selling for her own profit, should instead be given to the poor in the neighbourhood (RLH, LH/A/17/6, 4 February 1830). The cook appears to have retained her additional source of revenue, however, as in 1834 the house visitors noted in their report that she was making a large income by selling the bones and grease from the kitchen (RLH, LH/A/16/4, 134).

The patients of each ward who were not bedridden ate at dining tables located in the wards, and the nurses were given 2s 6d per bed under their care to maintain the supplies of cutlery for the patients' use. In 1830 the house governor accused them of failing in this task and pocketing the money (RLH, LH/A/17/6, 25 March 1830). W H Pepys of Poultry is known to have supplied the hospital with cutlery as well as surgical instruments (below, 5.11, 'Finds related to medical and surgical treatment'), and there were other suppliers, such as John Hinde of Whitechapel who, for example, supplied among other items '6 knives and forks and a gravey spoon' in 1799 (RLH, LH/F/8/11). After meals, the dirty dishes were washed in the lobbies between the wards, in sinks that were sometimes also used as a convenient receptacle for surgical waste. One of the governors highlighted this unhygienic practice in a letter to the house committee: 'the order for no compresses etc. being washed anywhere but in the Wash House is also neglected. I have been struck with the

impropriety of plates dishes of provisions being washed almost at the same instant as the above surgical Articles' (RLH, LH/A/5/17, 11 May 1824, 342).

The hospital catered for the dietary requirements of the local population, listing a 'Jews diet' of 'four pence per day with bread and beer when on full or middle diet; but when on low, milk or fever diet, no money' (RLH, LH/A/1/4, 36). Members of the Jewish community were generous donors to the hospital, some of them also being governors. They were well catered for at the anniversary dinner, and in 1831 the 'Hebrew Cook' was given a budget of £20 16s (RLH, LH/A/5/19, 51). By 1837 there were around 40 Jewish patients in the hospital at any one time, and the allowance given to Jewish patients in lieu of food had risen to 9d a day. Wealthier members of the Jewish community lobbied the governors to provide facilities for a Jewish kitchen and cook (RLH, LH/A/5/21, 28 November 1837, 29–30). The governors decided that the present funds of the hospital did not allow them to do so, but promised to reconsider the matter when the hospital was in a better financial position (RLH, LH/A/5/21, 20 December 1837, 43).

The house committee minute books list the annual tenders from suppliers to the hospital (Fig 121) and show that large quantities of bread, oatmeal and linseed meal (presumably for gruel), milk and potatoes were purchased, along with soaps and candles of various different kinds (RLH, LH/A/5/18). Payment was also made for fish (ibid, 166).

The supply of provisions was not without its problems. In January 1825, the governors noted that the decision to provide 'extra diet' had led to the 'consequent and necessary addition of servants in the kitchen (RLH, LH/A/5/18, 10). Although the extra diet had been carefully defined in 1810, by June 1827 the medical officers had been prescribing more and more luxurious and expensive items to patients as part of the extra diet, and the house governor complained to the house committee that 'when these indulgences begin to be included to such delicacies as Lemon Ice, it does appear formidably extravagant' (RLH, LH/A/17/5, June 1827). There was a constant battle to keep the hospital's expenses down and by October that year the

Table 66 Diet of the patients in 1810 (RLH, LH/A/1/4)

Common diet		Breakfast	Dinner	Supper
Sunday	12oz bread, 1½ pints beer (men), 1 pint beer (women)	gruel	8oz beef baked	1 pint broth
Monday	"		8oz mutton with boiled rice or potatoes	"
Tuesday	"		8oz potatoes & soup with vegetables	"
Wednesday	"		8oz beef	"
Thursday	"		8oz mutton with boiled rice or potatoes	"
Friday	"		8oz beef baked	"
Saturday	"		8oz potatoes & soup with vegetables	"
Middle diet	as above	as above	as above but 4oz meat	as above
Low diet	8oz bread, 1½ pints beer (men), 1 pint beer (women)	as above	broth	gruel or broth
Fever diet	no bread, 1½ pints beer (men), 1 pint beer (women)	as above	broth	gruel or broth
Milk diet	12oz bread	as above	1 pint milk	1 pint milk

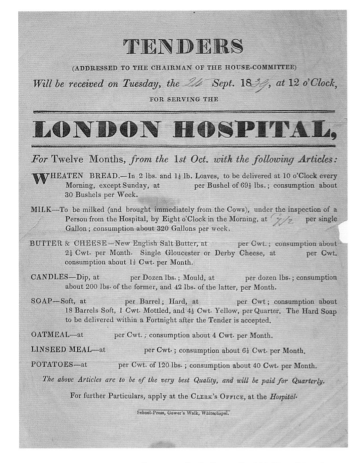

TENDERS

(ADDRESSED TO THE CHAIRMAN OF THE HOUSE-COMMITTEE)

Will be received on Tuesday, the 24 Sept. 1839, at 12 o'Clock,

FOR SERVING THE

LONDON HOSPITAL,

For Twelve Months, *from the 1st Oct. with the following Articles:*

WHEATEN BREAD.—In 2 lbs. and 1½ lb. Loaves, to be delivered at 10 o'Clock every Morning, except Sunday, at   per Bushel of 69½ lbs.; consumption about 30 Bushels per Week.

MILK—To be milked (and brought immediately from the Cows), under the inspection of a Person from the Hospital, by Eight o'clock in the Morning, at 7/2 per single Gallon; consumption about 320 Gallons per week.

BUTTER & CHEESE—New English Salt Butter, at   per Cwt.; consumption about 2½ Cwt. per Month. Single Gloucester or Derby Cheese, at   per Cwt. consumption about 1½ Cwt. per Month.

CANDLES—Dip, at   per Dozen lbs.; Mould, at   per dozen lbs.; consumption about 200 lbs. of the former, and 42 lbs. of the latter, per Month.

SOAP—Soft, at   per Barrel; Hard, at   per Cwt; consumption about 18 Barrels Soft, 1 Cwt. Mottled, and 4½ Cwt. Yellow, per Quarter. The Hard Soap to be delivered within a Fortnight after the Tender is accepted.

OATMEAL—at   per Cwt.; consumption about 4 Cwt. per Month.

LINSEED MEAL—at   per Cwt.; consumption about 6¼ Cwt. per Month.

POTATOES—at   per Cwt. of 120 lbs.; consumption about 40 Cwt. per Month.

The above Articles are to be of the very best Quality, and will be paid for Quarterly.

For further Particulars, apply at the CLERK's OFFICE, at the *Hospital.*

School-Press, Gower's Walk, Whitechapel.

Fig 121 A poster inviting tenders to supply the hospital, 1839 (Royal London Hospital Archives, RLH, LH/A/23/33)

committee 'resolved that no extra diet shall in future be allowed except rice pudding, gruel made from grits and beef tea' (RLH, LH/A/5/18, 175). A further attempt to exert greater control over the allowances given to patients was made by the house committee in 1840, when they resolved that instead of the term 'extra diet', the specific additional articles required by the patient should be written on the ticket. In November 1830 they 'resolved that the supply of table beer to the Hospital at 10/ per barrel be discontinued' and replaced by 'fair wholesome beer' of one (cheaper) quality for general use (RLH, LH/A/5/18, 381). In 1835 the expense of providing the extra diet to patients for the three months up to 30 September was £237 1s 2d (RLH, LH/A/5/21, 149).

Water needed in the house was drawn from a pump in the garden (RLH, LH/A/5/18, 365), but the hospital had its own beer cellar (RLH, LH/A/5/19, 204); the rules concerning the consumption of alcohol within the hospital were strict, if not always adhered to. In 1822 the house committee resolved that no porter or spirits should be allowed in the hospital except when prescribed by the medical staff. The porter, wine and spirits in the hospital were kept under the care of the apothecary in the dispensary, and measures were purchased for administering the correct quantities (RLH, LH/A/5/17, 72). However, it seems that the patients were not above supplementing their diet with items brought in from outside.

A complaint was made against the nurse of Mellish ward (RLH, LH/A/5/19, 222) for:

having suffered a Pint of Ale to be given to a Patient by his friends, contrary to the Laws of the Hospital. The Nurse (who denied all knowledge of the circumstance and pleaded as an excuse, that the extent of the wards which she had to superintend rendered it impossible that she could be aware of what was brought to every Patient by visitors) was informed that any recurrence of such complaint would subject both herself and the assistant nurses to dismissal.

It was clear to the house governor, however, that some patients might benefit from the consumption of items that the hospital's funds could not stretch to supplying to all patients, and in 1829 he recommended to the house committee that patients who would benefit from porter, but for whom it was not absolutely necessary and prescribed, could be given tickets to allow their family and friends to supply it to them (RLH, LH/A/17/6, 2 June 1829). This relaxation of the rules could give rise to problems, however. In 1836 a relative of a patient by the name of John Weldy, admitted with a fractured tibia and resident in the hospital for six months, complained to the house committee about the lax control of the items, particularly alcohol, supplied to patients. He claimed that if a patient had the means, 'he may eat and drink as much as he pleases'. After undertaking to supply John Weldy with wine, on the advice of his surgeon, at a rate of two bottles a week, this relative had been sent a bill for 32 bottles of wine only two months later from a local publican, who sent into the hospital regularly for orders from the patients. Weldy had also been supplied with gin by one of the assistant nurses (RLH, LH/A/5/21, 256–8). This practice, although not sanctioned, was evidently fairly common, as in May 1834 two assistant nurses were dismissed for bringing spirits into the hospital through the railings (RLH, LH/A/5/20, 312). In the case of John Weldy, the house committee came to the conclusion in May 1836 that his leg had not healed after six months as a result of 'the ill judged kindness of his Friends in the supplying him with large quantities of wine, which was unfortunately sanctioned by the house visitor of the day' (RLH, LH/A/5/21, 261–2). These events suggest that although the hospital sometimes took action to prevent strong alcohol being brought in, by the mid 1830s a blind eye was being turned to patients who attempted, if they possessed the finances to do so, to supplement their diet and drink with provisions brought in from outside.

Numerous complaints about bad food, including potatoes and bread, were recorded (RLH, LH/A/5/19, 12, 63). The Metropolitan Alderney Dairy Company wrote to apologise in October 1825 after such a complaint against the milk they supplied (RLH, LH/A/5/18, 51). In Janaury 1826 the matron reported 'that the butter was not generally good' (ibid, 63); in 1830 bad meat was returned to the supplier (RLH, LH/ A/5/18, 311); and there were complaints about both butter and oatmeal in December 1831 and the butter and bread in March 1832

(RLH, LH/A/5/19, 147, 210).

The hospital was also supplied by the local dock companies. In 1831 West India Dock House sent the following items for the use of the patients (RLH, LH/A/5/19, 30), though at least some of the provisions were probably sold on by the hospital (above, 5.2):

1 bag ginger weighing		54 lb
1 bag coffee	"	98 lb
1 cask sugar	"	178 lb
1 cask molasses	"	127 lb
1 parcel cocoa	"	5 ½ lb
1 parcel pimento	"	11 ¼ lb
1 parcel cloves	"	5 ½ lb
1 parcel arrowroot	"	43 ½ lb
1 parcel nutmegs	"	27 1/6 lb
1 jar Balsam To[??]	"	2 1/6 lb
1 jar wine		2 gallons
2 casks rum		45 gallons

Given that those who were buried in the hospital cemetery would have presumably been fed such a diet for only a limited period of time, the osteological evidence of nutritional deficiency or excess provides information about the lifestyles and backgrounds of those served by the London (Chapter 7.8, 'The status of the buried population'), rather than the diet of the patients. Other strands of archaeological evidence can, however, provide significant additional information.

Crockery

Nigel Jeffries

Ceramics used for serving and possibly storing food were recovered from the cemetery deposits during the excavation in area A; they would have been used in the hospital during the second and third quarters of the 19th century (Figs 122–3; Chapter 3.4). These wares included commissioned pottery bearing the underglaze blue transfer-printed (TPW2) image of

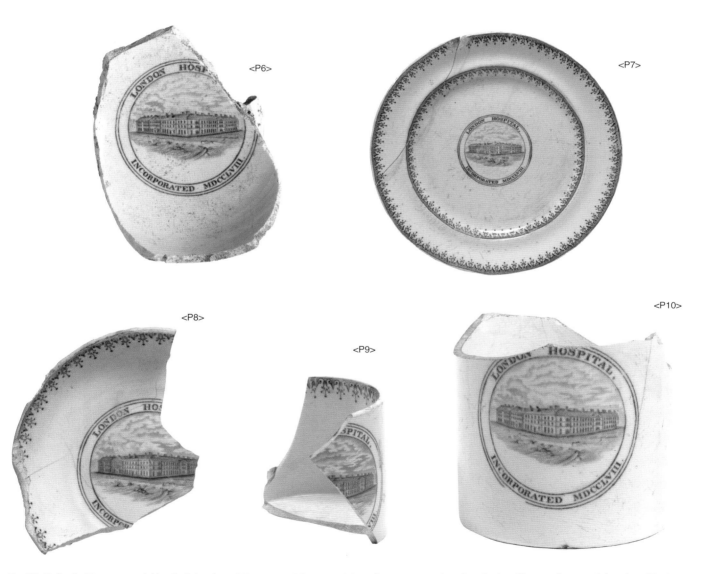

Fig 122 Refined whiteware rounded bowl <P6>, plate <P7>, saucer <P8>, mug <P9> and jar <P10>, each with underglaze blue transfer-printed (stipple and line) decoration including the image of the London Hospital (scale c 1:2)

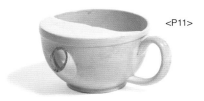

Fig 123 *Invalid feeding cup <P11> in plain refined white earthenware (scale c 1:4)*

the hospital, viewed from the north-west. Spooned foods were served in rounded bowls (<P6>; up to 2 vessels found), with main meals provided on plates (<P7>; 3 vessels). The single saucer (<P8>) suggests that matching tea cups and saucers were also supplied, with a small mug (<P9>) for taking either hot or cold beverages. A cylindrical jar (<P10>) could have had a variety of storage functions. The group is completed by a plain refined white earthenware feeding cup (REFW; <P11>, Fig 123) used for serving those patients who could not easily sit up with semi-liquid pap, a mixture of bread or flour soaked in milk.

Manufactured in either a pearlware or a heavier refined whiteware body, many of these ceramics bear the impressed monogram of Staffordshire potter Thomas Dimmock junior (who operated 1828–59) on their base (<P12>, Fig 124; see Godden 2003, no. 1300, 208). Also of note are the numbers, ranging between 1 and 4, underglaze-painted on the base on some, but not all, of this group (<P13>–<P16>, Fig 125). These pieces fulfilled a variety of functions within the hospital, and can be matched to a small collection of (complete) pottery curated in the Royal London Museum that includes a teacup and saucer (RLHINV/120); two dinner plates (RLHINV/116; /117: both have Pekin stoneware printed on the base); a butter dish (RLHINV/109); three sugar bowls and lids (RLHINV/110; /111; /112: these have the number 4 underglaze blue-painted on their base); and a soup bowl (RLHINV/118). Only the two dinner plates in this collection provide any variation in the printed design used when compared against the archaeologically recovered pieces. Here the base of these plates bear the printed 'Pekin stoneware' mark, a pattern listed in Coysh and Henrywood's 1982 dictionary of blue-and-white printed

pottery as associated with a small group of Staffordshire manufacturers, including Thomas Dimmock (ibid, 279), thereby strengthening the association with this Staffordshire potter.

The sequence of numbers (1 to 4) underglaze blue-painted on the bases of many of the archaeologically recovered pots (mostly the sputum mugs, plates and rounded bowls) and the Royal London Museum's sugar bowls and sputum mugs is consistent (Chapter 5.8). This numbering appears to be related to a predetermined accounting system employed by the hospital that enabled these pots to be easily traced, though exactly how remains unclear. A similar precedent of numbering pottery can be observed on the 'mess wares' used on ships of the period (Coysh and Henrywood 2001, 135).

Before the excavation, the manufacturer and dating of the Royal London Museum's crockery on display was unclear (none of it bears distinguishing features such as Dimmock's monogram), but combining these collections significantly adds to our understanding of the range of pottery vessels circulated in the London Hospital during the early Victorian period and of the commissioning of Dimmock's factory in Albion Street, Hanley, Stoke-on-Trent, to make pottery bearing the image of the London Hospital. The view of the London Hospital from the north-west depicted on both the archaeologically recovered vessels and those of the Royal London Museum is strikingly similar to the 1832 engraving made by its surveyor, Alfred Richmond Mason (RLH, LH/S/2/4, Fig 126), which presented a conjecture of the hospital before the extension of its east and west wings. Dimmock's engraver first copied and sized this image on to paper before tracing the outline on to thin oiled tissue paper and then, on carbon tissue, reproduced it on to the copperplate prototype of this print. Before the Copyright Act of 1842 prevented potters from using these resources, Staffordshire potters drew much of their inspiration from various books, in particular topographical works, and engravings (Coysh and Henrywood 1982, 10–11). Engraving a new copper plate took a minimum of six weeks to complete (Neale 2005, 10), and was therefore a costly process.

The London Hospital's treasury ledgers for this period record a significant increase in expenditure on 'glass and earthenware' for the years 1843–4 (RLH, LH/F/1/8, 135) (Table 67). This appears to have been linked to a decision recorded in the house committee minutes for 14 June 1842 (RLH, LH/A/5/23, 253):

<P12>

Fig 124 *Monogram of Staffordshire potter Thomas Dimmock junior <P12> (scale c 1:2)*

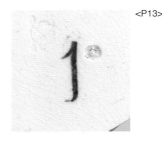 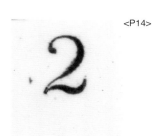 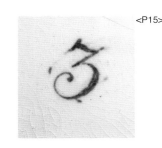 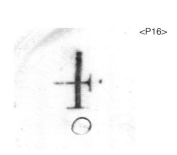

Fig 125 *The numbers 1 to 4 applied to the bases of a selection of vessels in refined whiteware with blue transfer-printed (stipple and line) decoration (<P13>–<P16>) (scale c 1:1)*

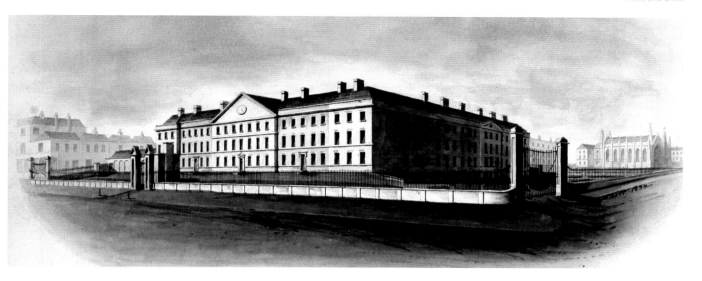

Fig 126 Alfred Richmond Mason's engraving of the proposed development of the London Hospital, 1832 (Royal London Hospital Archives, RLH, LH/S/2/4)

Resolved that a sufficient quantity of earthenware of the patterns now approved be provided as a stock to be issued from time to time to the nurses as required and the cost to be charged to them, and that J Scott Smith [James], I Currie jnr [Issac] and S Rohde [Samuel] Esqs be requested to act as a Subcommittee to undertake the arrangement of the requisite details.

No further references to this subcommittee are made, but the commissioning of this pottery can nevertheless be placed in the period when the London Hospital developed what could be crudely considered a corporate identity: in 1833 10 dozen engraved medals for the hospital staff were ordered at a cost of between 4s and 4s 6d each. The 'distinguishing medals' were to be worn 'on the left side of the dress, & outside, at all times when engaged in the business of the Hospital, either at home, or abroad' (RLH, LH/A/5/20, 74). In 1836 100 rugs with

Table 67 Summary of money spent by the London Hospital for its 'glass and earthenware' account, 1836–50

Year	Amount expended			Reference
	£	s	d	
1836	32	4	4	RLH, LH/F/1/8, 70
1837	43	6	6	RLH, LH/F/1/8, 70
1838	42	17	3	RLH, LH/F/1/8, 70
1839	72	3	2	RLH, LH/F/1/8, 70
1840	43	16	9	RLH, LH/F/1/8, 70
1841	69	5	2	RLH, LH/F/1/8, 70
1842	85	11	8	RLH, LH/F/1/8, 135
1843	146	5	-	RLH, LH/F/1/8, 135
1844	103	12	1	RLH, LH/F/1/8, 135
1845	60	5	9	RLH, LH/F/1/8, 135
1846	71	3	2	RLH, LH/F/1/8, 135
1847	70	13	9	RLH, LH/F/1/9, 153
1848	97	1	7	RLH, LH/F/1/9, 153
1849	51	16	-	RLH, LH/F/1/9, 153
1850	51	18	8	RLH, LH/F/1/9, 153

'London Hospital' on them were ordered from Messrs Janson & Co (RLH, LH/A/5/21, 316).

It is easy to imagine the multitude of ways in which pottery could have been broken, not least because running water was not extended beyond the first floor of the hospital until the early 20th century, so that boxes of washing-up water had to be carried up and downstairs for the nurses to wash the crockery. Any breakages were taken out of the nurse's wages. The apparent emphasis placed by the hospital's administrators on the nurses to be provided with pottery to be paid for from their own pocket, be responsible for its use on the wards, and clean, account and curate these pots provides an informative insight into the relationship between them.

Pottery dating to the 19th century bearing the mark of other hospitals has been found at the Radcliffe Infirmary in Oxford (OX-RAD07; Braybrooke 2011, 40–2) and the Dreadnought Seamen's Hospital, Greenwich (DSH98; Bowsher 1998). Perhaps the most significant group of Victorian institutional wares currently known remains the chamber pots, plates, rounded bowls and mugs dumped into the Eagle Pond, Snaresbrook, in Epping Forest (north-east London) and marked 'Infant Orphan Asylum', referring to a building located close by (Hughes 1992, 382–7). However, blue transfer-printed pottery in domestic forms displaying general views of hospitals was manufactured throughout this period (eg, 'Greenwich Hospital', Coysh and Henrywood 2001, 98; 'The Hospital near Poissy, France', ibid, 107) and it has been assumed that, apart from the jug bearing the name 'Lancashire Asylum' (ibid, 123), these were not commissioned and used by the institutions named on them.

Cutlery

Beth Richardson

Ten knife or fork handles and knives (not illustrated) were recovered from the deposits that sealed the 1825–41/2 cemetery. There are only three knife blades, none of which has a maker's mark. The handles vary in form. There are two pistol-grip handles – one of scale-tang construction and made from bone with part of the knife blade intact (<S16>), the other of whittle-tang construction and made from ivory with decorative circular settings for inlays, either side of the handle (<S17>). These two handles, together with two bone (<S18>) and ivory (<S19>) straight, whittle-tang handles with slight bulges at the end, are forms that date to the early or mid 18th century (Thompson et al 1984, 100–5); a rectangular-sectioned ivory handle (<S20>), a square-sectioned handle (<S21>) and two flattened oval-sectioned bone handles (<S22>, <S23>), although different from each other, are stylistically more likely to date to the later 18th or early 19th century.

There are also two ivory knife or fork handles from the machined deposits in area B; one has a slightly bulbous end (<S24>) and is similar to the 18th-century handles, <S18> and <S19>, from the make-up levels over the burial ground; two other handles are cylindrical, one made from ivory and probably also from a knife or fork (<S25>), the other made from bone and faceted from carving (<S26>). A rectangular piece of ivory with a circular perforation may be from a scale-tang handle (<163>).

Meat

James Morris

Remains recovered from the hospital cemetery (OA6; period 4) and machined deposits (OA8; period 5) (Chapter 3.4, 3.6) originate from both the hospital's kitchens and the anatomy school, and the problems of separating this material are outlined in Chapter 1.7. The committee books record in 1825 the contracting of butchers to supply meat to the hospital. For example, 'Mr Cramp Contractor for Meat attended and proposed to take the enclosed Ground behind the Hospital for one Year at £30' (RLH, LH/A/5/18, 16). Later that same year Cramp won the contract to provide the hospital with meat, as the previous supplier could not be found despite a visit to Leadenhall market to search for him (ibid, 49).

By this period the processing of animal carcass in London had become much systematised, with market butchers being supplied by middlemen, carcass processors (Yeomans 2006). The market butchers would in turn supply specific cuts of meat to their customers. This is also highlighted in the committee minutes – for example, it is noted in March 1832 that 'the Butcher had this morning sent eight breasts of mutton which was a very improper proportion' (RLH, LH/A/5/19, 214).

The possible 'kitchen waste' material recovered is dominated by elements of sheep/goat (in all likelihood sheep) and cattle. These are the most common species represented in the faunal remains as a whole (excluding the ABG deposits associated with the anatomy school). Remains of other food species such as pig, chicken, goose, turkey, duck, gadid (fish from the cod family) and mackerel are also present but in small numbers (Table 68).

The pig remains consist mainly of femora and metapodials, with evidence of butchery indicating that joints of meat may

Table 68 Summary of the animal remains recovered from periods 4 and 5: figures indicate the NISP (number of individual specimens present); figures in brackets indicate how many of the bones came from ABG deposits

Taxon	Period 4	Period 5	Total
Mammal			
Cattle	177 (5)	65	242
Sheep/goat	245 (13)	135	380
Goat	1	0	1
Pig	35 (4)	4	39
Horse	13 (4)	3	16
Dog	760 (689)	29	789
Cat	72 (32)	19 (2)	91
Primate, *Cercopithecus*	118 (118)	0	118
Primate	3	1	4
Hare	3 (2)	0	3
Rabbit	328 (258)	2	330
Guinea pig	0	1	1
Hedgehog	37 (37)	0	37
Rat	3	1	4
Bird			
Chicken	16	4	20
Turkey	0	3	3
Goose	4	1	5
Mallard	1	0	1
Passerine	1	0	1
Fish			
Gadid sp	2	0	2
Conger eel	12	0	12
Mackerel	1	0	1
Plaice	39 (39)	0	39
Plaice/flounder	1	0	1
Amphibian/reptile			
Frog/toad	1	0	1
Tortoise	19 (18)	0	19
Unidentified			
Cattle-size	166	48	214
Sheep-size	183	28	211
Mammal	4	0	4
Bird	5	1	6
Fish	2	0	2
Total	2252 (1215)	345 (2)	2597

have been consumed in the hospital. However, given the number of bones such events appear to have been rare. The hospital kitchens supplied meals for both patients and staff, many of whom lived on site, and it is therefore possible that some of the more 'expensive' meats represent staff meals. Accounts of Christmas Day at the hospital in the late 1800s show that turkeys were carved by the residents in the lobbies at dinner time and a midnight supper was served to the scrubbers (Clark-Kennedy 1963, 102–3); this may explain the origin of the turkey bones found in machined deposits (OA8). It is also possible that the pig, poultry and fish remains (cod and conger eel) represent occasional patient consumption, particularly since patients' friends and family could bring them foodstuffs.

The dominance of sheep and cattle elements reflects the overall high proportion of mutton and beef consumed during the 1800s and corresponds with other sites such as the Greenwich Naval Hospital, where the pensioners ate beef or mutton, usually boiled (Boston et al 2008, 18). There is a distinct pattern in the sheep/goat elements from both the fills of the graves (period 4) and the redeposited material over the graves (period 5). For both the number of identified specimens (NISP) and minimum number of elements (MNE), pelvis followed by femur and lumbar vertebrae are the most common (Fig 127). The majority of long-bone, pelvis and vertebra elements from these contexts have evidence of butchery. Indeed, [100] appeared to contain a dump of butchered sheep/goat lumbar vertebrae split along the sagittal plane (Fig 128). The high percentage of sheep/goat pelvis and lumbar vertebrae would suggest that a mutton saddle, combining the 'best' and 'chump' end of the loin (Rixson 2000, 245), was often supplied to the hospital.

The most common cattle elements were also vertebrae, although not to the same extent as the sheep/goat remains, followed by roughly equally proportions of humerus, radius, pelvis and femur. Many of the cattle elements also have butchery marks present; in particular the long bones appear to have been segmented. With the higher proportion of limb-bone fragments the cattle remains appear to represent a higher quality

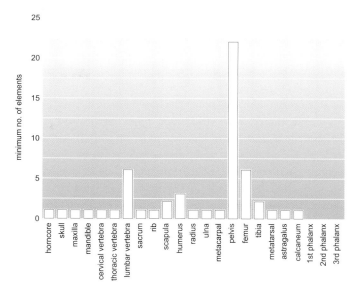

Fig 127 Minimum number of elements for sheep/goat for periods 4 and 5 combined

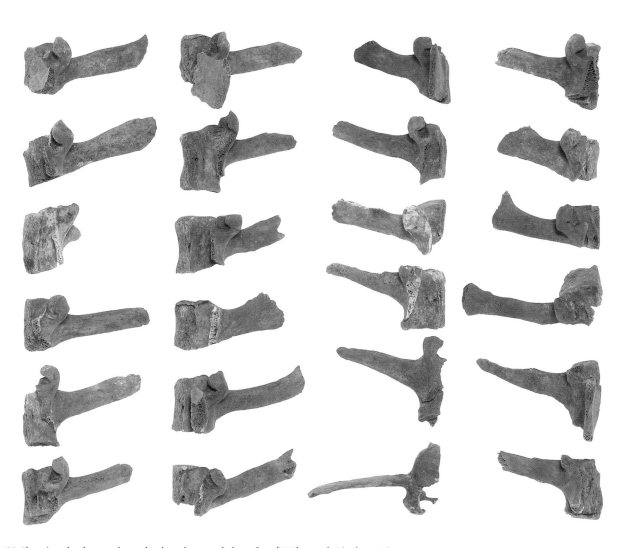

Fig 128 Sheep/goat lumbar vertebrae split along the sagittal plane, from [100], period 5 (scale c 1:2)

of meat compared to the sheep/goat elements, perhaps explaining the dominance of sheep/goat remains.

The committee records often indicate that the lowest costed tender was accepted for meat supplies and there were numerous complaints regarding the 'bad' meat: in 1821 a Mr Lintoff was awarded the contract to supply the hospital's meat, but in 1822 his tender was rejected, even though it was the cheapest, because the meat supplied was of such low quality (RLH, LH/A/5/17, 142). Perhaps some of the sheep/goat vertebral and pelvis fragments represent these low-quality meats. However, we must also take into account the fact that the faunal remains recovered represent only a very small fraction of the bone waste that would have been produced by the hospital's kitchens. Many of the bones may have been sold on by the kitchen, with the deposits recovered representing only sporadic dumping and redeposition of waste.

5.11 Treatment and care

Medical treatment

During the early 19th century, the science of medicine was still the subject of much experimentation. A belief in humoral theory continued and bloodletting was a common treatment, particularly for fever (Higgs 2009, 71). Agreement between different practitioners about appropriate medicines and doses was a matter of debate, trial and (unfortunately) error.

Higgs (2009, 73) classifies the drugs prescribed to patients in the early 19th century as falling into the following classes: laxatives, purgatives, emetics, bitters, tonics, expectorants and narcotics or opiates. Alkaloids of opium were regularly used, but at this time would not have been injected into the patient, the first morphine injection taking place in 1855 (ibid, 84).

It was not just professionals who prescribed drugs. In 1836, the expert opinion of Dr Frederic(k) Cobb, physician at the London Hospital, played a vital part in the conviction of Robert Salmon for causing the death of John McKenzie. Salmon, a 'Hygeanist', had prescribed huge doses of Morison's pills (a cure-all) to McKenzie, who was at the time in generally good health but had a severe pain in his knee. The pills contained asafoetida, aloes, gamboge and cream of tartar, the first three of which are powerful purgatives (Coventry 2000, 9); one drachm of gamboge has been known to kill. On Salmon's instructions, McKenzie had been taking 20 tablets at a time (though when he became too ill to administer this himself his wife reduced the dose to 10 tablets). Cobb had been called to McKenzie's aid in the latter stages of his affliction and treated him as best he could. He later attended the autopsy and noted widespread peritonitis, ulceration of the stomach and bleeding throughout the intestine with indications that gangrene had set in. Found guilty of manslaughter, Salmon urged that it was in the public interest that he was not convicted as 'if a monopoly in medical practice be upheld, no improvement can take place,

except from one of their own body' (*Old Bailey Proc*, April 1836, Robert Salmon (t18360404-906)).

An audit of drugs and suppliers was undertaken towards the end of 1829 to check on price and quality, following questions into how well this was being managed, and subsequently a drug committee was formed (RLH, LH/A/5/18, 294). From this audit we can see the many ingredients purchased by the house to treat the patients. These included castor oil, vinegar, 'Chlororat Soda, Epsom salts, cloves, Henbane, Myrrh, Rose leaves, liquorice, yellow flax, saspurilla [sarsaparilla], linseed oil, oxide of Bismuth, Liquor Ammoni, Muratic Acid [hydrochloric acid], Sulpur [sulphur], Ferri carboni' (ibid, 347, 350). Messrs A W McAndrew and Son of Pudding Lane supplied lime juice in 1829 (ibid, 295), whilst tenders for drugs from 1831 include 40 gallons of olive oil and 20 gallons of spirits of wine (RLH, LH/A/5/19, 9). In 1825, Messrs Wilson and Co of Snowhill supplied the London Hospital with drugs. During that year, James Cole forged a document purporting to come from Joseph Ward, the apothecary, in order to obtain 20lb of mercury and 2lb of opium, worth over £6 (*Old Bailey Proc*, February 1825, James Cole (t18250217-173)). Calico, lint and skins were also included in the lists of supplies (RLH, LH/A/5/18, 200; LH/A/5/19, 179), whilst 'spreading plasters' were made in-house until at least 1831, when the drug committee looked into buying ready-spread plasters to save time (RLH, LH/A/5/19, 131).

Leeches were an important tool for the physician and in October 1831 the committee recorded that the price of leeches had increased by 300–400%. The hospital's supplier, a Mr Hudson, had written to ask to increase the price he charged (6s 6d for 100 arranged at a fixed price contract), which was now so low that he could not afford to supply them – he was currently paying *c* 28s per 100. They awarded a new contract for him to supply them at 12s per 100 (RLH, LH/A/5/19, 121, 125). In November that year the committee negotiated a reduced rate of 10s 3d and a further reduction to 9s per 100 was achieved in December (ibid, 141, 158). By August 1832 the price had fallen to just 4s per 100 (ibid, 292). The medicinal leech (*Hirudo medicinalis*) lives in shallow pools or ponds where it attaches itself to a passing host animal to feed. They were often harvested by men who would wade in to the water and wait for the leeches to attach themselves to their bare legs, before heading back to the shore. Over-exploitation in the 19th century, coupled with the drainage of land for agricultural use and introduction of troughs for livestock (rather than open ponds), was responsible for a dramatic reduction in the leech population (Sawyer 1981; Whitaker et al 2004, 136).

Mental health care

Hospital policy precluded the admission of 'lunaticks' (above, 5.5). Those suffering from insanity were to be cared for in asylums such as St Mary Bethlehem (Bethlem or Bedlam) in Moorfields, St Luke's Old Street or a number of private asylums that admitted those paid for by private income or parish charity (Lane 2001, 98–100). However, in December 1832, the house governor reported that there were three lunatics in the hospital. Mary Brown was recorded as suffering temporary insanity from a particular cause (though it was not stated what this was) and her admission was therefore not considered to be in breach of the by-laws. Mary Macknell (who was having fits) and Mary Benden, however, were 'still suspected to be lunatics' (RLH, LH/A/5/19, 427).

Realistically, the London Hospital could offer little treatment to such patients, beyond rest and food. The report seven years later of the trial of the Hanoverian John Frederick Jordan, who was prosecuted for attempting to murder his wife, indicates how a disturbed patient was treated. Jordan appears to have been paranoid and delusional, accusing others of trying to steal his money, wandering the streets and threatening to drown himself. When his wife, Mary, tried to stop him leaving again, he stabbed her six times in the face and neck, causing her to lose the use of her limbs and putting her in the London Hospital for five weeks and under medical care for a further three. At the time of the trial she had still not regained all movement. Her husband was also brought to the London Hospital, where a medical student, Stephen Henry Ward, treated self-inflicted throat wounds. Jordan was extremely agitated about his wife and tried to reopen the wound on his neck. The staff placed him in a 'strait-waistcoat' and gave him a dose of opium to quieten him. Jordan spent two days in the strait-waistcoat, was given a further dose of opium, a dose of 'opening medicine' (presumably to counteract the digestive effects of the opium) and was monitored by the ward nurse. As he was in custody, a policeman sat by Jordan's bed at all times (Jordan reporting to the officer that the doctors had given him poison). He remained in the hospital for two weeks, during which time he was kept on a low diet for the first few days, then on a full diet. Jordan was found not guilty by reason of insanity (*Old Bailey Proc*, July 1839, John Frederick Jordan (t18390708-2101)). Clearly the hospital had a straitjacket on hand for dealing with violent or delusional patients to protect the staff (and other patients on the open wards) and also to prevent the patient from self-injury; Ward stated that he would have used the jacket again if he had known that Jordan was trying to reopen his wound.

The specific needs of patients who were not considered to be lunatics but were suffering from depression or had suicidal tendencies were also recognised by the hospital staff. In February 1822 the surgeon Richard Headington suggested in a letter to the house committee that such patients might be better off kept on separate wards (RLH, LH/A/5/17, 90):

…can such an individual be calculated for the general Ward of an Hospital where his recovery may be likely to be retarded by the laugh of vulgar thoughtlessness or the jeer of inconsiderate levity? The mind of the poor Man is as finely framed as that of his Superior and his susceptibility is often more acutely raised from the supposed hopelessness of his condition. They require the medicine of the Mind and that lenitive the common Ward of an Hospital is but ill calculated to supply. A Hospital besides has often within its walls those unfortunate individuals who have known better days and

whose situation is often embittered by a deep reflection on the consequences of their folly or by lamenting on the tortuous obliquities of their fortune. To such individuals certainly some little distinction might be shown.

The task of soothing the depressed was also amongst the spiritual duties of the house governor (RLH, LH/A/5/22, 25 August 1840, 410–16). In 1828 Valentine reported to the house committee that in his opinion extra attendance should have been given to a man who was brought into the hospital as an accident after trying to commit suicide. Although the man had received counselling from Valentine, who had taken the time to write a letter to the man's abandoned wife on his behalf, he had subsequently seized an opportunity to run away from the hospital when no one was watching him (RLH, LH/A/17/5, 29 April 1828).

Spiritual care

As indicated by the central role of the chaplain in the running of the hospital, the spiritual and moral care of the sick was considered as important as their physical care. At the London Hospital, it was recorded in 1830 that testaments and prayer books were kept on the wards together with 'cards with prayers for the heads of the beds' (RLH, LH/A/5/18, 322–3). Patients were not to play cards or dice, smoke, swear, spit or curse in the wards. If they did they could be expelled and refused further entry (1810: RLH, LH/A/1/4, 14–15). In October 1841 a patient on Gloucester ward by the name of Perkins was dismissed by the house committee, at the request of the surgeon Mr Luke, for using obscene language (RLH, LH/A/5/23, 142).

The hospital showed a pragmatic attitude towards religion. In August 1829 'the Chairman gave permission to George Freare … to attend his place of worship on Sundays he being a Quaker' (RLH, LH/A/5/18, 278) and the hospital also catered for the Jewish community (above, 5.10, 'Diet and provisioning'). Dissenting ministers were allowed into the hospital to visit members of their congregation, although there were limits. In 1840 a Mr William Fry of Liverpool wrote to the hospital enclosing a cutting from the *Morning Chronicle*, which reported the case of a dissenting minister being thrown out of the hospital. The committee replied in April 1840 that 'in the case alluded to in your letter the Minister was rather preaching to the Ward than praying by the Patient, who was not one of his usual congregation and the latter is always permitted under proper restrictions, the house committee cannot consent to allow the former' (RLH, LH/A/5/22, 352).

Surgical treatment and amputation

Hospitals were not the only places where surgeons practised at this time, and surgery would also take place in the home (Higgs 2009, 10), but from the beginning of the 19th century the number of surgical patients admitted to the London Hospital steadily increased (RLH, LH/A/5/18, 29 May 1827, 147–8) (Fig 129).

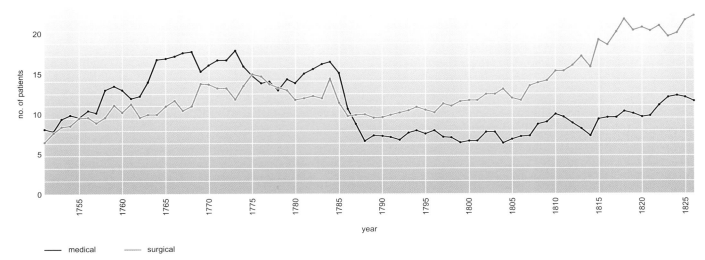

Fig 129 Evidence from the house committee minute books of the increase in surgical patients in the early years of the 19th century (RLH, LH/A/ 5/18, 29 May 1827, 147–8)

Surgery took place in the operating theatre, under the curious eyes of as many as 70 students. In 1822 the theatre was altered to provide more storage space for instruments, together with a step in the front row to give the audience a better view of the operations (RLH, LH/A/5/17, 141). In 1835 the surgeon James Luke raised the crowded state of the operating theatre with the house committee and suggested that alterations should be made to provide more room and enable the accommodation of more students. The house committee declined to spend the estimated £200 to increase the capacity to 100, as there was not considered to be sufficient benefit to the hospital in doing so. By June 1840 the theatre was lit with gas (RLH, LH/A/5/22, 367). A painting was made of it before it was demolished in 1889 (Fig 130).

A contemporary operating theatre survives at St Thomas's Hospital, where the pupils were raised on a series of steps to improve their view of the operation in progress. However, a contemporary account of St Thomas's indicates that in spite of this measure there was overcrowding and many spectators experienced difficulty in viewing the subject of the operation. This would suggest that the atmosphere of the operating theatre at the London Hospital was little different to that of the theatre at St Thomas's (South 1970, 128):

the first two rows ... were occupied by the other dressers, and behind a second partition stood the pupils, packed like herrings in a barrel, but not so quiet, as those behind them were continually pressing on those before and were continually struggling to relieve themselves of it, and had not infrequently to be got out exhausted. There was also a continual calling out of "Heads, Heads" to those about the table whose heads interfered with the sightseers.

Treatment of fractures with an open wound before the discovery of antibiotics was a precarious business. Antiseptics such as vinegar and iodine were used (Higgs 2009, 78), but there

was no general understanding of the transmission of infection and a surgeon would wear the same coat for every operation or intervention, with no gloves to form a protective barrier between him and the patient. It was not until 1864 that Louis Pasteur would propose his theories on the transmission of disease (ibid, 82). Thus when, in 1838, the elderly James Ginns broke his femur during a minor altercation with the 20-year-old William Law, he languished for seven weeks in the London Hospital before dying from 'mortification' of the wound. John Adams, giving evidence at the subsequent trial, was quick to emphasise that everything possible had been done to treat the injury, two pupils who were overseeing the admission of accidents at night having set the injury (*Old Bailey Proc*, August 1838, William Law (t18380820-1794)).

The healed but non-united fracture of the right scaphoid seen in adult [412] (Fig 59) would have required at least six weeks' immobilisation from the time of injury to assist union (Resnick 2002, 2842–6; McRae 2003, 331–2). Since this injury pre-dates the use of plaster casts to facilitate healing, the only options available would have involved various kinds of splints, or simply pads and bandages (Radley 1835). Splints seem to have formed a significant component of the treatments used at the London Hospital – from 4 March 1828 the committee decided that to save money the in-house carpenter should make all the required splints (RLH, LH/A/5/18, 201). In April 1832, the surgeons' library was fitted out as a store for splints, surgical instruments and so forth and at the same time changes were made to the pupils' regulations regarding their eligibility to dress patients (RLH, LH/A/5/19, 235, 241).

A healed Duverney fracture of the ilium suffered by 36–45-year-old probable male [138] (Fig 60) suggests that he had been given considerable care, as more than half of modern patients with such an injury will die. Whether this care took place in a formal medical context (ie, on an earlier visit to the hospital) or in his home cannot be determined. Regardless, luck is also likely to have played a part in his recovery.

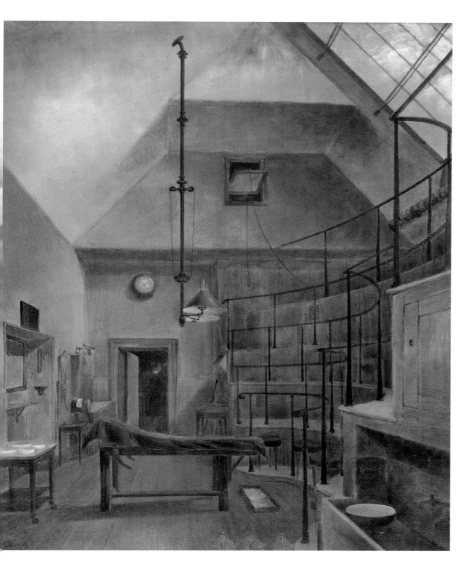

Fig 130 The old operating theatre at the London Hospital by F M Harvey (oil on canvas), painted before its demolition in 1889 (Royal London Hospital Archives, RLHINV/59/1)

In 1834, two surgeons, Bond and Gale, described in a letter to *The Lancet* a similar injury to that observed in male [124] (Bond and Gale 1834). A young man had fallen from a cart, fracturing the 'upper part of the lower third' of his right femur. The extreme obliqueness of the broken ends of the bones hampered efforts to keep them in apposition during extension of the limb using standard techniques. This problem is attested to by the position in which the remains of the limb of [124] were found, with the fractured ends of the femur noticeably overlapping (Figs 65–6). Bond and Gale resorted to fixation in a trough of plaster of Paris and the young man survived thanks to this innovation, partly perhaps because of his relative youth, and probably because of some amount of good fortune. The lack of apposition in the case from the London Hospital suggests that permanent or semi-permanent fixation techniques were not employed, which may indicate that the case pre-dated that reported in *The Lancet*, or perhaps that it was simply not possible to reduce the fracture to a position where such fixation would have been of value.

Amputation carried even greater risks for the patient than did fracture treatment: between the 1840s and 1870s a post-operative death rate of 35–65% was usual, depending on the location of the amputation (Higgs 2009, 76). At the London Hospital, the risks can hardly have been alleviated by the damp reported in the operating room in January 1825 (RLH, LH/A/5/18, 6). Such treatment would therefore be seen as a last resort, as a report on the treatment of one unfortunate man at the London shows. On 9 October 1832 a man aged about 44 years was admitted with a serious leg injury, having been run over by a cart. His femur was broken and he appeared to have lost a considerable quantity of blood before admission. After 'considerable persuasion', not to mention 'sixteen ounces of wine and several ounces of gin', he agreed to the limb being amputated. However, the journey to the operating theatre proved too much for him and 'he fell back exhausted … and the heart's action became a mere flutter, under these circumstances it was considered impossible to perform the operation'. In fact, so concerned were the surgeons that they moved a bed from the wards to the theatre rather than risk moving him again. The next morning he seemed a little better and Blizard ordered that the operation proceed at once. Mr Luke was called for and the limb removed at the thigh 'by the circular incision'. With a liberal dose of laudanum, the patient fell asleep and 'lingered on till six o'clock the following morning, when he died' (*The*

Lancet, 27 October 1832, Fractures of the leg and thigh –
amputation – death, 19(478), 160). Interestingly, after his death
the surgeons dissected the removed limb. They concluded that
the fracture was such that if placed in apposition, the ends
would have been locked together; without amputation he
might have survived.

Since amputation would have been considered a last resort
for only the most serious disease or injury, it would be
reasonable to expect some bony evidence of the underlying
reason for *in vivo* surgery to be present, at least in some instances,
in the human remains. Certainly a distal limb segment (ie, the
amputated portion) should show some underlying clues as to
the reason for its removal. Without this, distal limb segments
can be considered indicative of dissection or practising surgical
techniques on cadavers rather than as representing surgical waste.

All examples of possible *in vivo* amputation (proximal limb
portions) or the resultant surgical waste (distal limb portions)
identified from observations of the diagrammatic recording
forms for the articulated assemblage were evaluated and evidence
for concurrent pathological changes noted. Limbs from 49
contexts were considered to have possible evidence of surgery,
based on the location of single saw cuts through a limb segment.

Eight contexts contained proximal limb segments (primary
inhumations [152] and [242] and portions [27202], [28410],
[28503], [32910], [32911] and [58702]). No concurrent
pathology was noted in any instance with the exception of male
[242], who had a healing rib fracture and so may conceivably
have suffered an accident that also damaged his left hand, which
had been removed. The direction of the cuts to his forearm
(distal radius and ulna) indicate that the limb was in supination
during this process. It is not clear whether this procedure was
the result of post-mortem dissection or of surgery, but the
location of the cut (distal to the insertion of the pronator radii
teres) would preserve the power of pronation and supination.
No further evidence of dissection was present and he had not
apparently undergone autopsy (though the cranium was absent,
preventing observation). This individual therefore remains the
best evidence of the burial in the hospital cemetery of those
who did not survive surgery (Fig 131). Death subsequent to
amputation is suggested by the presence of fine patches of
woven bone on a segment of proximal and mid right humerus
(sawn midshaft to remove the lower arm) found disarticulated
within [391].

Forty distal limb segments were catalogued and considered
as possible evidence of surgical waste. In 24 of these (60%) no
pathological bone changes were present, suggesting that these
represent practice amputations or part of the dissection process.
Practising surgical techniques on cadavers was certainly
encouraged by those at the London Hospital (Chapter 7.3). It is
interesting, therefore, that of the 40 possible examples of
surgical waste, active infection was noted in the cut bone or an
adjacent element in eight instances (20%), including portion
[22302] (Fig 132), as this seems to have a parallel in the results
from Newcastle Infirmary where infection was the most
common concurrent pathological change noted (Boulter et al
1998, 148). In two further limbs healed infectious lesions were

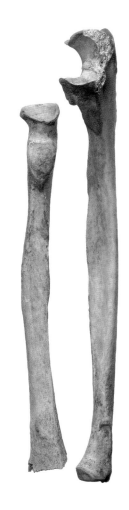
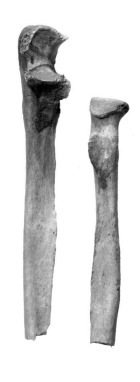

Fig 131 Probable in vivo *amputation of
the left lower arm and hand, male [242]
(scale c 1:2)*

noted, and as these represent conditions that were recovered
from some time prior to death, the removal of the limbs is more
likely to be the result of classes at the medical school than of *in
vivo* surgery. In contrast, traumatic lesions were present in only
three instances: a healed Colles fracture in the left ulna of adult
female [396], aged ≥46 years, healed impaction injuries in the
foot of an adult of undetermined sex from [24602] and a healed
patella fracture in another adult of undetermined sex from
[28408]. The eight examples of likely amputation waste
consisted of seven lower leg and/or foot portions and one left
wrist and hand. One subadult, [19202], was affected, with a
possible circular amputation technique used to remove the right
lower leg and foot at the mid thigh (femur).

The remaining affected limbs were from adults of
undetermined sex and represent a minimum of three
individuals, though they are more likely to have originated
from seven separate adults. The possibility that such limb
segments might also have been retained as specimens during an
anatomy class should also be considered as pathological bone
can frequently be found in museum collections, and the
overlying soft tissues may have had gross manifestations of
disease of interest to the student or surgeon. The posterior to
anterior direction of saw cuts in [35410] is highly suggestive of
the latter interpretation since this would be an unusual position
for a leg to be placed in for the purpose of *in vivo* amputation.
Further details on the direction of saw cuts can be found in

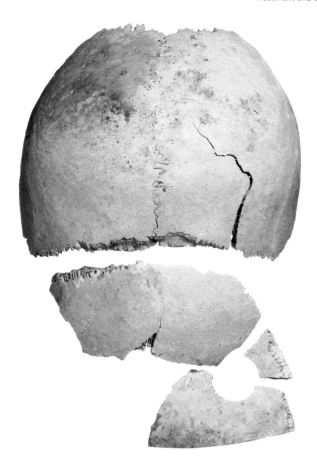

Fig 133 Trephination in a disarticulated adult left frontal from [174], showing the marks of the drill on the external surface (scale c 1:2)

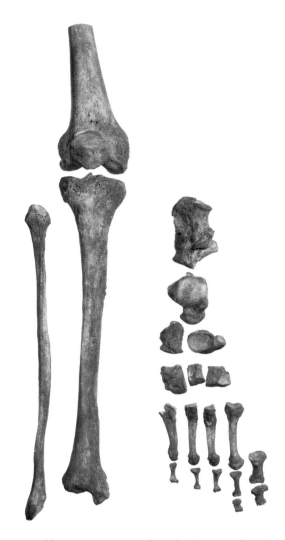

Fig 132 Possible in vivo *amputation of an infected right leg, [22302] (scale c 1:4)*

Chapter 7.8, 'Tools and techniques'.

Male [408], aged ≥46 years, revealed somewhat enigmatic evidence of possible surgery with the removal of the right femoral head together with evidence of autopsy. Amputation by the removal of the femoral head was a technique under development in the first half of the 19th century (Kaufman and Wakelin 2004), and it is possible that this is an early example of experimentation with such a technique (on either the living or the dead). No indications of the reason for such a procedure remained.

One example of trephination, usually carried out to relieve pressure on the brain, was also noted. Located on the left frontal of adult [174] was a neat hole 24.5mm in diameter. The tooth marks of the drill used were visible on the ectocranium and show a clockwise drilling action (Fig 133). As this bone came from the disarticulated material it is not possible to say with certainty whether it represents the non-survival of this patient or the practising of surgical techniques on cadavers, as is the case with numerous burr holes – a similar technique that was also used to relieve pressure – noted in the assemblage (Chapter 7.8).

It is notable that amongst the articulated burials from Newcastle Infirmary, just five individuals were identified who were believed to have undergone medical amputation, together with a probable male with an unhealed trephination in the superior cranium (Boulter et al 1998, 139). The disarticulated bone from the site provided further evidence for two or possibly three trephinations (3/384 adult crania; 0.8%), each cranium containing a single drilled hole. Two subadult long bones (2/32:6.3%) were interpreted as showing indications of amputation; in the adult assemblage 7.7% (171/2231) of the long bones observed had evidence of distal amputations and 1.4% (29/2132) had proximal amputations (ibid, 135). It should be stressed that this definition (by location only) does not preclude the possibility that the amputation was a procedure performed after death to aid surgical practice. At Worcester Royal Infirmary 214/1458 fragments showed evidence of medical intervention (14.7%, deriving from a minimum of 24 individuals) and one healed frontal trepanation was identified (Western 2010, 31–3).

Finds related to medical and surgical treatment

Nigel Jeffries and Beth Richardson

A small assemblage of items used in the treatment of patients was recovered during the excavation, although some of the

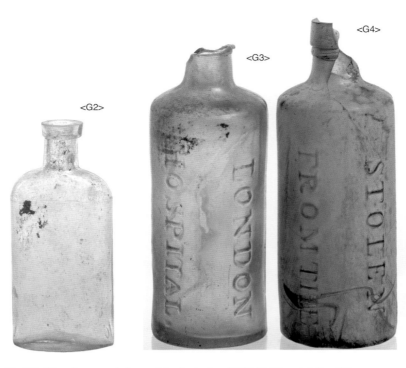

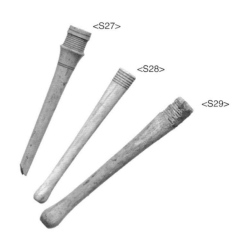

Fig 134 *Glass pharmaceutical or medicine bottles from [100] (OA8, period 5): <G2> – aqua-coloured, oval-shaped pharmaceutical or medicine bottle; <G3> and <G4> – green-coloured and aqua-coloured, respectively, cylindrical prescription bottles (scale c 1:2)*

Fig 135 *Three bone syringe applicators or 'pipes' <S27> <S28>, <S29> (scale c 1:2)*

finds date to later in the 19th century, after the cemetery of c 1825–41/2 (OA6, period 4) had gone out of use.

In the 1830s, bottles, jars and pots for the dispensary were purchased from Richard and Sons (RLH, LH/A/5/19, 97); in May 1832 old and dirty bottles and jars were sent to a broker for disposal 'at the best prices they can bring' (ibid, 244). From within the disturbed ground overlying the burials in Open Area 6, [100] (OA8, period 5) contained four glass bottles dating to the second and third quarters of the 19th century. The first, an aqua-coloured, oval-shaped bottle made in a two-piece mould with an applied finish (where the seam ends abruptly at the upper neck at the rim) and patent rim (<G2>, Fig 134), would have contained tonics, bitters and other remedies. Two identical cylindrical glass prescription bottles (<G3>–<G4>, Fig 134), which would have been filled with drugs from the hospital's dispensary, have the relief moulded text 'STOLEN FROM THE LONDON HOSPITAL' applied vertically down the side. Similar warnings on bottles from this period (for example, 'NOT TO BE TAKEN') are commonly observed, and companies sometimes prosecuted individuals for illegal reuse (Lucas 2002, 7). Sufficient of one of the bottles survived to reveal an applied mineral rim finish, and both were made in a two-piece mould.

A number of medical implements was also recovered during the archaeological excavation. Three bone syringe applicators or 'pipes' (<S27>–<S29>, Fig 135), which are accessories from enema syringes, used for rectal irrigation, were found within the deposits overlying the cemetery in area A. The syringes were made of brass, pewter or glass with a rubber or twine-bound plunger, and a silk-covered rubber 'elastic' tube ending in a brass tube with a screw fitting. The hollow bone pipes had

screw fittings at one end that screwed directly into the brass tube – as in Read's or 'Reed's' patent hydraulic syringe, which dates from the early years of the 19th century (Fig 136) – or into another small brass fitting, which might be straight or right-angled – as illustrated in Weiss's 1831 catalogue (Weiss 1831; Fig 137, upper). The collections of the Old Operating Theatre Museum (Guy's and St Thomas' NHS Foundation Trust) contain a similar set, advertised as a stomach pump and

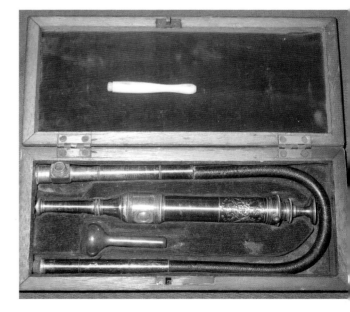

Fig 136 *J Read's patent hydraulic syringe, early 19th century (Royal London Hospital Archives, RLHINV/209)*

enema kit and containing two slightly different-sized bone applicators; this particular set was manufactured by or purchased from Krohne and Sesermann of 8 Duke Street.

Enema syringes are known to have been in common use in the early and mid 19th century, and were widely illustrated in books, tradesmen's journals and advertising leaflets of the time. A pamphlet dated *c* 1826 by J Read advertises his patent syringe and the many attachments (two bone pipes were supplied as standard) that could be used with it. Catalogues by Savigny (*c* 1798) and Weiss (1831) (Fig 137, upper) have detailed drawings

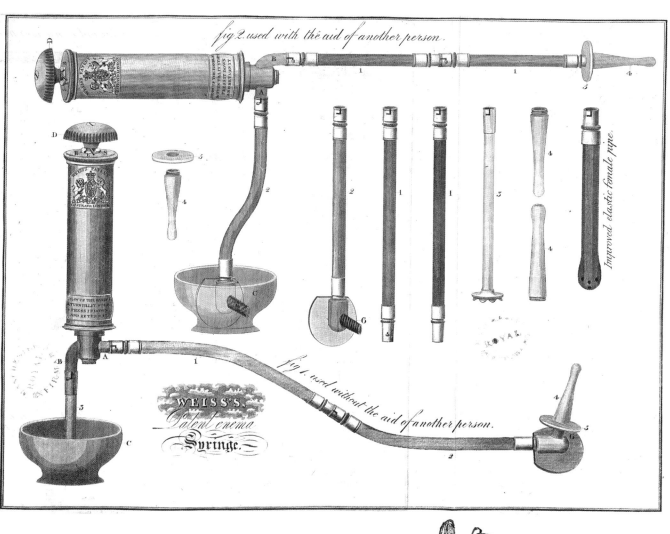

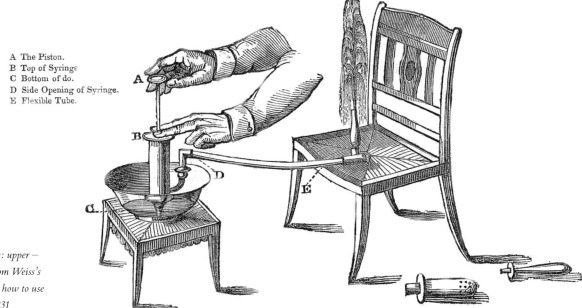

A The Piston.
B Top of Syringe.
C Bottom of do.
D Side Opening of Syringe.
E Flexible Tube.

Fig 137 Enema syringes: upper — patent enema syringe from Weiss's 1831 catalogue; lower — how to use a syringe, from Jukes 1831

of the pipes, which are very similar to those excavated, whilst illustrations in a book by Read's rival, Edward Jukes (1831), also give a good impression of the use of the enema syringe (Fig 137, lower).

Cassell's *Science and art of nursing: Vol 2* (n d [*c* 1905–10]), compiled nearly a hundred years later but essentially discussing Victorian practices, describes the process of enemata (injections into the rectum) as those to be returned (using a syringe) and those to be retained (using a catheter and funnel). Examples are given of solutions to be used with the syringe, including salt and water for children with threadworms, soft soap and water as a purgative and turpentine and water for flatulence.

In the early 19th century, the syringes used by the London Hospital were supplied and repaired by W H Pepys of Poultry, surgical instrument-maker and cutler (above, 5.10, 'Diet and provisioning'). The tradesmen's ledgers, two of which list hospital purchases from 1798 to 1807 and 1808 to 1814 (RLH, LH/F/8/11; /12), contain pages of medical instruments supplied including elastic syringes costing 11s (1798), an elastic syringe and three pewter syringes (1800), one dozen elastic urethra syringes costing 2 guineas (1811) and 12 elastic syringes with stopcock costing 15s (1812). In 1832, the surgeons requested a trial of the instruments made by Messrs Weiss and Sons, and

they are later mentioned as suppliers to the hospital (RLH, LH/A/5/19, 338, 343, 352–4). Material displayed at the Old Operating Theatre Museum shows that in *c* 1840 Weiss and Sons were situated at 62 The Strand.

Read's patent hydraulic syringe could also be used 'for removing poisons from the stomach' (Fig 138), and the bone syringes may have been put to this use within the hospital. A number of cases are reported in which the hospital's 'stomach pump' was used. The friends of a man who had overdosed on laudanum knocked on the house governor's private door for help one night. As the apothecary, holder of the key to the room in which the pump was kept, had left the building, the door to the room had to be forced open. Then 'the Assistant Apothecary and one of the pupils attempted to introduce the tube of the pump in vain – the Apothecary returned at half past one or two o'clock, then he attempted to use the pump but failed' and the man died (RLH, LH/A/17/6, 14 April 1829). The pump was also used to treat Thomas Combes, a labourer employed at the rum quay at the West India Docks, who was brought to the hospital 'in a state of insensibility' after drinking a large quantity of rum, and subsequently died (*Morning Post*, 28 September 1837, issue 20833). The syringes may also have had a function in anatomy classes (Chapter 7.8, 'Tools and

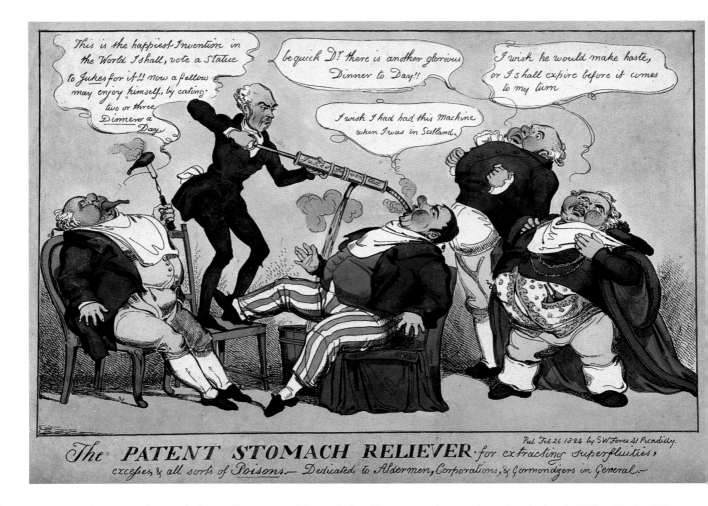

Fig 138 Dr Jukes pumping the stomach of Sir William Curtis, while several other aldermen wait to be operated on; coloured etching by William Heath, 1824, satirising the gross appetites of some civic dignitaries and dedicated to 'Aldermen, Corporations, & Gormandizers in General' (Wellcome Library, London, V0011337)

techniques').

The deposits sealing the later (post-1841) cemetery also produced a small number of items that may have had a surgical use (Fig 139). A tapering copper-alloy tube, broken at the wider end, may have been part of a medical or surgical instrument (<S30>). An implement with a broken blade (<S31>) may be the handle from either an amputating knife or a bone saw, used in the hospital. Its large scale-tang handle, made from bone, is heavily inscribed on both faces with a 'checkered' pattern that made it easier to grip; the blade is broken and appears from the radiograph to be forked (hence the possibility of it being a D-shaped saw) but this may be a result of breakage. Surgical knives and saws for amputation had 'checkered' handles in this period, as did butchers' knives and steels; the earliest general English tool catalogue (Smith 1816, fig 2) illustrates several, but there is no surviving text or price list. A long and narrow curved brush with a handle (<S32>) may have had a specific medical use. It is very similar to a brush illustrated on a page with surgical and other knives (ibid), but it could also have had a cleaning use, such as dusting or cleaning crumbs from tables. A handle and knife (<S33>, <S34>, not illustrated) found in the deposits sealing the earlier *c* 1825–41/2 cemetery may be tools rather than eating utensils.

Worryingly, in October 1831, 'Several of the instruments sent in by the manufacturer for the use of the surgeons, were not in a fit state for the purposes intended' (RLH, LH/A/5/19, 134).

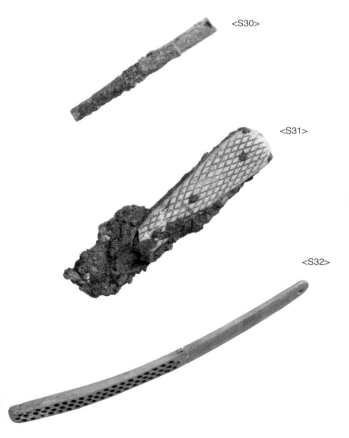

Fig 139 Items with a possible surgical or medical use (from period 5 deposits): <S30> – tapering copper-alloy tube; <S31> – implement with a broken blade, possibly from a surgeon's knife or saw; <S32> – curved brush (scale c *1:2)*

Accusations of malpractice

A number of complaints relating to treatment were recorded by the committee and it is interesting that there seem to have been few occasions when investigation within the hospital concluded that the medical staff were at fault.

In June 1828 a letter from Mr Toley of Bermuda Street complained that his son had died from an 'improper bleeding' (RLH, LH/A/5/18, 216). Then in September 1830 'Mr Cooper attended (on the part of Miles Stinger Esq) to complain of the treatment which a Patient named Ezra Westneat was stated to have received … on application being personally made by Mr Kemble Esq to several Patients [on George's ward] as to the existence of the practice alleged it was proved, to the satisfaction of Mr Cooper that the complaint was entirely unfounded' (ibid, 367). The details of the complaint remain a mystery.

A letter of complaint was received from Mr George Childs of Bread Street on 28 April 1831 claiming that the hospital delayed in attending his infant child, who had suffered an accident. This delay was blamed on the current lack of an assistant surgeon (RLH, LH/A/5/19, 52).

In May 1836 the chairman of the house committee received a letter from a relative of John Weldy, a dock worker injured after falling down the hold of a ship in the London docks. In addition to concerns about the standard of the treatment that Weldy had received (above, 5.9, 'The dressing pupils'), his relative was concerned that it was too easy for the patients to obtain large quantities of alcohol, including gin, if they could pay for it. Although Mr Weldy had been 'discharged cured', his leg again broke whilst he was in bed not long after he had left the hospital. His relative notes that 'If his limb had gained strength and he had recovered, the Hospital would have credit for his cure, if he had died, or lived a Cripple, the Committee I address thro [sic] you would never have heard, had he been as friendless as the great majority of the recipients of your Charity'. Again the house committee determined that the hospital was not at fault, that a surgeon had seen him on the evening of his admission and that the reason for the leg not healing was 'the ill judged kindness of his Friends in the supplying him with large quantities of wine' (RLH, LH/A/5/21, 256–62; above, 5.10, 'Diet and provisioning'). However, the house committee shortly afterwards passed a number of resolutions in an attempt to improve the medical provision available at night (above, 5.9, 'The dressing pupils').

Such incidents could perhaps be considered inevitable by-products of the fact that medical science was still in its infancy, though some of the individuals involved seem to have had a somewhat lackadaisical attitude to care. Potentially far more damaging to the reputation of the London Hospital, which from its inception had relied on the continued financial support of the public, were those complaints that were reported in the press.

In 1826 a coroner's inquiry was held into the death of John McCall following bleeding treatment at the hospital. The coroner concluded that he had died from the use of a poisoned (dirty) lancet. The results were published in a number of newspapers and the governors decided it was necessary to hold their own inquiry. They found that since someone else had been bled at the same time (though whether with the same lancet is unclear) and had no ill effects and since the lancet was new and specifically used for venesection, the hospital was not at fault. The inquiry also mentioned that the operation had been performed by pupils (RLH, LH/A/5/18, 72, 76). In November 1832, *The Times* published a report that the hospital had neglected a deaf and dumb boy. This was rebuked with the statement that he had suffered only a slight head injury and that, despite this, they had kept him in overnight out of kindness (RLH, LH/A/5/19, 355–6).

In 1833, the hospital was again in the papers, accused of neglect in the case of William Roberts, a sawyer working at the London docks, who was admitted after a piece of timber fell on his leg and who died two weeks later. None of the medical staff of the hospital were present to give evidence at the inquest, in spite of having been summoned by the constable. The nurse was eventually called for, and she conceded that although the wound was dressed (presumably by one of the pupils) when Mr Roberts was admitted, it was not until Mr Andrews the surgeon saw it some days later that it was recognised as having been broken and put into splints. The jury returned a verdict of accidental death and fined the medical officers for not attending the inquest (*Morning Post*, 13 September 1833, issue 19584). Letters were published calling for an inquiry, and the house committee called a special meeting to investigate the case. They decided (quite possibly erroneously) that Mr Roberts's eventual death could not be attributed to the initial delay in his diagnosis and treatment, and resolved that he had been 'treated with every possible attention + surgical skill, & that not the slightest blame can be attached to the surgeons or the other Officers of the Hospital' (RLH, LH/A/5/20, 134). The statement was published in several papers, some of which were paid to publish it as an advertisement. The hospital kept a scrapbook of newspaper cuttings relating to the case (RLH, LH/A/26/1).

6

Medical teaching and anatomy in the 19th century

To examine the causes of life, we must first have recourse to death.
(Shelley 2004, 61)

6.1   Introduction

During the 16th and 17th centuries, Italy lay at the forefront of anatomical teaching. A century later, Paris was the main centre for study (Richardson 2001, 35), but from the early 18th century, an aspiring medical student could take classes at one of a number of medical schools in London (Lane 2001, 27). A functionalist and mechanistic approach became more favoured during the 17th century and led to an increase in the desire to understand human anatomy through experimentation (Cherryson 2010, 135).

In the separation of the Surgeons from the Barbers in 1745 (previously the Company of Barber-Surgeons), the by-law that prevented private dissections without prior permission from the Company was removed and this, together with an absence of formal classes run from 1745 to 1752, led to a rise in private anatomy schools (Lawrence 1996, 86). Although William Hunter attempted to set up a central, government-funded anatomy school in 1765, he met with insufficient support, so instead opened premises on Great Windmill Street (Richardson 2001, 37), just one of the many schools that operated in the metropolis in the late 18th and early 19th centuries (Table 69). During the late 18th and 19th centuries, hospitals increasingly played an active role in medical and surgical study. The London Hospital was at the forefront of this movement. Sir William Blizard passionately believed that medical staff should be trained in hospitals, and because of his efforts when the London Hospital Medical College opened in 1785, it was the first such school in London to be associated with a hospital (Clark-Kennedy 1962, 165–7). By 1800, the school was one of only three associated with hospitals and much medical teaching in the capital still took place in private schools (Higgs 2009, 112). An estimated 250–300 pupils were taught at Grainger's school in Webb Street each year in the 1820s (Wise 2004, 27, 167), and students were able to 'shop around', taking classes in different subjects at a number of different institutions, both private and hospital-based (Lawrence 1996, 171).

Legislative changes in 1823 and 1824 stipulated that to obtain a medical qualification students were to study anatomy at a school or university that was recognised by the Royal College of Surgeons, and only during the winter season (Richardson 2001, 101). This resulted in an influx of students to the hospital schools of London and by 1828 the Report from the Select Committee on Anatomy noted that there were 800 students at anatomy schools in London, 500 of whom practised dissection. The select committee estimated that these students had access to 450–500 bodies, less than one per student (Blake Bailey 1896, 70).

Before the Anatomy Act of 1832, the only legal method for obtaining a body for dissection was to acquire that of an executed criminal (after 1832 those in charge of workhouses and hospitals were authorised to send the remains of the unclaimed dead for dissection (Lane 2001, 29)). The demand for bodies for dissection created a lucrative market in illicitly obtained corpses, many of which were supplied by 'bodysnatchers' or 'resurrection men'.

Whilst there appears to have been a 'professional silence'

Table 69 Private anatomy schools in London operating in the late 18th and early 19th centuries

Location	Dates	Key staff (in date order)	Reference
Great Windmill Street [1]	1765–1828	William Hunter, Cruikshank, Matthew Baillie, James Wilson, Benjamin Brodie (1807–14), Charles Bell (1811–; broken up on foundation of London University), Herbert Mayo, Caeser Hawkins, Babington, Gregory Smith, Bushell, William Hewson, Mr Thomas (1800–3), Shaw (1815–20)	Power 1895a, 1389; Lawrence 1996, appendix III; Richardson 2001, 37, 287
Great Windmill Street [2]	–	Benjamin Brodie (property taken after sale of [1] to Charles Bell), John Shaw	Power 1895a, 1389
Little Windmill Street	1833–7 or later	George Derby Dermott J Gregory Smith*	Scripps 1837, 181; Power 1895b, 1452; Richardson 2001, 287
Webb Street	1819–42	Edward Grainger, Richard Dugard Grainger, Armstrong	Power 1895a, 1389; Wise 2004, 27
50 Dean Street [1], Soho	1805–c 1831	Joseph Carpue	Power 1895a, 1389; Lawrence 1996, appendix III; Richardson 2001, 287
Dean Street [2]**	1834–41	G J Guthrie	Westminster Hospital Medical School records (http://www.aim25.ac.uk/cgibin/vcdf/detail?coll_id=2852&inst_id=3&nv1=search&nv2=basic)
Little Dean Street	1826	Bennet, Armstrong	Power 1895a, 1389
Chapel Street	?1830s	George Derby Dermott (move from Little Windmill Street)	Power 1895b, 1453; Richardson 2001, 287
Howland Street	–?1834		Richardson 2001, 287
Aldersgate Street	1825–49		Richardson 2001, 287
Blenheim Street	1800–c 1830	Joshua Brookes	Power 1895b, 1452; Lawrence 1996, appendix III; Richardson 2001, 287
Grosvenor Place	?	Samuel Lane	Power 1895a, 1389
Gerrard Street, Soho	?	George Derby Dermott (move from Chapel Street)	Power 1895b, 1453
Charlotte Street, Bloomsbury	–1845	George Derby Dermott (move from Gerrard Street)	Power 1895b, 1453
Bedford Square	1845–7	George Derby Dermott (move from Charlotte Street)	Power 1895b, 1453
Great Russell Street, Bloomsbury	1763–8	David Bayford	Lawrence 1996, appendix III
Finsbury Dispensary*	1805	Mr Taunton	Lawrence 1996, appendix III
10–11 Leicester Square*	1807–10	Charles Bell	Lawrence 1996, appendix III
Theatre of Anatomy, 18 Berwick Street, Soho	1818–20+	Herbert Mayo	Lawrence 1996, appendix III
22 Spring Garden*	1818–20+	Mr Pettigrew	Lawrence 1996, appendix III
13 St Saviour's Churchyard, Southwark	1820–	Edward Grainger	Lawrence 1996, appendix III
11 Gregory Place, Southwark	c 1820–	Mr Mason (Sir Astley Cooper, secondary/occasional staff member)	Millard 1825

* lecturing in anatomy or anatomy and surgery (dissection on-site is unclear from reference)

** became the Westminster Hospital Medical School

over the details of the practice of dissection (Richardson 2001, 98), anatomy classes were openly advertised in the press during the 18th and early 19th centuries. Lawrence (1996, 194) states that the newspaper-reading public did not pay much heed to where the corpses required for the many advertised lectures were obtained.

It seems that during the second decade of the 19th century the increase in student numbers led to a greater number of people trying to ply the 'resurrection' trade. This, in turn, raised public awareness of their practices (Cooper 1843, 345).

6.2 The dissection of criminals

In 1540 the newly formed Company of Barber-Surgeons was granted the annual right to the bodies of four hanged criminals (later raised to six) for the purposes of dissection (Richardson 2001, 32, 36). In 1565, the right was extended to the College of Physicians and Gonville Hall, Cambridge. Public dissection at

the Surgeons' Hall took place only a few times each year (the decision to move executions from Tyburn to Newgate was in part a result of the proximity to the Hall (ibid, 75)), but it was possible for individuals to request permission to carry out private dissections. The passing in 1752 of the 'Murder Act' (25 Geo II, c 37, 5) confirmed dissection as an alternative post-mortem punishment to display on the gibbet (Lane 2001, 27; Richardson 2001, 35; Cherryson 2010, 142), but shortages of bodies led to reports of surgeons bribing prisoners to sign over their corpses after execution (Richardson 2001, 52).

Following the formation of the Royal College of Surgeons in 1800 (Richardson 2001, 35), it had become customary for the conservator of their museum to carry out a token dissection, although bodies were often 'anatomised' elsewhere (Dobson 1951, 112). This means of obtaining subjects was available to the surgeons at the London Hospital and, indeed, the diaries of William Clift Snr, the first conservator of the museum of the Royal College of Surgeons, record that in January 1832 the body of the murderess Elizabeth Ross was delivered following her execution. Superficial cuts were made from the sternum to pubis and through muscles of the chest, after which the body was sewn up and 'ordered to be delivered to Mr Luke or his assistants at the London Hospital at six o'clock in the same evening precisely' (Dobson 1951, 120). A delicately rendered pencil sketch of Elizabeth on the mortuary table, by William Clift Jnr (William Home Clift), portrays her with technical accuracy but also with great humanity, including details down to her pierced ears (Fig 140).

The 38-year-old Ross was herself accused of disposing of her victim, an old woman called Caroline Walsh, to the anatomists, a rare example of a woman being directly involved in the procurement of bodies for dissection (the wife of the resurrectionist 'Patrick' being another: Chapter 8.1). Another convicted murderer, however, Bishop (below, 6.3) stated that he was sure that the murder had not been committed with the express purpose of selling the body as at that time of year (August) all the schools were closed and the price obtained would be very low. Selling the body on after the event might have seemed like a good way to cover up the murder or perhaps the anatomy schools were simply a convenient way for the authorities to excuse the fact that Walsh's body was never found (Dobson 1951, 120).

Importantly for the interpretation of the osteological evidence for dissection, Clift also noted that the hyoid was rarely broken despite hanging and, frighteningly, that several criminals' hearts had been beating when their chests were opened. This suggests that there would be no osteological indicators that a corpse had come from a legitimate source.

The association of dissection with capital punishment presented it as a 'fate worse than death' (Richardson 2001, 32)

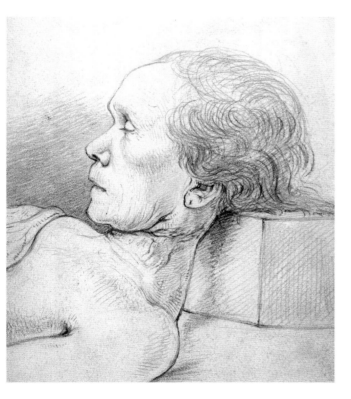

Fig 140 The body of Elizabeth Ross awaits dissection, 1832, drawn by William Home Clift (RCS, MS0007/1/6/3)

and may go some way towards explaining the public attitude towards dissection, which seems to have differed from that seen in continental Europe. A visitor in 1791 noted that the aversion of the English to dissection had resulted in both clandestine practices and great expense on the part of the surgeons (Lane 2001, 26).

6.3   Notorious practices?

Bodysnatching may have taken place in the late 17th century and certainly did so in the early 18th century, when Edinburgh medical students were required to pledge that they would not become involved in exhumations and bodies were more regularly bought and sold (Richardson 2001, 54–5). In 1795 a group of 15 resurrection men were exposed. They worked only in the winter, supplying eight surgeons and an 'articulator' from 30 burial grounds (ibid, 57). Because a body could not legally be owned, resurrectionists were prosecuted for stealing the clothes or belongings of the dead. Whilst stealing clothes was a felony, to steal a corpse was only a misdemeanour and so was a bailable offence (*The Times*, 15 October 1819, issue 10751, p 2, col A).

The mass graves of the poor may have provided easy access to multiple individuals, but class and wealth offered little protection from a strong-minded resurrectionist. Thomas Wakley, founder of *The Lancet*, stated that class paid no part in the decision to raise a particular body, whilst Sir Astley Cooper claimed to have little doubt that a determined resurrectionist would steal his body should they wish to (Richardson 2001, 61, 127, 117). If no digging were needed to obtain a body (expending effort and risking discovery) then so much the better. Bodies did not have to be 'resurrectionised' to make their way to the dissecting room illegally. In 1822, the undertaker of Horsemonger Lane jail was jailed for six months and fined 20s for selling on the body of an executed prisoner called Lees. Having taken money from the county for burial (3s) he proceeded to sell the body to Joshua Brookes and buried a coffin filled with rubbish (*Examiner*, Sunday 30 June 1822, issue 753). Another way to obtain a body for dissection was to pose as a relative and have the corpse signed over for private burial (Wise 2004, 33). Sextons and servants could be bribed and bodies could be taken whilst laid out before a funeral ceremony (Richardson 2001, 64–5). In 1831 a body was reportedly stolen from a wake (ibid, 102–3), and a police officer who gave evidence to the Select Committee on Anatomy claimed that he had recovered 50 bodies stolen from private houses (ibid, 22). Bodies were reportedly also stolen from coroners' offices and undertakers (Wise 2004, 41).

During the early 19th century there were several dramatic cases involving resurrectionists. The press appears to have been keen to portray the most sensational aspects of events, particularly in the years leading to the introduction of the Anatomy Act. Regardless of this, the general fear of the anatomists – a fear that crossed the boundaries of class – was such that watchers might be hired to protect a recent burial (Richardson 2001, 22, 99). Technology too could be used to combat bodysnatching, with the invention of the mortsafe (an iron cage that would surround the grave, used in Scotland), and a locking coffin, patented in 1818 (ibid, 81), an example of which can be found in the church crypt of St Bride's Fleet Street (Fig 141). Metal bands and multilayered coffins (one containing an undertaker!) used at Christ Church Spitalfields were also thought to have been intended to counter attempts at theft (Molleson and Cox 1993, 204–5). Such expensive deterrents were not widely used, however. Some burial grounds applied more generalised defences. Recalling his childhood, Thomas Catmur wrote in the *East London Observer* in 1914 that at Sheen's burial ground, Whitechapel, 'A big notice was displayed in the ground. "Beware of spring guns". This was to prevent "Body-snatching"' (THLHLA, *East London Observer* 1914, no page). Such methods were not always effective (Cooper 1843, 379).

Our subsequent view of the profession of body-dealing, for undoubtedly that was how it was seen by at least some contemporary observers (Cooper 1843, 345), has been somewhat coloured by reports of these events, which build up a picture of

teams of amoral resurrection men from the dregs of society, at any time just a hair's breadth from committing murder, skulking around cemeteries at night to hunt out the best prize, often to order, and fighting to sell it for the highest price. This may be partially accurate, but to suggest that it is the whole picture is to underestimate both the perceived necessity for human dissection, and the character of the (mostly) men who rose to supply such a demand.

Bransby Cooper (Sir Astley's nephew) stated that the 'gangs' were led by two men, (Ben) Crouch and Murphy, who operated in London during the second and third decades of the century respectively, with the other main protagonists named as Butler, Harnett, N——— (?Naples), Holliss, another Crouch (the younger brother of Ben), 'Patrick', L——— and Vaughan. Others who were from time to time involved were not professionals, but rather 'Spitalfields weavers and thieves' (Cooper 1843, 359, 410). Cooper had personal experience of some of the men working in the trade, and acquired further information about them from Sir Richard Owen, who stated that all the men had originally been part of one gang, splitting into two groups after an argument about prices (Richardson 2001, 66). Ben Crouch was a pock-marked prizefighter who worked at Guy's Hospital and dropped dead in the bar of a

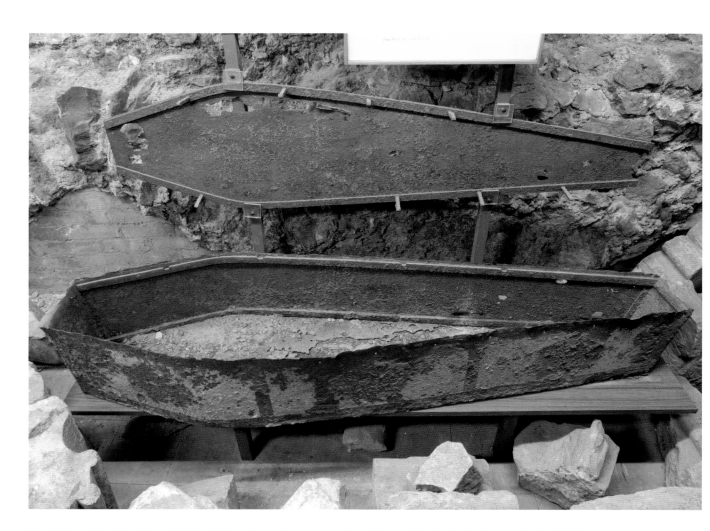

Fig 141 Iron coffin with a locking lid, believed to have been used to prevent bodysnatching, and found in the church crypt of St Bride's Fleet Street

public house in Tower Hill. Jack Harnett invested his earnings wisely and left 6000 guineas to his family, whilst Bill Harnett was a favourite of Cooper and worked with N———— (?Naples), himself employed by a Scot called White who did not engage directly in resurrection but made his money through trading), as a rival team to that of Crouch and Jack Harnett (Cooper 1843, 413–21). Murphy was clever, although uneducated, invested his earnings in property and left his wife and child well provided for. L————, on the other hand, is described as a gentleman's servant and a cheat (ibid, 435–6). 'Patrick' (a pseudonym for Cornelius Fitzgerald) was at one point apprehended in the burial ground of the London Hospital, a case that is discussed further in Chapter 8. By the late 1820s the select committee appointed to investigate the need for legislative change recorded that 'petty common thieves' were entering into the resurrection business (Richardson 2001, 116).

The resurrection men were sometimes commissioned to steal the corpses of particularly interesting subjects (Cooper 1843, 402–4). In 1823, the stolen corpse of a young boy was found already partially dissected at St Bartholomew's Hospital. The child had been suffering from an undiagnosed disease and upon his death the 'eminent medical practitioner' who had been caring for him asked to perform an autopsy. The boy's father reluctantly agreed and after examination the child was buried at Fish Street Hill (London EC3). Two days later it was noticed that his grave had been opened up and the body removed. It had been heard that St Bartholomew's had just received a fresh delivery and a search warrant was executed. When eventually permitted entry by the porter the party found the child in the dissecting room 'already in a state of fitness to be lectured on' ('Vice Chancellor's court', *Morning Chronicle*, 11 March 1823, issue 16814).

Most notorious of all are the reports of 'burking', murder to order, named after the infamous Edinburgh case of Burke and Hare, which came to court in 1828. Burke and Hare, when an old man died owing them money, had found that supplying bodies to a Dr Knox could be a lucrative business. They soon decided that they could cash in on the good prices obtained for a fresh corpse by creating them, and went on to murder 16 people (Richardson 2001, 132). This case led to widespread 'burkophobia' and the assumption that all bodysnatchers were potential murderers (ibid, 195). It was not just the public who feared that people were murdered for dissection (Fig 142). A Dr Thompson wrote during the rabies outbreaks of the early part of the century that he believed the state was sanctioning euthanasia of those suffering from hydrophobia, who would otherwise have died an agonising death, and that smothering these poor unfortunates provided a supply of bodies for dissection classes. This prompted the response in 1833 that since hydrophobia left no sign on the body, there was no need to dissect them (Pemberton and Worboys 2007, 17).

In London in 1830, Bishop, Williams and May were charged with the murder of an 'Italian boy' (Wise 2004). After their execution for the crime, Bishop and Williams were partially dissected by Sir William Blizard at the Royal College of Surgeons, before Bishop's remains were sent to King's College

London and William's to Little Windmill Street (Dobson 1951, 118). The use of dissection as a punishment in this case and after the execution of Burke strengthened public feeling against anatomical study (Richardson 2001, 143). Bishop had been a resurrectionist for 12 years before his arrest (Wise 2004).

In the early 19th century there was considerable confusion about the spiritual role of the body and there is little evidence for the attitudes of the general public or of family and friends of those whose bodies had been dissected (Richardson 2001, 15–17, 77). Public feelings at times ran high, as is evident from the near riot which occurred in Greenwich in 1832 after the arrest of one gang (Chapter 8.1) In the 1820s the family of one executed criminal in Carlisle had taken revenge on the anatomists who dissected him, killing one and shooting another in the face, but such extreme reaction was uncommon (ibid, 76). Some went as far as to suggest that the public were fairly indifferent to the practices of the medical men (letter of George Guthrie, 1829, quoted in Wise 2004, 175):

The doors of every dissecting-room in London are always open, there is nobody to watch them, they swing backwards and forwards on a pulley weight, they may shut of themselves, in case anybody leaves them open; every man may walk in and walk out wherever he please; many persons do, but no one gives himself any concern about what is going on. The neighbours care nothing about it, and unless, from some accident, the place becomes offensive, no one interferes … no one knows or cares what is going on, unless he is interested in it.

In 1843 Bransby Cooper noted that the resurrection men liked to keep the details of their work quiet, not so much from fears of public outrage as because there were 'considerably fewer persons than was generally supposed' carrying out this

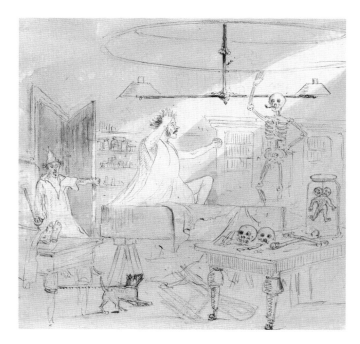

Fig 142 A man wakes up in his coffin in a dissecting room, in a drawing of the 1830s (Wellcome Library, London, L0039194)

work and that they wished to maintain this exclusivity. The resurrectionists were continually finding problems caused by people from outside the trade, who thought that bodysnatching sounded like an easy way to make money fast. The more secretive they were about their methods, the harder it was for others to steal the work (Cooper 1843, 353). To some extent, then, our view of the shady world of the resurrection men is a product of their own desire for commercial exclusivity.

Despite a notoriety that still inspires Hollywood today, there were actually comparatively few riots subsequent to arrests and indeed few prosecutions for bodysnatching. No medical practitioner was convicted for conspiracy or for possession of a stolen body until 1828, when a Liverpool anatomist was prosecuted for causing a body to be disinterred (Richardson 2001, 63, 59, 107). Richardson (ibid, 87) suggests that the scale of the trade must have been enormous in order to provide the schools with all they required but that if this were the case, discovery was rare (an efficient resurrectionist would leave no sign that a grave had been disturbed (ibid, 63)). This in turn supports the idea that most of the resurrection men were practised professionals, who knew and understood the market and were skilled at obtaining bodies from the least dangerous source possible (not always burial grounds), using methods that avoided detection.

6.4   The trade of the London resurrection men

Evidence presented to the select committee in 1828 demonstrated that it was possible for a sober man of good judgement to make a good living, if he supplied the schools (Richardson 2001, 58). The accounts of Joshua Naples show that the work provided a steady but relatively modest income (ibid, 68). Cooper (1843) also provides a fascinating insight into the men themselves and demonstrates that the resurrection trade could be a passport to financial security and respectability for the working classes, or a path to ruin.

The distances that the London resurrection men would travel for bodies appear to have been considerable. Vaughan was jailed twice, and seems to have moved around the country with his work (conveniently evading arrest: Chapter 8.1), whilst three members of the 'Borough gang' were charged with stealing a body from the churchyard at Seal near Sevenoaks in 1821. As they failed to appear at the Maidstone sessions to answer the charge, the report does not provide us with their names (*The Times*, 5 November 1821, issue 11395, p 3, col A). The body of Lawrence Sterne (the author of *The Life and Opinions of Tristram Shandy, Gentleman*) is reported to have been stolen from London and found in Cambridge (Richardson 2001, 60).

Some resurrection men would travel abroad to provide subjects for those in London. Writing in 1832, Lieutenant C Shaw, RA, recollected that during the Napoleonic campaigns he

had been stationed in northern Spain when his regiment had noticed a man wandering around their camp. The man spoke with their doctor, who later reported the stranger was a dissecting room attendant from London sent to the battlefields to obtain sets of teeth for London dentists. The man claimed that two colleagues had already returned home after obtaining many teeth following the battle of Vitoria (1813). Having missed this opportunity, he was anxious, and had been enquiring as to when the next action was likely to begin (Shaw 1832). Interestingly, this account is supported by the writings of Bransby Cooper, who states that Butler, a porter at St Thomas's Hospital, was sent to Spain during the Peninsular Wars to see what he could collect. Cooper had been in Spain in 1814 and was just re-entering France, at the village of Sarre, when Butler appeared with a message from Sir Astley. Butler was in some distress, having walked from Lisbon, and said, 'Oh Sir, only let there be a battle, and there'll be no want of teeth. I'll draw them as fast as the men are knocked down' (Cooper 1843, 401). This account corresponds so closely to that of Lieutenant Shaw that it leaves one to wonder if it might not refer to the same event, although Cooper further mentions that both Crouch and Harnett had worked in Spain, following behind the army (ibid, 414–15).

Back in London, at the start of each term the resurrection men would attend the hospitals they supplied and agree prices, implying that they would then work exclusively for the one institution, though it seems that no one really expected this exclusivity to last more than a week (Cooper 1843, 362). Cooper also refers to the 'moderate degree of circumspection' used by the resurrection men when delivering bodies to Sir Astley's rooms in St Mary Axe, whilst he was a pupil of Mr Henry Cline (ibid, 341). The accounts of the 'Italian boy' case provide insights into the trade in bodies. Bishop alleged that he had taken a hamper from just inside the gates of St Bartholomew's Hospital, where they were left out for the resurrection men for the transport of bodies for dissection (Wise 2004, 20). Bishop sold a woman to Appleton (Grainger's porter) for £10 and went to Webb Street when St Thomas's said they didn't need anything that day (ibid, 153). Much of the work was seasonal, running from October to April, though private schools also ran summer classes (ibid, 30). More money could be achieved for special cases, such as the brain of a lunatic woman who in the autumn of 1827 was the subject of an attempted bodysnatch from Wigginton's private burial ground, Golden Lane (ibid, 31).

The trade in 'stolen' bodies was only one part of the network that provided subjects for dissection, and within the medical profession it was not just tolerated but was seen as an integral part of restoring patients to health. Bransby Cooper spoke of how students sometimes accompanied the resurrection men, who were seen quite openly in hospitals at the start of term, whilst Sir Astley Cooper used his servant, Charles, as a go-between (Cooper 1843, 339, 440). The London Hospital was allegedly 'one of the most prolific sources from which to obtain subjects' (Millard 1825; Chapter 7.8).

The scale of the trade is still open to much debate. Bishop

claimed to have sold between 500 and 1000 stolen bodies to the London schools (Richardson 2001, 196). Research carried out by Elizabeth Hurren using records kept by St Bartholomew's Hospital indicates that in the decade after the passing of the Anatomy Act in 1832 anatomists there purchased 802 bodies for dissection, approximately 80 per year. These bodies came from a wide range of sources, predominantly from other hospitals, or from poor law infirmaries and workhouses, although the London Hospital is not listed as a supplier (Hurren 2012, 142, 145, 153).

Disagreements between hospitals and resurrectionists occurred. At St Thomas's Hospital in 1816 four resurrection men forced their way into the dissecting room, assaulted two students and cut to pieces two bodies that had been prepared for lectures. This was repeated a short time later when they destroyed the bodies of a man and a woman before being disturbed by the dissection room attendant. They then made their escape over the back wall of the hospital (*Morning Chronicle*, 25 December 1816, issue 14867). We can only guess that the motive for such an attack may have been financial (the hospital would now need more bodies, or perhaps they were not paying well enough), or that a change of supplier had left an aggrieved trader.

Despite the overwhelming documentary data, there is very limited archaeological evidence of bodysnatching. In part this is simply an effect of the fact that a coffin or individual removed from a busy cemetery would leave little trace, and that trace would be quickly dispersed by the arrival of new burials. Nonetheless, the published evidence is limited to an empty coffin recovered from the Quaker burial ground at Kingston-upon-Thames. Anna Barnard's burial had taken place in 1792, but her casket had been ripped open at the head end and only a blonde hairpiece remained. The vault was abandoned after Anna's burial and it is tempting to speculate that the theft of her remains may have played a part in this decision (Bashford and Sibun 2007, 111).

6.5   A necessary evil?

Many people held the view expounded by Thomas Wakley (*The Lancet*, Friday 15 May 1829, The Lancet, 12(298), 211) that anatomical study was 'an operation on the dead necessary for the benefit of the living'.

When a patient is admitted into the hospital, after having sustained a fracture of the thigh-bone, it will be of little good to that patient if the anatomist only correctly pronounces the nature of the injury received, points out the exact locality of the fracture, how many inches and lines it lies below the articulating head of the bone, at what distance it has occurred below the insertions of the psoas and iliacus muscles, and how the upper fragment rides above the lower one, which latter depends with the weight of the parts attached. This

knowledge, uncombined with some mechanical skill whereby he may obviate the false position of the parts implicated, will avail but little.

On the other hand, (and we need not remark upon it,) it is evident that the mere mechanical art, however perfect in itself, if it be unattended with a knowledge of the anatomy, will avail us little; whereas it is from a combination of both that the best mode of treatment is to be expected (Maclise 1846, 67).

The educational impetus behind dissection is emphasised by the 1801 statute of the Newcastle Infirmary requiring that 'an account of every case, operation, or dissection, which is rare, curious, and instructive, shall be drawn up by the physician or surgeon, under whose care it has been; and be entered in a register to be preserved as the property of the Infirmary' (Nolan 1998, 33). The registers there suggest that a quarter of the hospital dead went unclaimed (A Witkin, pers comm).

Anatomy lectures were not open for all. At the London Hospital, in 1832, the assistant apothecary, Blomfield, was censured for attending lectures when he was not permitted to do so (RLH, LH/A/5/19, 415) (apothecaries were considered the lowest in status of medical practicners and would be excluded from qualifying for a licence to dissect under the Anatomy Act (Richardson 2001, 213)). Expensive fees prevented all but the wealthy from study. A lecture course at Guy's Hospital cost £10 10s, as did a dissection course (Wise 2004, 162). George Birkbeck, however, presented a series of anatomy lectures at the London Mechanics Institute in 1827 that featured dissection and was open to the artisan class (Richardson 2001, 151).

Although dissection was presented as a vital branch of medical learning, there were alternatives available to the anatomists of the day. Prepared specimens (prosections) could be retained and used for numerous classes, whilst a wave of Italian migration after the Napoleonic wars brought a number of craftsmen who made, amongst other items, anatomical models (Wise 2004, 84–5).

If dissection were indeed an essential part of medical training, what alternative sources of supply were available? Sir Astley Cooper's discussions with fellow anatomists in 1823 considered all criminals dying in custody (not just the executed) to be a most suitable source, together with those dying in military and naval hospitals, suicides and the importation of bodies from abroad (Richardson 2001, 163). Hospitals caring for the poor were another obvious source of subjects (Lawrence 1996, 194). Voluntary donation was not considered a viable alternative by most, though a pledge initiated by a Dublin professor in 1828 had acquired 400 signatories by 1831 (Richardson 2001, 168), and small but significant numbers of both well-known and ordinary people are reported to have requested that their remains were dissected after death (ibid, 171, 172). There is at least one example where a donation was made by a relative on medical (rather than financial) grounds (ibid, 418). John Davis provides an example of a similar case at the London Hospital (Chapter 7.5).

6.6   The Anatomy Act

When Thomas Wakley, editor of the fledgling *Lancet*, wrote in 1824 of the necessity of dissection, he advocated a relaxation of the law to facilitate this (*The Lancet*, 8 February 1824, Resurrection men, 1(19), 194–5). Debate concerning the supply of bodies for dissection began in earnest in 1828, with the formation of a select committee. The committee was composed of members who were sympathetic to the draft Act and chose its witnesses carefully. Questioning was designed to present the resurrection men as the purveyors of an immoral trade whilst avoiding censure of the anatomists (Richardson 2001, 104, 109, 115). It was in the interest of the select committee to make a connection between bodysnatching and other criminal proclivities and this aspect was subsequently overemphasised (ibid, 70). The proposal was that the needs of the anatomists should be supplied by the unclaimed bodies of those who died in workhouses and hospitals (ibid, 198). Sir Astley Cooper felt that any change in the law would not reduce the theft of bodies, and that the increased risk would raise the price that was to be paid for them (ibid, 63). Wakley also expressed serious reservations over Henry Warburton's 'Unlawful disinterment and School of Anatomy Bill', which was read for the first time on 5 May 1829. Wakley thought that the Bill would 'neither facilitate the study of anatomy, put a stop to the disgusting system of exhumation, nor prevent the murder of human beings for the price of their corpses' (in this last point he was referring to the recent case of Burke and Hare, (above, 6.3). The fear of dissection after death was no deterrent for murder and so the dissection of the executed should be abolished in order to remove its association with criminality and the resulting stigma. This, Wakley felt, was 'throwing almost insuperable obstacles in the way of cultivating human anatomy' and that without equal and severe punishment of both resurrection man and medical receiver of stolen bodies, there would be little impetus for illegal trafficking to cease (*The Lancet*, Friday 15 May 1829, The Lancet, 12(298), 211–14).

The first Bill failed in part because it was seen as pursuing people after death and denying the poor a 'decent' burial (Richardson 2001, 157), but the case of Bishop, Williams and May – the London 'Burkers' – provided the Act with new impetus and it was passed on 1 August, despite the controversy over the emphasis it placed on dissecting the poor (ibid, 194, 292, 215). Little is known of how those in the workhouses reacted to the Act (ibid, 219).

An inspector of anatomy was appointed with an annual salary of £100 and the records show that there was considerable fluctuation in the available supply of bodies (Richardson 2001, 239, 245). The passing of the Anatomy Act did not have an immediate effect on the clandestine activities of the surgeons. The sexton of Cripplegate burial ground was caught transporting the body of a pauper to St Bartholomew's Hospital, but does not seem to have followed the procedures required by the Act in doing so. Richardson suggests that he was simply carrying on as he had done previously (ibid, 233). The Act did change the role of the resurrection men, though Joshua Naples's employment in the dissecting room of St Thomas's Hospital (ibid, 61) suggests that the surgeons still valued their skills. Crossland suggests that the new legislation perpetuated the differential treatment of strangers in a community because of the emphasis placed on the use of the unclaimed dead (2009, 104). In a diverse and fluid community such as that served by the London Hospital, however, defining a 'stranger' is somewhat problematic. The Act also led to the decline of the private schools in London from eight in 1826 to none by 1871 (ibid, 287).

Voluntary donation remained the exception and in the 1832 case of Charlotte Baume, who bequeathed her body and that of her child to London University, it was viewed with such suspicion that her brother was arrested for murder (Richardson 2001, 236). Wakley, meanwhile, claimed that 'Hospital surgeons know nothing of the law relating to dissection, and they appear to be desirous that it should be equally misunderstood by others' (*Morning Chronicle*, 2 March 1832, issue 19506).

7

Dissection and anatomical teaching at the London Hospital

Anatomy is studied with a view to perfect education … the happiness of many is to be confined to our care. (The Lancet, 8 October 1825, Mr Headington, 5(109), 64)

7.1   The medical school

From the time of his election in 1780, William Blizard emphasised his belief that the duty of a hospital was as much to teach as it was to care for the sick (Lawrence 1996, 34). In 1781 he requested permission from the house committee of the hospital to deliver two courses of lectures on anatomy and surgery, in the demonstrating theatre of the hospital. This was granted on his promise that no patients would form the subjects of anatomy classes (RLH, LH/A/5/10, 275). In 1782 the physicians and surgeons petitioned the committee to provide purpose-built facilities for anatomy lectures and it was agreed that a theatre could be built to the east of the house, but that the hospital would not contribute financially. Blizard and James Maddocks set about raising the finances required and the new theatre was opened in 1783. The college opened in 1785, and by 1799 Blizard was openly advertising the first practical anatomy classes associated with a London hospital (Lawrence 1996, 198, 202–4).

The school was built on land owned by the hospital but much of the money had been contributed by Blizard himself, and the school was essentially a private enterprise. On 24 February 1827, it was proposed that the hospital should take responsibility for the theatre in the medical school and should raise money 'for making such additions to the Building, the Museum, the apparatus, and the library as will render them more complete'. In addition, the governors noted that 'all preparations obtained from the Patients should be considered the property of the Hospital and added to the Museum' (RLH, LH/A/5/18, 128). This implies that it was regular practice to take specimens from the patients, though of course it does not state whether they were living or dead (Fig 143). In May 1831, the Society of Medical and Surgical Lecturers of the London Hospitals sent its rules to the house governor. This society's formative members included Mr Hamilton and Mr Adams, anatomical demonstrators (RLH, LH/A/5/19, 60–1). The death of Mr Headington (Chapter 5.9, 'The surgeons and physicians') in July 1831 gave the hospital the opportunity to buy the theatre and museum. The committee met on 4 August and 'unanimously resolved that any further consideration of the subject be for the present postponed' (ibid, 80, 91). After Blizard's death, the hospital governors recommended that all the staff should have a stake in the school. In March 1837 the house committee was informed that 'satisfactory arrangements had been made for the transfer of the Museum and other property connected with the Medical School In Trust for the Medical School of the London Hospital, the Lecturers in future to be elected by the Physicians and Surgeons of the Hospital' (RLH, LH/A/5/21, 413–14).

A letter written to *The Lancet* in March 1828 provides an insight into the workings of the classes. An anonymous student wrote to complain that the main incentive to study at the London Hospital was that you would receive your education from Mr Headington but that he had handed over his teaching to Mr Luke, who was such a poor teacher that many students

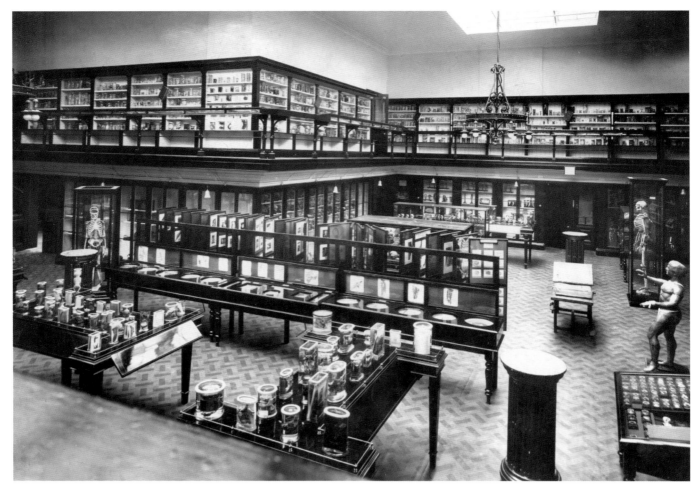

Fig 143   The pathology museum of the London Hospital Medical College, 1899 (Royal London Hospital Archives, RLHMC/P/4)

had given up attending (*The Lancet*, 29 March 1828, Complaints of a pupil against Mr Headington, 9(239), 944). The pupils subsequently held a meeting and, after discussing whether anyone of importance actually read *The Lancet*, decided that the best course of action was to reassure Mr Luke that they were all very happy with his teaching (*The Lancet*, 14 November 1829, London Hospital, 13(324), 250–1).

By 1833 lectures were offered in a wide range of subjects. Pupils could pay individually or attend all the courses of lectures for a fee of £50, 'qualifying for the Royal College of Surgeons' and Apothecaries' Hall' (Figs 144–5). In 1837 the courses offered over the autumn term were similar, with the addition of morbid anatomy, with practical illustrations, with Mr T B Curling, comparative anatomy, with Dr W J Little, and clinical lectures by Dr Gordon, Dr Davies, Mr Scott and Mr Luke (*Hull Packet*, 8 September 1837, issue 2753).

An introductory lecture from Mr Headington outlines the general structure of his course. The first classes 'shall make a few observations on animal matter in general', then blood; cellular membrane; bones; diseases; mycology, joints, ligaments and cartilages; the cardiovascular system; the lungs; arteries, veins and 'absorbents'; glands; brain and nerves; and finally the organs with specific mention of the stomach. The second part of the course concentrated on the practice of surgery and,

finally, issues of aftercare were addressed. Headington then moved to the anatomical part of the course stating 'there are many opportunities given us of treating on surgical cases, and this method relieves us from a sameness of description, and adds the charm of interest to that of variety' (*The Lancet*, 8 October 1825, Mr Headington, 5(109) 61–4). This suggests that we might not be able easily to differentiate the two in the osteological material and that the courses did not follow a strict pattern but were structured according to the available material and patients. He further stated that students needed to attend two courses of lectures, observing the demonstrations before they attempted to take notes and should only look at 'anatomical plates' once they had made 'considerable progress' in anatomy (ibid, 64).

It is clear that there was an opportunistic element to the structure of the classes, and with this in mind it is no surprise to find that the admissions policy of the hospital had a direct effect on what the pupils learnt. In 1846 there was a complaint from a student that despite the fact that syphilis was rife in the city, it was impossible to learn about the symptoms and treatments of the disease at the London Hospital as sufferers were excluded (*The Lancet*, 26 December 1846, Impossibility of studying syphilis at the London Hospital, 48(1217), 700). The osteological evidence, however, suggests that syphilitics were

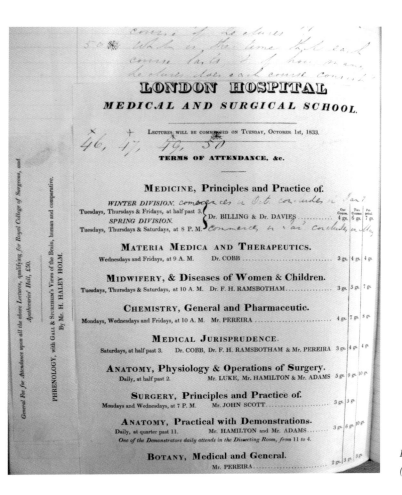

Fig 144 Flyer for the London Hospital lecture series, 1833–4 (Royal London Hospital Archives, RLH, LH/A/5/20, 299)

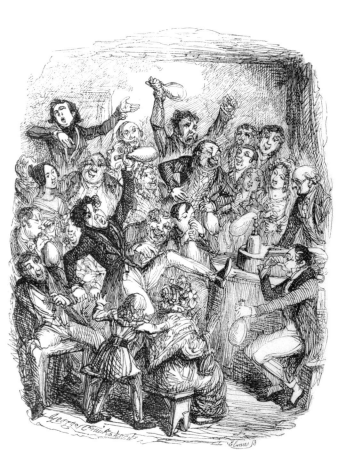

Fig 145 Students experimenting with laughing gas, drawn by George Cruikshank, from Chemistry no mystery *by John Scoffern, a lecturer at the London Hospital Medical College (London, 1839) (Wellcome Library, London, M0009666)*

probably occasionally dissected.

Writing in 1829, Wakley was keen to emphasise the, as he felt, inflated price of anatomical study, urging that 'the student should only be subjected to such an expense for bodies as must necessarily arise from their conveyance to the dissecting-room, and the expenses of "burying the remains"' (*The Lancet*, Friday 15 May 1829, The Lancet, 12(298), 213).

In 1832, the pupil's admission fee was reduced from 30 to 20 guineas (RLH, LH/A/5/19, 232). By 1834, the London Hospital was charging £5 5s or £10 10s for anatomy classes (6 months or a year); a physician's pupil had to pay 10 guineas for 12 months or 20 guineas for a perpetual position plus an apothecary's fee of 1 guinea; a surgeon's pupil paid 20 guineas for 12 months; and a dressing pupil paid 30 guineas (or 20 guineas for six months) plus a library fee of 1 guinea (*The Lancet*, 27 September 1834, Account of the hospitals and schools of medicine in London, London Hospital School and practice, 23(578), 9). Visiting pupils could access the surgical wards and operating theatre but

153

were not permitted to dress or direct any patient or reside in the hospital, whereas house or dressing pupils were permitted to do so (Chapter 5.9; RLH, LH/A/5/19, 235, 241).

It seems that studying at the London was very popular, possibly because of the ready supply of cadavers, for in November of the same year (shortly after the start of term), *The Lancet* reported in terse fashion that Valentine had instructed a beadle to be stationed at the door of the hospital to refuse entry to anyone who had not paid the appropriate fee (*The Lancet*, 8 November 1834, London Hospital, 23(584), 272) (Fig 146). The slant of the article, railing against the strictures placed on students, reflects the ongoing animosity between the editor, Wakley, and the staff of the London Hospital (in particular Blizard and Headington); during the early years of the journal, reports of cases from the London are notably absent.

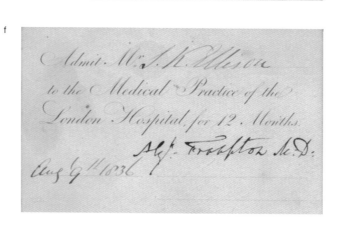

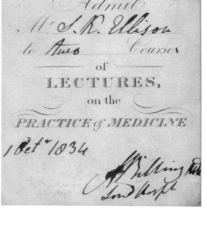

Fig 146 Samuel K Ellison's tickets for lectures during the 1830s (Royal London Hospital Archives, RLH, PP/KIT/1–4, 6, 8)

7.2 The surgeons' beadle and the hospital dead

In addition to his other duties (Chapter 5.9), the surgeon's beadle held the keys to the 'dead house' (*The Times*, 8 October 1823, issue 11996, p3, col D) and played a key role in the provision of bodies for dissection. The position was paid for by the staff and pupils, the latter paying 5s for six months' assistance in 1829 (RLH, LH/A/5/18, 291). The beadle also received 'a guinea a year from the Samaritans Society for taking care of and giving out when ordered the old clothes of deceased patients buried at the Hospital' (RLH, LH/A/5/18, 4 March 1828, 201). There were also other lucrative possibilities for the less scrupulous, and perhaps the most profitable activity that the surgeon's beadle engaged in, prior to the Anatomy Act at least, was the exhumation and supply of bodies to the pupils of the medical college, who, according to one observer, paid 6 guineas for each subject to the beadle and the attendant of the dissecting room (Millard 1825, 25). It is possible that it was the cessation for the surgeon's beadle of this means of remuneration on the passing of the Anatomy Act in 1832 that caused the difficulties encountered in retaining staff in the role during the later 1830s (Chapter 5.9)

An 1826 missive (RLH, LH/A/5/18, 85) from the parish of Whitechapel outlined:

Parish of St Mary White Chapel 29th April 1826

Gentlemen
The Trustees of this Parish have desired me to request that you will have the goodness to give directions to the proper officer in your establishment to forward to me early information whenever any unknown Corpse is brought into your Hospital in order that publick [sic] notice may be immediately given of the circumstance.

John Smith

The surgeon's beadle was instructed to provide the relevant information (RLH, LH/A/5/18, 86), indicating that he was the recipient of unknown corpses. He was also ordered to demand the warrant for burial before letting the coroner leave the premises with any body (ibid, 90).

Although the surgeon's beadle clearly played the pivotal role in the provision of subjects for dissection, his was not the only post with duties towards the dead. 'The Chaplain shall keep a list of all patients buried in the Hospital ground, and the Steward shall take receipt for each body taken away' (1810: RLH, LH/A/1/4, 16).

The (post-Anatomy Act) by-laws outline the revised duties of the beadle (RLH, LH/A/1/7, 66–7):

3. He shall take care after the death of any patient, that the body be removed from the ward, as soon as propriety shall admit.

4. He shall have the charge of the room in which the bodies are deposited, and take care that it be clean and in order: and he shall not allow any person admission, without the leave of a Physician or Surgeon.

5. He shall take care that no body be removed from the Hospital within 24 hours after death except by permission of the Medical officer, under whose care the patient may have been. The removal must be made in the summer, between six and seven in the morning or eight and nine in the evening and in the winter, between seven and eight in the morning or five and six in the evening; and no post mortem examination shall take place, but in the presence of one of the Medical officers of the Hospital. He shall take from the friends of the deceased, a certificate of the removal.

6. He shall supply the Chaplain with the name, age, occupation, and residence of such registered. And he shall not allow any corpse to be taken away from the Hospital without the Chaplain's [crossed out and replaced with House Governor] permission'

[Handwritten additions from 18 October 1832]: every body removed … for the purpose of anatomical examination, shall, previously to removal be placed in a decent coffin or shell and removed therin, and he shall give notice to the Chaplain, of every such removal, within six hours after it takes place.

The removal of the dead from the wards was supposed to be highly regulated but was 'constantly violated when it ought to be rigidly enforced and if it had been it is believed that the inducement to give bribes would be diminished' (RLH, LH/A/5/18, 200). Bodies were supposed to be rapidly sent to the dead house, wrapped in their bedsheets, presumably acting as a makeshift shroud, before the sheets were removed to be washed (ibid, 4 March 1828, 200). In 1832 the house visitors complained that 'dead bodies are not removed so early after death as they should be from the relative wards' (RLH, LH/A/16/4, 110–11).

7.3 Attitudes of those at the London Hospital towards their patients and the dead

There has been much discussion of the reflection of contemporary social attitudes provided by the subjugation of the poor by the upper-class medical men, collecting the destitute dead for their own ends. Richardson (2001, 50) goes so far as to suggest that the treatment of the poor in charitable institutions was simply a means of experimenting with medicinal techniques before treating the wealthy. Although it is difficult to piece together evidence for hospital governors' attitudes to the practice of dissection, Lawrence (1996, 194) identifies both 'outright ignorance' and 'tacit tolerance in exchange for discretion'. Crossland suggests that the practice of anatomy did not just objectify individuals, but even discriminated between them by treating different 'types' of body in different ways, removing the dissected dead from the context of funerary ritual and 'detaching the anatomised body from human relationships' (Crossland 2009, 102–3).

Contemporary writings shed a subtle and nuanced light on the outlook of the surgeons at the London Hospital. It is clear that attitudes towards the dead were as individual then as they are today. The principle of clinical detachment was still evolving in the early 19th century, whilst contemporary writers recognised the difference between dissection as an abstract concept and as a practice involving known people (Richardson 2001, 31, 77). We are fortunate to have been left a clear account of the attitudes of the man who was perhaps the most influential of the teachers at the London, Richard Headington (Fig 112).

A report of his introductory lecture for the winter series of surgical classes, given at the theatre of anatomy, on the evening of Wednesday 6 October 1824, outlined human dissection as a necessary evil saying (*The Lancet*, 9 October 1824, Mr Headington, 3(54), 35) that:

those who promoted it [the study of anatomy] rightly judged, that he who is best acquainted with the structure and functions of the human body, in a state of health, must be the best capable of detecting and curing disease … the movements of the animal machine are so various…without an accurate investigation of the machine itself, it is impossible they can ever be understood.

Without knowledge of 'minute' anatomy, Headington cautioned, surgeons could make terrible mistakes. He also emphasised the importance of listening to one's living patients and taking notes at the bedside, stating that 'an unfeeling heart, harshness of character, or insensibility to human suffering, should form no part of a surgeon's composition' (ibid, 35–6). These views were repeated in his introductory lectures: 'anatomy is studied with a view to perfect education, and … the happiness of many is to be confined to our care', though he admitted 'there are prejudices to surmount, and difficulties to overcome of a peculiar nature, but which even the anatomist would not wish to have entirely removed' (*The Lancet*, 8 October 1825, Mr Headington, 5(109), 63–4). Headington's writing clearly emphasises the humanity of the dead but values the health of the living as paramount.

Headington was not alone in expounding this view. Writing nearly a decade later, after his introductory lectures at the London Hospital, Dr Gordon (1833, 11, 14) advocated the 'careful cultivation of morbid or pathological anatomy', stating that 'the philosophy of pathological anatomy – a philosophy extracted from the loathsome pursuits of the dissecting-room – appears to me to consist principally in the necessity it inculcates of daily correcting our previous impressions of

disease, and adhering with unshaken firmness to the method of induction from observation'. Further, he was not just concerned with the fate of the poor on the slab: he compelled his students to 'cherish humanity and minute consideration for the comfort of the poor', urging, 'the physician learns to disregard the fictitious distinctions of rank, and to contemplate before him, simply, a human being, and that being suffering' (ibid, 16, 17). These words were backed up with action: many of the medical staff at the London sat on the committee of the Samaritan Society, itself founded by Sir William Blizard, which raised and distributed funds to assist patients and their families (Chapter 5.6).

Even Wakley felt that dissection was necessary, stating that if 'dead bodies cannot be procured, it will be impossible for the pupils to learn anatomy, and without anatomy, neither surgeons nor physicians can practise with the least prospect of benefiting their patients' (*The Lancet*, 25 January 1824, Dissection, 1(17), 135). This position seems to have had widespread public support: surgeons needed to practise and it was best that they did so on the dead (Richardson 2001, 120).

If we can be fairly sure that Headington and Gordon saw dissection of cadavers as preferable to the butchery of the living, and instilled the same values in their pupils, the relationship between the hospital and dead patients is not as easy to define. Staff and patients certainly seem to have attended the funerals of those who died on the premises (Chapter 3.2).

The views of the house governor and chaplain also had influence. Valentine was almoner of the Samaritan Society and a committed Christian who went out of his way on numerous occasions to help patients, sometimes at the expense of his relationship with the medical staff and the house committee. Initially, his views on the practices in the hospital's medical school placed him in conflict with both the school and with the governors: 'the subject was brought, incidentally, before the Committee in November [1822], + several present expressed their opinion that the Bodies of Patients unclaimed by their friends, should be devoted to the school; at that time I dissented from that opinion'; by the following year he 'could scarcely make up [his] mind between the claims of professional science, + the feelings of regret that such proceedings should be necessary' (RLH, LH/A/17/3, 75–7). It is clear from Valentine's comments that at least some of the governors knew both what went on within the school and how it was supplied with subjects.

We also know that Valentine made efforts to ensure that at least the patients who were devoted to the school received a funeral service. Richardson (2001, 17) defines a decent burial as that which followed an accepted combination of religious and community rituals – for example, the wake. When William Woodman 'died in the House during the past week in great penury', Valentine wrote that 'his family were left without even the means of giving his remains a decent interment'. The committee advanced 3 and a half guineas to pay for his funeral (RLH, LH/A/5/19, 282). The case implies that burial within the hospital ground wasn't considered 'decent' even by its own chaplain.

7.4 Supplying subjects to the dissecting room

Before the passing of the Anatomy Act in 1832, the dissecting rooms of most of the schools in London were supplied chiefly by the resurrection men (Chapter 6.4). At the schools attached to hospitals, the bodies of unclaimed patients sometimes ended up on the dissection table, but this was not in general the chief source from which they were supplied. Although Ann Millard, writing in 1825, claimed that staff at St Thomas's received money for handing unclaimed bodies over to the school, a student declared that during the early 19th century 'obtaining a subject from the dead-house was a matter of great rarity' (South 1970, 96). Contemporary observers, however, noted that there was one school in London where the reverse was true – the medical college attached to the London Hospital (Millard 1825, 25):

> the dissecting room of the London Hospital is *entirely* supplied by subjects, which have been their own patients: and that every facility may be afforded for this purpose, the dissecting room has a door opening into the burial ground of the Institution, where, those who have died in the Hospital are sometimes interred for the sake of appearances, and whence they may be easily transferred to the dissecting room, as occasion may require. During the winter, the professors of the London Hospital keep all who die, under their care, for *home consumption*; in the summer they have enough and some to spare; with which ... they accommodate their less fortunate brother professors.

Ann Millard's claims are also supported by an entry in the house governor's report book from 1823. After Valentine was pressed by the house committee to make enquiries of the medical staff he reported back to them that (RLH, LH/A/17/3, 78):

> I have had an opportunity of conferring with Mr Headington [surgeon and lecturer in the medical college], who informed me, that during the winter months in which dissections and Lectures are given, the School is supplied with subjects chiefly from the Burying Ground of the Hospital, + that <u>He himself</u> pays the Theatre + <u>Surgery beadle</u> for their trouble in procuring them from the Ground with as much secresy and delicacy as possible; that this is the practice of <u>other Hospitals</u>, + has been of <u>this</u>, ever since there have been Lectures and dissections here, + no obstacles have been thrown in the way by the house committee, but they had always calculated on their conviction of its necessity, + therefore on their affording every facility, except their <u>public</u> concurrence.

Ann Millard further stated that Hurst, the surgeon's beadle, and Cobley, the anatomy assistant, would charge the students 6 guineas for each body, which they would then 'resurrectionise' (1825, 5). She also notes that after her husband's arrest and conviction two other men were apprehended by vigilant police officers in the hospital burial ground. Dismissed by the magistrate, they returned to the burial ground to continue disinterring a body, which they removed to the hospital's dissecting room (ibid, 33). Ann Millard believed that the hospital had influenced the magistrate, and confronted Valentine when she petitioned the house committee, who replied that 'the governors might think proper "to wink" at what their servants did' (ibid, 49). Indeed, Valentine's reports and the minutes of the house committee confirm that this was the case.

The London differed from other hospitals in another important respect, too. At St Thomas's, which was presumably not alone in the practice, there were reports that bodies were transferred directly from the dead house to the dissecting room, and that sham funerals were performed over coffins full of nothing but stones, brickbats and sawdust (Millard 1825, 9, 56). What happened to the remains after they had been dissected was not recorded, but archaeological investigations have provided some evidence. Crossland states that most archaeological evidence for dissection was of discarded 'dumps' of human and animal bone found close to the anatomy schools through which they had passed, arguing that burial in a churchyard was clearly not thought 'necessary or suitable' (Crossland 2009, 107). Cherryson says that between 1751 and 1832 the subjects of dissection 'were unlikely to be afforded formal burial at all' and that only after 1832 would their remains be found within the burial grounds attached to those institutions from whom bodies could be legally sourced (2010, 137).

It seems likely that it was the personal efforts of William Valentine that changed the way things were done at the London. Millard wrote that 'he is a strenuous advocate for the rights of the church, and the strict observance of decency, seldom permitting a deceased patient to be dissected before burial, as such a practice would obviously tend to diminish the fees for interment' (Millard 1825, 27). What we know of Valentine's views about dissection (above, 7.3) suggests that Millard's assessment of his motivations was perhaps unfair. It is not clear whether he was in fact paid any extra fee for performing funerals (and in any case he would have received any fee payable whether he performed a funeral over an empty coffin or a full one). It is likely that John Flint South was referring to Valentine when he claimed that at one hospital in London, which supplied its own school with subjects, the chaplain eventually decided that 'he would not read the service over coffins full of stones any longer' (South 1970, 96).

Whether those at work in the London Hospital saw the obtaining of subjects (by definition unclaimed) from the hospital burial ground as morally preferable to obtaining them from other cemeteries, we will never know. The hospital was not above examining its own staff after death (below, 7.8, 'Coroner's inquests and autopsy'), but the London was certainly not the only hospital to obtain subjects for dissection from within its own walls. The burial registers from Newcastle Infirmary show that, in general, the interval between death and burial was two to three days. A longer interval gave rise to suspicions that the individual was being dissected (Nolan 1998, 56).

Although unclaimed bodies from the London were the main source of supply for its school, there were others. Sometimes, for a particular lecture, they might require a subject that could not be supplied from within the school: 'Cobley, the dissecting room man at the London Hospital, came to St Thomas's from Mr Headington, with his compliments, requesting a young subject for the blood vessels' (Millard 1825, 24). There were also legally acquired bodies, such as that of the executed murderess Elizabeth Ross (Chapter 6.2). It is also clear that at times the hospital had a surplus of unclaimed patients, and was involved in supplying other schools of anatomy with subjects.

7.5   The donation of John Davis

Richardson has described in depth the feelings of the poor towards the prospect of dissection, which violated traditional views about what should happen to the body after death. She records a number of unusual cases in which people offered their bodies for dissection in the years leading up to the passing of the Anatomy Act, for motives such as atheism, 'enlightened self interest', those 'with some axe to grind' or 'with some trait of eccentricity, or which rendered their gesture newsworthy' (2001, 171–2). They include a woman who was a patient at St Thomas's Hospital in 1828 and a patient at Bristol Infirmary who bequeathed his body for dissection in the same year (ibid, 172–3). More than a decade previously, in January 1816, a patient at the London Hospital by the name of John Davis donated his body after his death to Headington, who had once treated him (RLHMC/PM/6/33):

> Mr Headington
> London Hospital
> January 26 1816
>
> Sir,
> I take the liberty of addressing these few lines to you, being of a curious subsistence, having had my legs brook ten different times, and was a patient in the London Hospital three different times under Mr Greenland and once under Sir W Blizard and once under Mr Thos Blizard, and was once under Mr Haddington [sic] and once under Mr Yelloly and six different times under Mr A Cooper the Helder [sic], once under Mr A Cooper in Guys Hospital, and once under Mr Lucas in Guys Hospital, and Mr Forster of (?).
>
> Therefore, Sir, I hope you will excuse the liberty I have taken in this way being in the greatest distress, it is my wish to dispose of my Body, after the departure of this life, to you, therefore Sir, I request your final answer as I remain your
>
> Most Obedt and
> Humble Servt
> John Davis

This man is again a patient in the London Hospital for the eleventh Broken Leg.

Although it contains errors and spelling mistakes the letter is written in a good hand, and paints a curious picture. Davis seems to take a certain pride in the long list of eminent surgeons and physicians under whose care he had been placed, and their interest in him as a patient. Perhaps he hoped to achieve a kind of immortality by maintaining that interest after his own death. We cannot know his precise motivations, but his letter is certainly unusual.

7.6   The influence of the Anatomy Act

In September 1832, the house committee resolved to hold a special meeting (RLH, LH/A/5/19, 325):

> on Wednesday next the 3rd day of October at 11 o'clock precisely; to take into consideration those clauses in the new Act of parliament relative to the Anatomical Dissection of the dead bodies, which affect the Surgical Schools of this Hospital; and to pass such Resolutions as may be deemed advisable, respecting the disposal of the remains of those Patients who may die in the House, and be unclaimed after their decease by friends or relatives.

This special meeting seems to have involved discussion of whether or not they could ignore the Act as (ibid, 326) they:

> resolved that it is the imperative duty of the House Committee to defer to that which has now become the law of the land. The Surgery Beadle was called in and the above Resolution having been read to him, he was enjoined to attend to the instructions of the Medical Officers of the Institution, as to the most unexceptionable mode of carrying it into effect.

On 4 October 1832 'Reverend W Valentine made an enquiry respecting the interment of bodies after having been submitted to anatomical examination but a reply to the question was deferred until there should be a larger number of the Committee in attendance' (RLH, LH/A/5/19, 328). Then on 11 October (ibid, 339):

> The Chaplain repeated a request that the Committee would take into their most serious consideration whether the Burial Service can with propriety be performed at the interment of the remains of such bodies of Patients as may have been submitted to Anatomical examination; and if so what possible provisions may be made, with a view of precluding such a performance from being a desecrating of that most solemn and affecting service of the Church. Resolved that the particular attention of the Surgeons and Assistant Surgeons be

called to Section 13 of the Act … and that they be informed the Committee can only permit such anatomical examination as is consistent with the said section and for the purpose the remains of each body must be kept separate and distinct.

Following this the standing orders were changed to require that the bodies be contained within coffins and that the surgeons should provide a certificate of identity for each patient to William Valentine (RLH, LH/A/5/19, 340). Section 13 of the Anatomy Act was then copied into the minutes (ibid):

Provided always and be it enacted that every such Body so removed as aforesaid for the purpose of examination shall, before such removal, be placed in a decent coffin or shell and removed therin and that the party removing the same, or causing the same to be removed as aforesaid, shall make provision that such Body after undergoing anatomical examination be decently interred in consecrated ground, or in some public Burial Ground in use for persons of that religious persuasion to which the person whose Body was so removed belonged and that a certificate of the interment of such Body shall be transmitted to the Inspector of the District within 4 weeks after the day on which such Body was received.

Alfred Hamilton, assistant surgeon and lecturer in anatomy at the London Hospital, wrote to James Somerville, the inspector of anatomy, to complain that the particulars of the Anatomy Act as they related to burial were not being observed by the anatomist Lane: 'the Coffin from your School containing the remains of a body for interment, if opened, as sometimes happens, by the Parish Authorities would have led to exposures and to results the occurrence of which it is not possible to contemplate without serious alarm' (Richardson 2001, 364). Richardson suggests that Hamilton's letter may have been a calculated move to discredit one of the private anatomy schools that was in competition for students with the London, but it is equally possible that Hamilton's misgivings about the practices of Lane's school were genuine.

In December 1832 the new Act was used to facilitate the dissection of Mary Ann (Polly) Chapman at the London Hospital, against the wishes of her friends. Polly, a prostitute in her 20s, had drowned herself, her suicide having been precipitated by being thrown out of her lodgings because she could not pay her rent. Mr Holiday, the churchwarden, asked the coroner, Mr Baker, whether he could pass her body to the hospital since it remained unclaimed. Baker agreed to this, seeing the move as a deterrent to others contemplating suicide. Polly's friends were much distressed by this, having raised £3 to pay for her burial, but the coroner was adamant and used the Anatomy Act as justification (Richardson 2001, 234–5). It is likely that Polly's remains are amongst those that were excavated.

The Whitechapel workhouse refused to cooperate with the new Act and it seems that the parish beadle took matters into his own hands, coming to an illegal arrangement with the London Hospital to circumvent the workhouse master (Richardson 2001, 243).

In the years immediately following the Act, some medical schools found that they did not have sufficiently good parish connections to enable them to obtain bodies, and it seems that those who had a surplus were not always willing to assist, preferring to bury bodies rather than pass them on (*The Lancet*, 6 December 1834, Supply of subjects for dissection, 23(588), 394–6). Whilst there is evidence that at Newcastle (end date 1845) the Anatomy Act was the catalyst for a reduction in the number of anatomised bodies over time (Crossland 2009, 109), this reduction does not seem to have been repeated at the London Hospital. Data from the inspector of anatomy's returns in fact show a slight increase in the number of bodies obtained from hospitals in the years immediately after the introduction of the Act, from 135 bodies in 1832–3 to 206 in 1835–6 (Fig 147).

In September 1833 (post-Anatomy Act), someone accused the teachers at the London Hospital of dealing with bodysnatchers and appropriating funds from the pupils to buy bodies for the lectures. In the previous winter the price the pupils paid for bodies had been fixed at 4 guineas, with any surplus to be divided and given back at the end of the season. In response J Luke, Alfred Hamilton and John Adams wrote to *The Lancet* to outline the financial position (*The Lancet*, 21 September 1833, Vindication of the teachers of anatomy against the charge of making a profit on subjects for dissection, 20(525), 826):

actual cost of bodies used by lecturers – £5 19
Payment by lecturers to general fund – £13 11
Payment more than actual cost – £7 12
actual cost of bodies used by pupils – £31 1
Payment by pupils to general fund – £20 0
Actual cost more than payment – £11 1

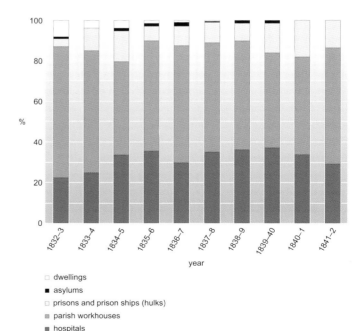

Fig 147 Origins of bodies obtained for anatomical dissection; taken from the inspector of anatomy's returns for 1832–3 to 1841–2 (Richardson 2001, 293)

The information suggests that the students had only five bodies that year. The hospital also sent £41 11s 4d worth of bodies to other schools, receiving £44 8s 0d in payment for them (and therefore making a small profit). 'Should it be asked why so many bodies were sent away, it may be answered that, no applications for bodies from our own pupils were on the list, and that the want of bodies at other schools was very great' (ibid).

7.7   Vivisection and comparative anatomy

James Morris with Natasha Powers

They who object to the putting of animals to death for a scientific purpose, do not reflect that the death of an animal is a very different thing from that of a man. To an animal, death is an eternal sleep; to a man, it is the commencement of a new and untried state of existence (Dr Blundell, quoted in Cooper 1843, 145).

Animals were viewed as essential tools in anatomical and medical training. Bransby Cooper described the necessity of surgeons working on 'the lower classes of animals' (Cooper 1843, 143). In part this represented the continuation of a tradition deeply rooted in the history of anatomy – Aristotle had undertaken animal dissections in the 4th century BC and Galen in the 2nd century AD (Hart et al 2008, 18). William Harvey, a surgeon at St Bartholomew's Hospital, outlined in the mid 17th century how his experiments on circulation had been elucidated by the vivisection of numerous species including pigs, dogs, toads and frogs, snakes, fish and shrimp and even 'house-snails' (Keynes 1928, 19). The early 1800s was also the time of the 'polite' gentleman scientist (Walters 1997), with individuals such as Samuel Johnson, William Stukeley and John Hunter interested in many aspects of natural philosophy. When Richard Owen posthumously published John Hunter's (1861) *Essays and observations on natural history, anatomy, physiology, psychology and geology*, it was noted that some 500 different species were represented by the 13,683 specimens in the Hunterian Museum (Dobson 1962). Animals were also examined and experimented upon as part of public anatomy 'shows' alongside human cadavers (Lansbury 1985; Guerrini 2004; Kalof 2007, 124).

For those individuals whose primary interests were anthropocentric, the greatest use of comparative anatomy was to throw light upon human anatomy. Two contemporaries of Blizard wrote (Cooper and Travers 1818, 112):

In collecting evidence upon any medical subject, there are but three sources from which we can hope to obtain it; from observation on the living subject from examination of the dead; and from experiments upon living animals. By the first, we learn the history of disease; by the second, its real nature,

so far as it can be certainly known; and by experiments upon living animals, we ascertain the processes resorted to by nature for restoring parts which have sustained injuries, and then apply that knowledge to accidents in man.

James Douglas (1760, 199–205) recommended comparing quadrupeds with humans, particularly the digestive system of ruminants, the action of the diaphragm in a rabbit, the uterus of a cow and, notably, the internal and external structures of the ear (Douglas advised looking at this structure in seven or eight different animals). A hen and a cockerel were to be dissected for observations on the reproductive and urinary systems. The circulatory system was to be demonstrated and compared to that of a whiting, whilst oyster, skate and lobster were also to be examined. Throughout his text Douglas noted the differences between human physiology and that of the dog.

Sir Astley Cooper kept as many as 30 dogs and other animals in the hayloft of his London house. His servant, Charles, coordinated the obtaining of these animals and Sir Astley would pay half a crown per dog, which his nephew Bransby feared meant that people were inclined to steal dogs to sell on for profit. Sir Astley also secured specimens from other sources, obtaining exotic animals from the Tower menagerie once they had died (he once dissected an elephant in public) and specimens of unusual fish and poultry from the more mundane markets of London (Cooper 1843, 334–8). Dogs appear to have been commonly used in vivisection. The Wellcome collections, for example, hold three specimens of bone prepared by Henry Cline (who was Astley Cooper's tutor), which were etched with designs (including his name!), then fed to a dog (Fig 148). After nine hours Cline cut open the dog's stomach and removed the bone to demonstrate to students at St Thomas's the corrosive properties of gastric acids.

Comparative anatomy classes were certainly held at the London Hospital (below, 7.8), but Shaw, writing in 1822, felt that 'more use should be made of the bodies of animals than is generally done' (1822, iv). As attitudes began change, the Royal Society for the Protection of Animals was formed in 1824. By 1870, little vivisection took place in Britain, and the rise of the antivivisectionist movement led to a Royal Commission report in 1876 and the subsequent Cruelty to Animals Act of the same year (Boddice 2011, 216).

Many of the faunal remains recovered from the London Hospital consisted of complete or partial associated bone group (ABG) deposits, in association with dissected human remains (Chapter 3.4). Overall there is a predominance of dog remains, with 13 ABGs recovered, three almost complete and the rest consisting of partial skeletons.

There is considerable archaeological evidence for animal dissection in the 18th century. Excavations at the Old Ashmolean Museum, Oxford (built 1683) found the remains of a North American raccoon and the radius of a manatee (Bennet et al 2000, 55–6), but it was apparently dogs that were most commonly used for dissections and vivisections. At least 24 dogs were recovered from the Old Ashmolean and dog bones were also numerous at Craven Street, London (Hillson et al

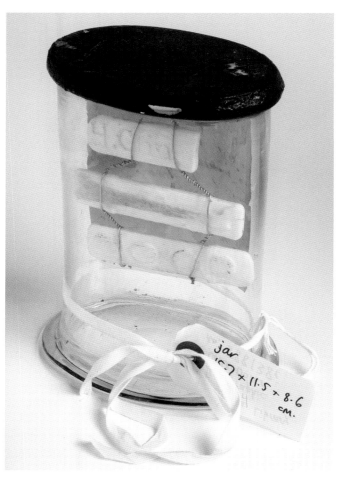

Fig 148 Specimens of bone fed by Henry Cline to a dog to demonstrate digestion; Cline's name can be seen on the top bone (not to scale) (Wellcome Library, London, L0044245)

1999; Hamilton-Dyer 2003). In his volume on canine pathology, Blaine (1817, 1) suggests that the anatomy of dogs and humans, in particular the digestive tract, is so similar that 'to study one is to gain an acquaintance with the other'. Interestingly no dog remains, or evidence for the dissection of animals, were found at Newcastle Infirmary (Hammon 1998).

The partial dog remains from the London range from a deposit of the first four cervical vertebrae from burial [262] in group 22 to 79 elements – including the head, body and forelimbs of an adult dog – in grave [622], group 20 (Chapter 3.4). There does not appear to be a discernible pattern regarding which body areas are present. Deposits of head, body, hind- and forelimbs are all well represented. Partial ABG deposits of the same species were examined to try and ascertain if the remains from the same individual animals had been placed into different grave fills, but no matches were noted. This may be a reflection of the difficulty in matching often-fragmented animal bones to the same individual animal.

Analysis of the human remains identified that 12.3% of the articulated contexts contained intrusive animal bone (78/636). Inhumations were more frequently accompanied (55/173: 31.8%) than portions (23/463: 5%). In most cases just one or two intrusive bones were found, but some burials contained the

major part of an animal skeleton. Thus while human and animal remains may normally have been kept apart for the purposes of burial, there were certainly exceptions and there seems in some instances to have been little consideration for the niceties of separating the human from the animal in death. However, these remains probably represent only a small proportion of the animals used by the school – forming the exception, perhaps, rather then the rule, in the school disposal strategy. It is possible that many of the animal remains were simply disposed of along with the kitchen waste.

Cut marks were rarely seen on the bones and were noted in just two of the dog ABGs. An almost complete adult female (identified as such because of the lack of baculum) from grave [553] had some fine cut marks present (Fig 149). Very fine knife marks were noted on the medial aspect of the distal shaft of the left humerus. Further fine cut marks were also noted on the posterior of the left femoral head and just below the left tibia proximal epiphysis. The sharpness of the cut marks compares well with the scalpel marks noted on the human remains. The location of these cut marks close to major joint surfaces would suggest that the bones had been marked whilst the joint's connective tissue was cut. The complete nature of the ABG deposit, however, suggests that some soft tissue remained to keep the skeleton in articulation. Perhaps the marks represent dissection so that the anatomical structure of the joints could be observed, as also seen in the human remains (below, 7.8, 'Tools and techniques'). Similar marks were noted on an individual dog femur fragment recovered from grave [419]. It is likely this fragment also came from a dissected animal, but no other dog remains were present in the grave.

A partial dog ABG recovered in association with the second burial to be placed in grave [220] had very different marks. The head, body (vertebrae and ribs), upper fore- and hindlimbs were present but the lower limbs were missing. The majority of the skull was also missing except for a fragment of partial and occipital bone, with saw marks along the midline and across the skull just before the orbit. These marks are similar to those observed on human craniotomy, and represent a proportion of the skull being opened so that the brain can be examined or removed.

Several rabbit and cat ABG deposits were also recovered. Like the dog remains, the composition of the rabbit ABGs was variable. A complete skeleton of a juvenile rabbit was recovered from the fill of grave [207], but the other five ABGs consisted of partial remains. These range from the almost complete deposit in the first burial of grave [332], from which just the skull was missing, to the eight elements representing the head and forelimbs in the third burial of grave [207]. As with the dog remains there appears to be no overall pattern in which body areas were deposited in the graves. Dissection marks were noted on the almost complete ABG in grave [332]. The skull was missing but both the right and left premaxilla were recovered with the upper incisors still present. The premaxilla had been sawn through at a vertical angle at the point where it fuses to the rest of the skull. Both mandibles were present but the rest of the skull was missing. It is unlikely the skull would have been

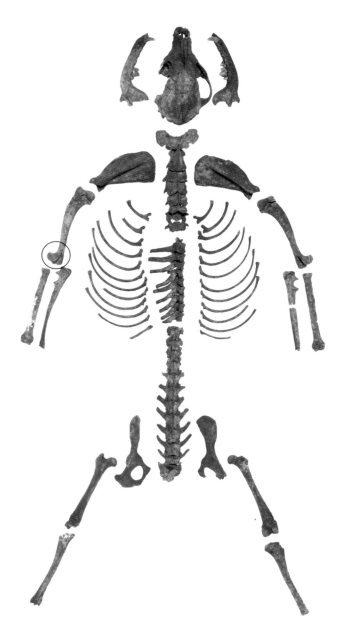

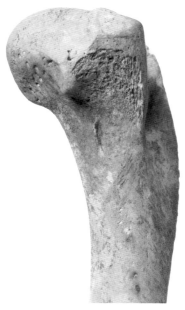

Fig 149 Left – dog skeleton recovered from grave [553] (scale c 1:5); right – fine cut marks are present on the distal humerus (scale c 2:1)

missed during the excavation, as even small foot bones had been recovered, so it seems that the rabbit carcass was placed in the grave minus the majority of the head. This is part of an interesting trend observed amongst the animal remains of ABGs lacking the skulls. The rabbit remains come from a mixture of age ranges, with both juvenile and adult animals present. One of the notable aspects of the rabbit assemblage is the large size of many of the elements. Measurement of both the adult and juvenile long bones suggests the rabbits were similar in size to the Flemish giant, which can weigh from 5kg to 8kg and grow to around 0.9m long, toe to toe (S Hamilton-Dyer, pers comm). The elements from the London Hospital therefore come from domestic rather than wild or feral rabbits and may represent one of the first instances of this large breed being identified

archaeologically. Records of Flemish giant rabbits being introduced to Britain are dated to the 1860s, so these remains may represent an earlier introduction.

In contrast to the dog and rabbit remains, the four cat ABGs recovered from the grave fills all consisted of partial skeletons from juvenile or neonatal animals. Adult remains were present, but consisted of individual fragments and the remains from a wired skeleton recovered from [100]. The presence of mainly young animals is interesting; perhaps they represent the use of unwanted and stray litters. The majority of the cat ABGs consisted of limb-bone elements, the exception being a skull with cervical vertebrae recovered from the last burial in grave [16], group 22. Cut marks were not noted on any of the cat remains, but the presence of partial cat ABGs amongst the human remains does suggest they originated from the anatomy school. We know that cats were used at the London Hospital. In 1844 Henry Leatherby, an assistant lecturer in the chemical department at the London, testified at the trial of a husband suspected of murdering his wife by prussic acid poisoning, outlining how he had restored a poisoned cat in ten minutes (*Old Bailey Proc*, August 1844, James Cockburn Belaney (t18440819-1920)).

There is also evidence for the use of horse at the anatomy school. The dissected remains of a horse's head and first three cervical vertebrae were recovered in association with the first burial in grave [220] (Fig 150). Only the posterior aspect of the skull was present. A number of saw marks are present on the skull. The occipital condyles have each been diagonally sawn – the right-hand side has been completely sawn through, the left-hand side partially sawn. The partial bone has also been sawn through on the medial, anterior and posterior sides. Like the procedures discussed above this may have been in order to access the brain matter. The sawing of the occipitals could have been undertaken to remove the head from the neck. The cervical

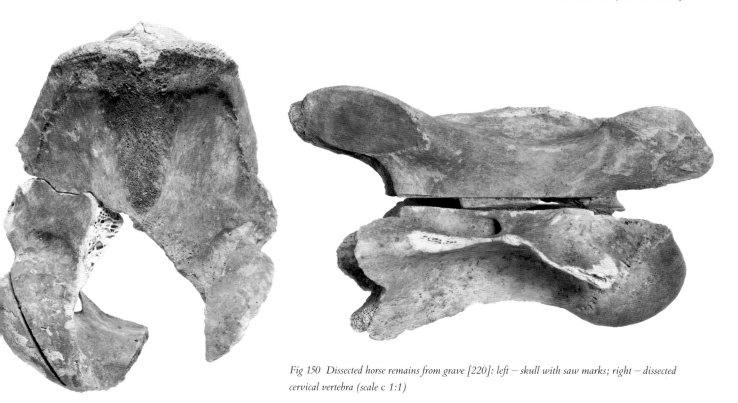

Fig 150 Dissected horse remains from grave [220]: left – skull with saw marks; right – dissected cervical vertebra (scale c 1:1)

vertebrae present also show signs of dissection having taken place. The tubercula have all been sawn through along the dorsal to ventral plane. There is evidence of false starts on all three vertebrae. Fine knife cuts are also present on the foramen transversus of the third cervical vertebra. It is likely the dissection of the vertebral column was undertaken to examine the horse's spinal cord. The horse may have been sourced from a local knacker's yard. From the lack of other horse elements we can theorise that the school procured a horse's head and neck rather than a whole animal.

Evidence for the dissection and use of other common domestic mammals in the school comes from some of the individual fragments recovered as well as from the ABGs. Remains such as the cow first phalanx recovered in association with partial human skeleton [440], from grave [464], cleanly sawn along the achsial-peripheral plane (Fig 151), show some of the clearest evidence for dissection and use in the anatomy school. Individual fragments also illustrate the comparative anatomy practices undertaken at the school, in particular the dissected cow periotic bone from [251] (see Fig 156) and the sheep/goat mandible from [650], one of the layers above the grave (below and Chapters 1.4, 3.6). Other individual fragments from group 20 include a primate fibula with numerous cut marks from grave [331] and a dissected horse mandible from [805].

Some graves contained more than one specimen. For example, as well as the cow periotic bone and the human remains, grave [251] contained the almost complete skeleton of a monkey belonging to the genus *Cercopithecus* (old world monkeys), possibly a mona monkey (*Cercopithecus mona*), which is found in western Africa. This represents the first

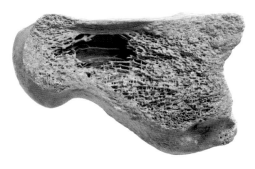

Fig 151 Dissected cow first phalanx from grave [464] (scale c 1:1)

archaeologically recorded find of this species from the United Kingdom (Fig 152). Only the distal humerus epiphysis is fused, indicating the animal was between 1 and 2 years old (Washburn 1943; Bolter and Zihlman 2003). Evidence of infection was seen on the medial aspect of the right clavicle and a healed greenstick fracture in the left fifth metacarpal. The skeleton is almost complete, with the exception of the skull, mandible and first six cervical vertebrae. The excellent bone preservation suggests that these elements had been removed prior to deposition, rather than destroyed by post-depositional factors. This corresponds with the evidence from the other ABGs, where apparently the skulls were often removed; possibly they were retained by the school.

A monkey humerus (*Cercopithecus* sp) was also recovered from a disturbed layer, [660] (Chapters 1.4, 3.6); again, this element was from a young animal. Two fine knife cuts were present on the anterior aspect of the shaft above the distal epiphysis (Fig 153). The fragmented skull and maxilla of a

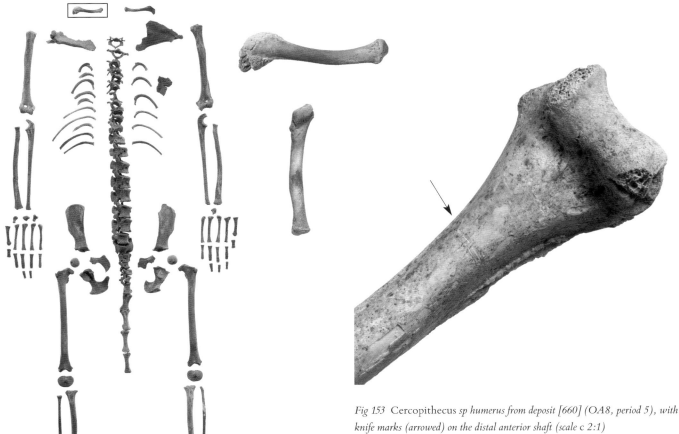

*Fig 152 Possible mona monkey (*Cercopithecus mona) *from grave [251]: left – almost complete skeleton (scale c 1:5); right – details showing (upper) the pathology on the left clavicle and (lower) the fracture of the left fifth metacarpal (scale c 1:1)*

Fig 153 Cercopithecus sp humerus from deposit [660] (OA8, period 5), with knife marks (arrowed) on the distal anterior shaft (scale c 2:1)

guinea pig (*Cavia porcellus*) were recovered from the same deposit (Fig 40).

A distal left fibula shaft from an adult primate around the size of a barbary ape was recovered from grave [331], along with dissected human remains. The fibula had fine horizontal cut marks that appear to have been made by a scalpel, running down the lateral aspect of the shaft. Two further monkey bones were recovered from grave [327]. These consisted of right first metacarpals with the distal epiphyses unfused. It was only possible to identify the elements as non-hominid Simian but they are morphologically distinct and appear to come from different species, both comparable in size to the mona monkey. Their presence in the same deposit suggests that the remains may be from monkeys dissected in the same way and at the same time, perhaps part of a comparative study.

Other non-native species include a partial skeleton of a Hermann's tortoise (*Testudo hermanni*) from grave [231] (Fig

154). As with many of the other ABG deposits the skull is missing, as well as the carapace and lower foot elements. Dating to the early 1800s, this represents one of the earliest archaeological finds of tortoise in the United Kingdom. Remains of the same genus have been recovered from Stafford Castle and date to the late 1800s (Thomas 2010). The Stafford tortoise is thought to have been kept as a pet, whereas the remains from the London Hospital were exploited for scientific endeavour. A single tortoise humerus was also recovered from grave [458] (Fig 155). The element appears to be too large to be from any of the European species of tortoise and may be from an African or Asian species (C McCarthy, pers comm).

An almost complete plaice was recovered in association with the Hermann's tortoise and graves [207] and [220] contained two possible examples of fish used in the anatomy school. The complete head and first three vertebrae of a congar eel were present from [220] (along with a partial dog).

The London docks brought in traders from across the British empire. The London Hospital clearly treated many sailors and dock workers (Table 62) and it might have been through these connections that exotic animals were obtained. Menageries containing monkeys and other unusual animals (such as were already present at the Tower of London, which became in 1834 London Zoo, and at Exeter Exchange) were clearly used by some surgeons as a source of supply (above) and exotic species would frequently arouse the interests of the medical profession. In December 1805, Mr Cline, William Blizard and Everard Home, as the professors of anatomy to the Royal College of Surgeons,

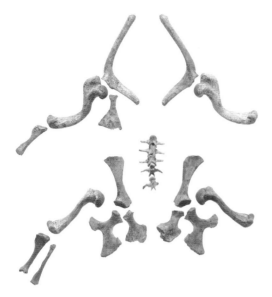

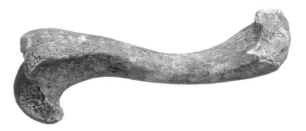

Fig 155 *Tortoise humerus recovered from grave [458] (scale c 1:1)*

Fig 154 *Partial skeleton of a Hermann's tortoise (*Testudo hermanni*) from grave [231] (scale c 1:2)*

heard that a camel 'in a dying state' was for sale and bought it for the purposes of dissection. The animal had been imported from Arabia and had resided in England for some 20 years. The surgeons had to wait until the following year for the animal to die (Home 1806). In his detailed account of the dissection, Home describes how the medulla oblongata was cut through by passing a blade between the cranium and the first cervical vertebra. He contrasts this to the method used for 'pithing' cattle, which cut only the medulla spinalis and, in his view cruelly, prevented brain death (ibid, 359). The body was suspended upright to maintain the position of the organs, particularly those of digestion, which were thoroughly examined and discussed by comparison with those of a bullock (ibid).

Although rare, other remains of exotic animals have been recovered archaeologically. Elements of barbary ape (*Macaca sylvanus*) have been recovered from post-medieval deposits in London (Pipe 1992), a South American capuchin monkey jaw (*Cebus nigrivittatus*) from a 17th-century layer at Brooks Wharf (Armitage 1981), turtles and terrapins from the 17th-century Limehouse site (Armitage et al 2005) and remains of barbary lion (*Panthera leo leo*) and leopard (*Panthera pardus*) from the royal menagerie at the Tower of London (O'Regan et al 2006). As mentioned above, the remains of a North American raccoon and the radius of a manatee were recovered from the 18th-century assemblage excavated at the Old Ashmolean Museum, Oxford (Hamilton-Dyer 2003). Guinea pig was found in dumping/machined deposits at Hill Hall, Essex (Hamilton-Dyer 2009).

Cercopithecoid monkeys and tortoises were certainly being used in comparative anatomy at this time. The skeleton of a mona monkey is illustrated in Grant's *Outlines of comparative anatomy* (1841, 116) and the anatomy of tortoise and terrapin discussed. John Hunter (1861, 10) discusses the anatomy of a green monkey (*Chlorocebus sabaeus*), the skull of which was kept as part of the Hunterian collection. Several tortoise and terrapin species are discussed in the volume and it is often noted that the

skulls and carapaces were kept as specimens in the Hunterian Museum (1861, 357–64).

In 1831 Blizard donated his collection (previously used in lectures delivered at the London Hospital) to the Hunterian Museum. Amongst these, and still present in the Hunterian Museum at the Royal College of Surgeons in London, are a preserved portion of cow liver with lymphatic vessels injected with mercury (object number RCSHM/K 467.2), a cow heart with abscess on the left ventricle (RSCPC/HC 17.1), a pig foot with syndactyly (RSCPC/HC 18.2), a sheep foetus with extreme reduction of face and cranium (RSCPC/T 20D.14) and twin hares with cranio-thoraco-abdominal union. It is interesting to note that the soft-tissue specimens preserved by Blizard derive mainly from the common domestic mammals, rather than more exotic species. This suggests that day-to-day teaching was best served by using easily available domestic mammals.

One of the interesting aspects of the human and animal assemblages is that similar techniques appear to have been used on both. This is likely to be in part a reflection of the school's comparative anatomy teaching. The dissected cow periotic bone from grave [251] and the similar dissected human temporal bone from [100] may be evidence of this comparative anatomy (Fig 156). Further evidence of comparative anatomy comes from the dissected sheep/goat (probably sheep) mandible from deposit [650]. The majority of the lingual aspect of the mandible has been removed, exposing the teeth root cavities (Fig 157). A slot has also been cut in the coronoid process, with some copper staining indicating that the mandible may have been part of a wired skeleton or hung as part of a comparative collection.

More evidence for wired animal skeletons – in addition to the wired cat hind limb from [100] (above and Chapter 3.6) – comes from the cat pelvis and femur also recovered from deposit [650]. Small holes have been drilled in the acetabulum and copper-alloy wire attached to the femoral head (Fig 158).

7.8 Human dissection at the London Hospital

Introduction

As early as 1746, the house committee at the London Hospital had resolved that a room in which to 'open such extraordinary

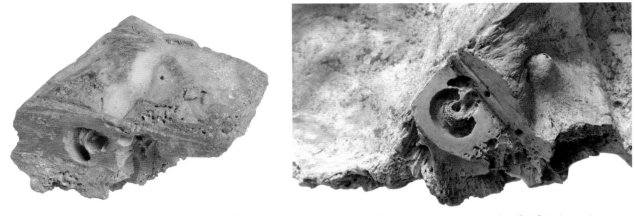

Fig 156 Left – dissected cow periotic bone from grave [251]; right – the same area of bone in disarticulated human remains from [100] (scale c 2:1)

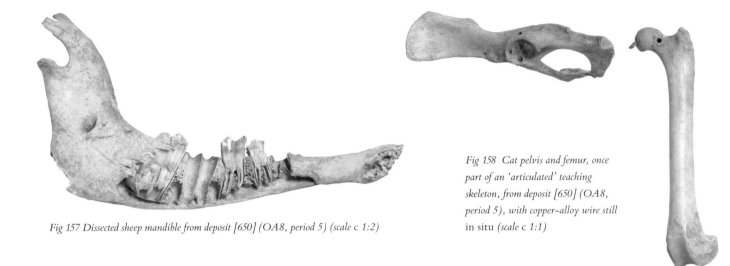

Fig 157 Dissected sheep mandible from deposit [650] (OA8, period 5) (scale c 1:2)

Fig 158 Cat pelvis and femur, once part of an 'articulated' teaching skeleton, from deposit [650] (OA8, period 5), with copper-alloy wire still in situ (scale c 1:1)

bodies as are directed by the surgeons' should be created above the dead house, and this was created in the late 1750s at a cost of £50 (Clark-Kennedy 1962, 143). Although there are no contemporary descriptions or representations of the dissecting room at the London during the early 19th century, the dissecting room at St Thomas's Hospital was described by John Flint South (1970, 28–9) as it was in 1813:

The dissecting-room in 1813 was a squarish room above the eastern half of the laboratory, lighted by two windows eastward and a square lantern in the ceiling; the west end of the room was fitted from top to bottom with glass cases for the preparations, and like cases were fixed high up wherever room could be found for them. A large fireplace and copper, used to prepare the subjects for dissection, was on the south side, and a large leaden sink under the windows was indiscriminately used for washing hands and washing subjects and discharging all the filth. In this room were usually standing about a dozen tables with their corresponding burdens, and six or eight pupils to each, so that on average the room was crammed with seventy or eighty people, clad in filthy linen or stuff dissecting gowns, so that there was literally scarce possibility of moving; nor was it much needed, for subjects were plentiful then, and pupils infinitely more

industrious in dissecting than for many years they have been, though partly I must admit from lack of subjects, caused mainly by the operation of the Anatomy Act.

In the autumn of 1834, anatomy classes at the London were taught by Luke, Hamilton and Adams each day at 2.30pm, with Hamilton and Adams leading the dissection classes (*The Lancet*, 27 September 1834, London Hospital School and practice, 23(578), 9). It was not just anatomy lectures that required human subjects. Surgery lectures were held each Monday and Wednesday at 7pm by John Scott, whilst 'lectures on phrenology, with demonstrations of gall and Spurgheim's view of the brain, human and comparative', which were led by Mr H Haley Holm, would have required animal specimens as well as human (ibid). Medical students and the dissecting rooms feature in photographs from the early 20th century (Fig 159); Donald Hunter, who was curator of London Hospital Medical College for many years, figures in Fig 160.

Osteological evidence for surgical intervention

One of the perennial questions raised when human bone with evidence of surgical intervention is encountered in archaeological contexts is whether the intervention was the result of *in vivo*

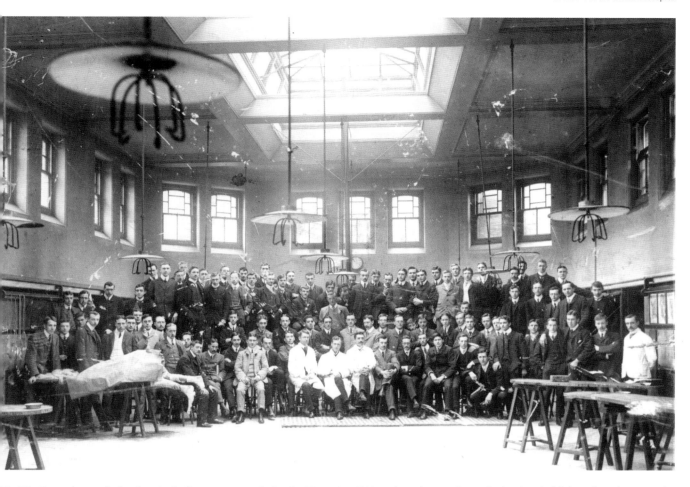

Fig 159 *Group photograph of students in the dissecting room at the London Hospital in 1904, with a cadaver on the wooden bench to the left (Royal London Hospital Archives, RLHMC/P/1)*

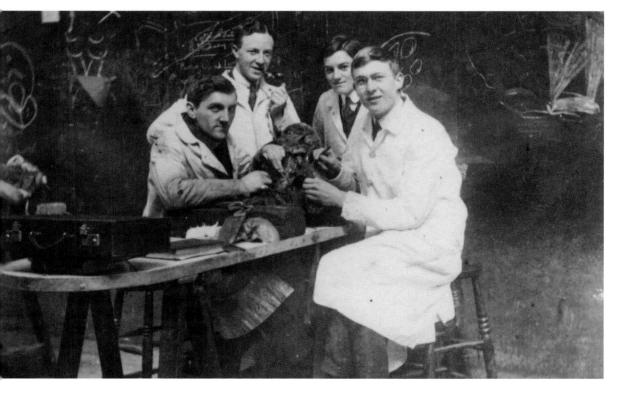

Fig 160 *Students in the dissecting room at the London Hospital in 1916, featuring (far right) Donald Hunter, subsequently curator of London Hospital Medical College (Royal London Hospital Archives, RLHMC/P/1)*

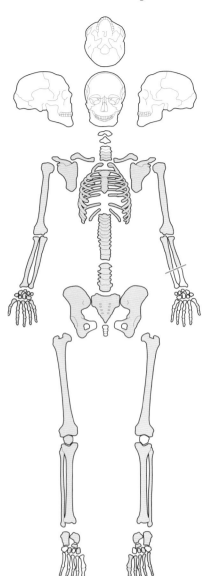

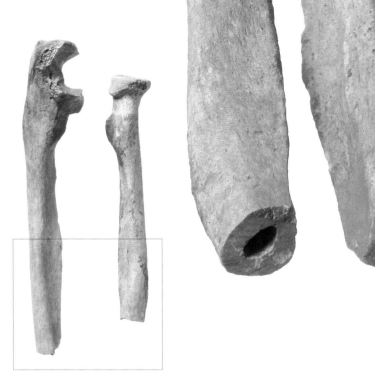

Fig 161 Diagram and view of possible in vivo *left forearm amputation in 36–45-year-old male primary inhumation [242] (scale c 1:2, detail not to scale)*

surgery, post-mortem dissection or autopsy. The remains from the London Hospital are most certainly derived from a combination of the three: discarded amputated limbs and the poor unfortunates who did not survive surgery in the house; those whose corpses were used in anatomical teaching and to provide materials on which pupils could practise, safe in the knowledge that their inexperience could cause the individual no further physical harm; and individuals upon whom autopsies were conducted to understand the cause of death.

A particular problem at the London Hospital is the high number of individuals subject to post-mortem intervention and with sawn limbs, which creates a level of 'background noise', possibly masking evidence of unsurvived *in vivo* amputation. What appears to have been an amputation may in reality have resulted from a training amputation performed by a student on a cadaver (Fig 161). In the absence of definable features within a saw or knife cut with which to characterise *in vivo* amputations securely, and thus distinguish between them and post-mortem modification, the osteologist cannot assign each case with certainty either to the surgeon's or to the student's table.

Nevertheless, certain surgical techniques and locations of saw or cut marks are consistent with post-mortem intervention and the location may provide evidence for the type of intervention (dissection or autopsy). For example, bisection or removal of the sternum (below) is unlikely to have been used for autopsy as it prevents the cosmetic reconstruction of the thorax (Shaw 1822, 245).

Visual examination of the patterns of surgical intervention was carried out for all articulated remains, using diagrams produced during recording (eg, Fig 161 left). Information from those remains that did not have accompanying diagrams was also added to these observations the better to establish the proportion of surgical interventions that could be ascribed to dissection as opposed to autopsy or surgery.

Amongst the disarticulated material from Open Area 6 (Chapter 3.4), the high numbers of frontal, parietal and occipital elements with indications of surgical intervention certainly reflect material that had resulted from craniotomy (Fig 162), though a large number of mandibles had also been subject to (post-mortem) intervention. In [224], all observed cranial cuts ran horizontally through the vault and were consistent with the removal of the calvarium using a saw as part of either autopsy or dissection, with the exception of a right parietal that had been sawn vertically through the midline. A larger number of vertical saw cuts were noted in [457], affecting one supraoccipital, one right parietal and an associated left parietal and left frontal and suggesting an assemblage that contained both autopsied and dissected remains. The pattern in the remaining disarticulated assemblage was more complex. Whilst 145 cranial elements or

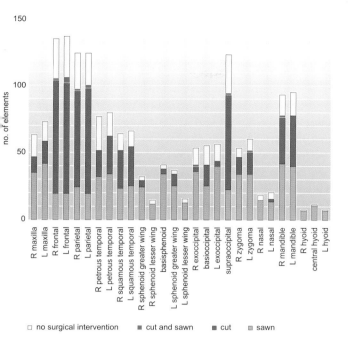

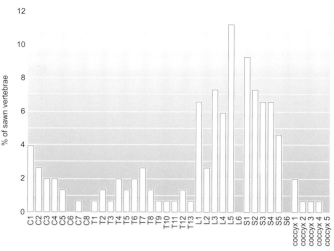

Fig 163 Percentage of sawn vertebrae from each location as a proportion of the total number of sawn vertebrae (n=152)

Fig 162 Number of disarticulated cranial elements with evidence of surgical intervention

portions had been sawn in a manner consistent with craniotomy, a variety of other saw or knife cuts were consistent with patterns expected in dissection. Nineteen right and 19 left mandibles (not necessarily pairs) showed vertical saw or knife cuts, most often in the midline (through menton), the premolar or molar area, or through the ascending ramus. One cranial portion from [204] showed horizontal cuts consistent with craniotomy but a vertical cut that had bisected the skull, through the base; context [433] contained maxillae that had been saggitally sawn in the midline; the left maxilla of [229] showed a similar saw cut, and a further cut lying medial to the junction with the zygomatic appeared to have been made to expose and examine the maxillary sinus. Vertical saw cuts were also seen through orbits (eg, [237]).

In all, 722 disarticulated vertebrae were present and 153 (21.2%) had been sawn or cut. When expressed as a percentage of the total number of sawn vertebrae, a greater percentage was from the lower spine than any other area (Fig 163). In the neck, the first cervical vertebra had most frequently been sawn, presumably to remove the head during dissection. Overall, the greatest proportion of disarticulated sawn vertebrae was from the lumbo-sacral border, a pattern also noted in the articulated body portions. A peak was also seen at the level of the seventh thoracic vertebra, suggesting the bisection of the body during dissection and possible evidence of cadaver sharing (below, 'Tools and techniques').

Amongst the disarticulated long bones of the upper limb, the clavicles showed the highest proportion of saw cuts, indicating that in the individuals from whom the remains originated the thorax had been opened to examine the viscera. This interpretation is supported by the fact that of the 632 disarticulated ribs recovered, 238 had been sawn (37.7%) and 12 of them also showed knife (cut) marks.

Demographic composition of the dissected remains

The most prized bodies for the study of anatomy were those of the young and fit (Richardson 2001, 248). Male corpses were reportedly preferred to female, since they 'offered greater scope for the study of musculature' (Wise 2004, 30). The contemporary textbooks provide some information to support this, with Shaw writing that 'the dissection of the parts in the female perineum is not very interesting, in a surgical view' (1822, 102). Others have suggested that a male bias is the result of obtaining remains from the gallows (Bennet et al 2000). The dissection of women by men was also seen by some as indecent (Richardson 2001, 95).

The male:female sex ratio in the portions was identical to that of the primary inhumations (2.7:1), although the large number of portions of undetermined sex may mean that the similarity is coincidental. There were many more males when compared to females, indicating that males made up a greater proportion of the burial population than can be explained by 'normal' demographic biases. However, a male bias is also seen in the patient statistics for 1841, noted at Newcastle Infirmary 'in both the documented admissions, discharges and burials, and the excavated remains' (Boulter et al 1998, 25), and seen in the smaller assemblage from Worcester Royal Infirmary, which was 66% male and 34% female (Western 2010, 16). At Newcastle, the 210 articulated burials consisted of 97 males and 47 females, a ratio of 2.1:1 (Boulter et al 1998, 21, 43), whilst at the Old Anatomy School at Trinity College Dublin, by contrast, 77 females and 40 males were identified, a ratio of 0.5:1 (Murphy 2011). At the London Hospital, the (admittedly limited) data from the primary inhumations suggest that the burials were reasonably representative of the documented demographic profiles of the patients (Chapter 5.4), but that a 'filtering' was occurring for those who were selected for post-mortem examination (Fig 164).

The presence of neonatal remains in the buried population does not necessarily reflect the admission of pregnant women

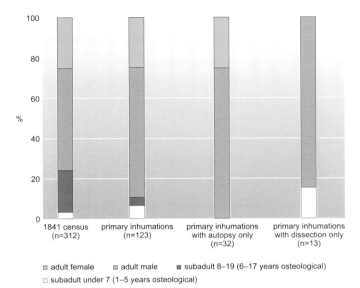

Fig 164 Comparison of the demographic profile of the 1841 census (TNA: PRO, 1841 England census, parish St Mary Whitechapel), the primary inhumations and the primary inhumations with evidence of surgical intervention

(Chapter 5.5, 'Pregnant women'), as such 'subjects' might have been specially purchased for a particular class, though supply from within the hospital is also possible.

Primary inhumations

The crude prevalence rate for primary inhumations with sawn bones, cut marks or other forms of post-mortem bone modification (including fixing and patterned staining) was 32.9% (57/173) (Table 70). Three subadults (3/13: 23.1%), including one perinate, and 54 adults (54/160: 33.8%) were affected. Approximately half of males were involved compared to about a quarter of females, although the difference was not statistically significant. There was no identifiable variation in adult prevalence rate by age (Fig 165). Of the 57 primary

inhumations with peri- or post-mortem modification, 55 (96.5%) contained at least one sawn bone element.

Males from the primary inhumations may have been more likely than females to have been subject to peri- or post-mortem bone modification, but there was no statistically significant evidence to confirm this. The comparison of mortality profiles gives no indication, at least in the primary inhumation sample, that any particular adult age category was more likely to undergo such modification than any other. The small number of subadults within the assemblage prevented comparison with adult rates of involvement. The mortality profile of aged adult primary inhumations affected by peri- or post-mortem modification was compared to that of unaffected individuals (Fig 166); no variation between the two groups was observed.

The youngest affected individual from the primary inhumations was perinate [476] (*c* 38 weeks *in utero*). Two other subadult primary inhumations showed evidence for post-mortem

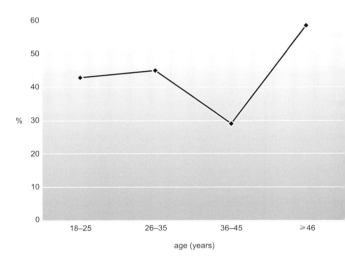

Fig 165 Crude prevalence rate of peri- or post-mortem modification in adult primary inhumations, by age

Table 70 Crude prevalence rate of peri- or post-mortem modification in the primary inhumations

Age	Female n	Affected	%	Male n	Affected	%	Intermediate n	Affected	%	Undetermined n	Affected	%	Subadult n	Affected	%	Adult n	Affected	%	All individuals n	Affected	%
<4 weeks	0	0	-	0	0	-	0	0	-	0	0	-	5	1	20.0	0	0	-	5	1	20.0
1-6 months	0	0	-	0	0	-	0	0	-	0	0	-	0	0	-	0	0	-	0	0	-
7-11 months	0	0	-	0	0	-	0	0	-	0	0	-	0	0	-	0	0	-	0	0	-
1-5 years	0	0	-	0	0	-	0	0	-	0	0	-	3	0	-	0	0	-	3	0	-
6-11 years	0	0	-	0	0	-	0	0	-	0	0	-	1	1	100.0	0	0	-	1	1	100.0
12-17 years	0	0	-	0	0	-	0	0	-	0	0	-	4	1	25.0	0	0	-	4	1	25.0
Subadult	0	0	-	0	0	-	0	0	-	0	0	-	0	0	-	0	0	-	0	0	-
18-25 years	4	0	-	6	3	50.0	3	2	66.7	1	1	-	0	0	-	14	6	42.9	14	6	42.9
26-35 years	10	4	40.0	25	13	52.0	1	0	-	2	0	-	0	0	-	38	17	44.7	38	17	44.7
36-45 years	9	1	11.1	27	10	37.0	0	0	-	2	0	-	0	0	-	38	11	28.9	38	11	28.9
≥46 years	3	1	33.3	9	6	66.7	0	0	-	0	0	-	0	0	-	12	7	58.3	12	7	8.3
Adult	4	2	50.0	13	5	38.5	1	0	-	40	6	15.0	0	0	-	58	13	22.4	58	13	22.4
Total	30	8	26.7	80	37	46.3	5	2	40.0	45	7	15.6	13	3	23.1	160	54	33.8	173	57	32.9

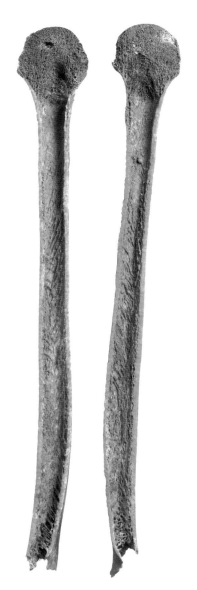

Fig 174 Probable disuse atrophy in a disarticulated humerus from [344], which had also been longitudinally sawn to observe the inner structure of the bone (scale c 1:2)

Cadaver sharing

John Collins Warren, writing in 1799, observed that 'Dissection is carried out in style: twelve or fifteen bodies in a room; young men work on them in different ways' (Jonathan Evans, pers comm). An 1828 Select Committee on Anatomy agreed that an average of three bodies was required per student (Wise 2004, 292). It seems, however, that this did not reflect the experience of the students at the London Hospital in the early 19th century. Headington wrote,'I regret that … the enquiries of most gentlemen are restricted to the examination of one, or at furthest two, subjects, and the dissection of the muscles and vessels of the two, (or one chiefly)' (*The Lancet*, 8 October 1825, Mr Headington, 5(109), 64). Other contemporary writers detailed methods by which a body could be effectively worked on by more than one pupil. Shaw (1822, 66) outlined a technique whereby some students worked on the upper body

and some on the lower, sawing the body in two. Bodies may also have been shared for educational reasons. Shaw suggested that first-time students should pair up to make dissection easier (ibid, 1). At St Thomas's Hospital, bodies were shared by groups of four students who paid £1 1s each (Millard 1825, 12).

To examine the possibility that one cadaver was shared between several students, the pattern of dissection was visually examined using diagrams that had been created during recording (Fig 175). Consistent patterns were noted of sawing through the cervical vertebrae to remove the head and through the lower spine to divide the upper and lower body (eg, Figs 167, 176). As this reflects the advice of the contemporary texts (above), it was taken to be good evidence that cadaver sharing was a standard practice. The number of head, upper body and lower body portions was quantified for each burial group, based on the presence of vertebral cuts (Table 75). Clearly this is an

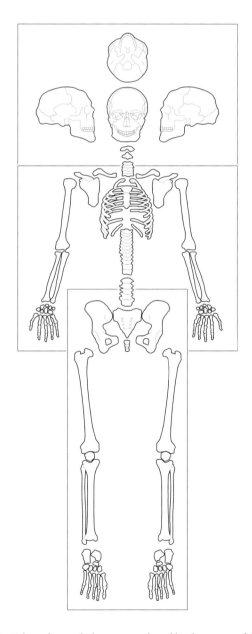

Fig 175 Cadaver sharing: body portions indicated by observations of the osteological assemblage

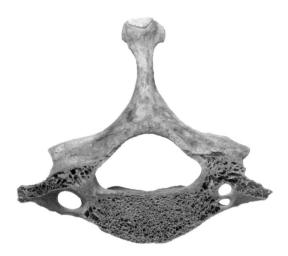

Fig 176 Sawn cervical vertebrae in adult portion [50804] (scale c 1:1)

underestimation of the number of shared corpses, as once further dissection or dispersal had occurred (eg, the removal and dissection of limbs) it was no longer possible to observe the standard portioning of the remains. Sections of vertebral column with cuts in the same locations were not counted where no other remains were present as the possibility could not be excluded that these originated from the same individuals. Nonetheless, the results suggest that the sharing of subadult remains was not commonplace and also seem to indicate that the cranium was under-represented, either because of the subsequent further dissection of the head, resulting in numerous disarticulated fragments, or perhaps because of the retention or sale of head and neck specimens. In particular, the probable retention of the head was noted in eight instances, including burial [301], an adult who had otherwise undergone only autopsy, with no further signs of dissection.

The possibility that heads were removed to send to dentists was considered because, during the scandal surrounding the public decapitation of the recently executed Thistlewood and his companions, who had plotted to assassinate the prime minister (Chapter 8.2), it was mentioned that the man who carried out the task 'was in the habit of cutting off nobs [heads] for the purpose of obtaining nackers [teeth]' (Wakley and Sheriff Parkins, *Morning Post*, 29 September 1820, issue 15456). This probably referred, however, to the activities of a bodysnatcher. Anecdotal accounts suggest that only sets of teeth would be collected and sold on by the medical schools (Shaw 1832).

In the wake of the 'Italian boy' murder case (Chapter 6.3) St Thomas's Hospital received a letter from John Jeffrey raising his concerns about the frequent practice of purchasing 'detached parts of bodies' as this was just one of the ways in which the practices of the dissection room might disguise the commission of an earlier crime (LMA, H01/ST/A/076/005). It seems likely that the London Hospital sold bodies and body parts on to other hospitals (including St Thomas's), and this could account for the under-representation of some areas of the body. Interestingly, a shortage of heads was also noted in the faunal assemblage (above, 7.7).

Table 75 Evidence of cadaver sharing with counts of body portions present in each group

	Group		
	20	21	22
Head & neck			
Male	1	0	0
Female	0	0	0
Other adult	0	0	0
Subadult	0	0	0
Total	1	0	0
Head, neck & upper body			
Male	0	4	0
Female	1	0	0
Other adult	2	0	0
Subadult	0	0	0
Total	3	4	0
Upper body			
Male	1	0	0
Female	2	0	0
Other adult	8	2	3
Subadult	0	0	0
Total	11	2	3
Upper & lower body			
Male	0	0	0
Female	1	0	0
Other adult	0	0	0
Subadult	0	0	0
Total	1	0	0
Lower body			
Male	6	8	2
Female	2	1	4
Other adult	2	0	0
Subadult	0	0	0
Total	10	9	6
Estimated min no. of shared bodies	14	9	6

Microscopic examination of the tool marks

Jenna Dittmar-Blado and Andrew S Wilson

Ten individuals with evidence of post-mortem modification were examined using an FEI Quanta 400 scanning electron microscope (SEM) at the University of Bradford. Male [349] had undergone autopsy and the remaining nine individuals had been dissected (Table 76). The observed post-mortem modification had been caused by two tool types, knives and saws, and examination of the marks made by the use of such tools resulted in the positive identification of the tool class in all the examined samples. In some cases it was possible to be more specific in the identification of the medical instrument used.

Male [349], who died aged 36–45 years, presented clear evidence of autopsy, with multiple sawn elements (n= 20), including evidence of a craniotomy and thoracotomy. The craniotomy had been performed using an alternate set (ie, the teeth are bent outwards slightly in alternate directions) handsaw together with a specialised cranial saw, used to sever the cranial

Table 76 Summary of individuals examined using scanning electron microscopy

Context no.	Age (years)	Sex	Element/s	Description of trauma	Procedure inferred
[225]	adult	-	splanchnocranium, partial frontal & portions of R & L temporals	craniotomy, saw marks on maxillae & zygomatics	dissection
[349]	36–45	male	complete skeleton	craniotomy, sawn clavicles & sawn ribs	autopsy
[522]	adult	-	L distal femur, L proximal tibia & fibula	all elements transversely sawn	dissection
[19202]	subadult	-	R distal femur, R fibula	femur transversely sawn, with cut marks posterior to sawn surface	dissection
[24301]	adult	-	R distal $^1/_3$ of femur, proximal $^2/_3$ of tibia & fibula	tibia & fibula transversely sawn, linear series of cut marks on anterior of fibula	dissection
[27201]	36–45	male	R proximal femur	transversely sawn	dissection
[29401]	18–25	-	R humerus, radius, ulna, clavicle & lateral portion of scapula. L proximal humerus, distal radius & ulna, complete L scapula & clavicle	humeri, radii & ulnae transversely sawn at midshaft	dissection
[34301]	adult	-	L distal $^2/_3$ of tibia & fibula, & pedal elements	both elements transversely sawn, cut marks inferior to sawn surface of tibia	dissection or possible medical waste from an amputation
[43303]	26–35	male	complete L os coxae, sacrum, medial portion of L ilium	R ilium severed, cut marks on ala, neural arches of sacrum removed	dissection
[50804]	adult	-	R proximal $^2/_3$ of humerus, R scapula, medial portion of L clavicle, L portion of manubrium & 1st sternebra, 3 vertebrae, 2 ribs	transversely sawn humerus & vertebrae, sawn manubrium, ribs & clavicle	dissection

muscles as well as bone. According to contemporary literature, craniotomies were performed by making a circumferential incision through the scalp with a knife, 25mm above the supercilliary ridge of the orbit and close above the protuberance of the occipital (Ellis and Ford 1876). The skin was then retracted and a hacksaw used to saw carefully through the elements of the skull while constantly repositioning the blade to avoid affecting the dura mater or the brain (Ellis 1840). In this instance, a cranial saw was used alongside the hacksaw to sever the cranial muscles and was possibly used to complete the initial incision made by the hacksaw; the cranial saw is considerably more delicate and easier to manoeuvre in confined areas.

Multiple false starts on the occipital of [349] indicate that sawing started on the posterior aspect of the occipital and progressed anticlockwise, terminating at the entry point on the occipital where a bone spur on the ectocranial surface is present (Fig 177). The location of these kerfs (grooves/slits cut by the saw) suggests that the scalp had been retracted well below the incision or removed entirely. The practitioner then continued sawing in an anticlockwise progression making multiple short cuts without penetrating the dura mater.

According to Ellis (1840), 'after the outer table has been divided a chisel and mallet should be used to cut through the inner table', but no evidence of this was seen. 'The calvarium should then be removed, exposing the dura mater' (ibid). After the removal of the brain, the fossae and the dura mater in the base of the skull would be visible.

Along the superior and inferior border of the incision there are short kerf marks that show the epicranial muscles and the aponeuroses. On the left frontal and temporal, saw marks indicate that the temporalis muscle was sawn through. To judge from the pattern of the kerf marks present on the craniotomy of

[349], an instrument was used in a sawing motion to create the marks, but the wavering of the blade suggests that this cut was made using an instrument with multiple cutting surfaces (teeth) with decreased stability. Based on the striations on the kerf floor, an alternate set saw was used with a blade width of 3.0mm, as determined by the narrowest point of the kerf. The false-start kerfs on the parietal and inferior occipital are consistent with a cranial saw with an alternate set blade (Fig 178). The linear striations on the occipital and the withdrawal marks found along the circumferential sawn surface are consistent with an alternate set hacksaw. It is likely that two different saws were used.

Craniotomies are also used in the initial stage of dissecting the head, as was seen in [225]. The degree of destruction to the skull is dependent on the structures under examination by the practitioner. When dissecting the head, this procedure allows for the study of the cranial nerves in the base of the skull, the vessels in the base of the skull, contents of the orbit, including vessels and nerves, the superficial muscles and the lachrymal gland. The length of the striations on the frontal and parietal elements of [225] indicates continuous movement of the saw (Fig 179), in accordance with the standard practice (Valentin and d'Errico 1995). Throughout this procedure the head would have been repositioned from side to side, or removed by severing the cervical vertebrae (as seen in [50804], Fig 176) to facilitate sawing.

The complex process of cranial dissection can be appreciated by examining contemporary (Ellis and Ford 1876; Fig 180) and modern anatomy texts. The recovered portion of the splanchnocranium of [225] indicates that there is extreme fragmentation associated with dissecting this portion of the body. The removal of the mandible and the multiple saw marks

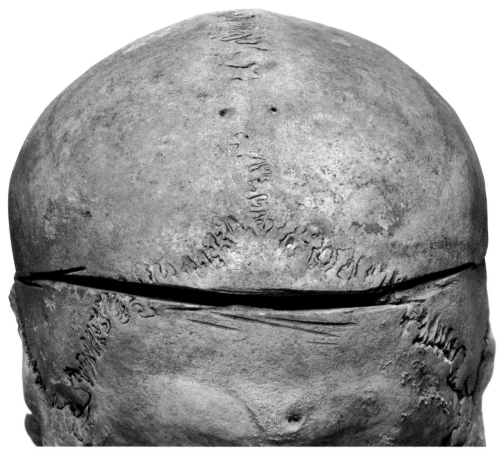

Fig 177 *Posterior aspect of the skull of 36–45-year-old male [349], showing multiple saw cuts that indicate the starting and finishing points of a craniotomy (scale c 1:1)*

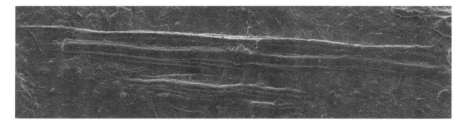

Fig 178 *SEM image of part of the left parietal of 36–45-year-old male [349]: composite micrograph showing a series of false-start kerfs with significant wavering of the kerf (x25 magnification) (© J Dittmar-Blado/University of Bradford 2011)*

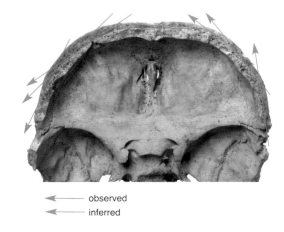

observed
inferred

Fig 179 *Craniotomy on [225] showing the repositioning of the saw (scale c 1:2) (© J Dittmar-Blado 2011)*

on the maxillae and the zygomatics suggest that the skull of [225] was examined thoroughly, including the brain, spinal cord, internal structures of the skull and ear, the muscles of the jaw and face and the inferior aspect of the nasal cavity. From the description by Ellis (1840), however, the orbits were not dissected.

There is no evidence for the use of a cranial saw in [225], indicating a difference in the tools that would have been used to perform an autopsy and those used to dissect the head. As a specialised tool, a cranial saw is not generally part of a post-mortem instrument kit (Fig 181). It is not used in other types of surgical procedures and would therefore need to be purchased specifically to conduct craniotomies. If a practitioner did not have this tool, a craniotomy could still be performed by using a different sawing instrument.

Body portion [43303] presented with a false start on the

progress from the superior surface of the sacrum on to the anterior surface. The lateral cut is 13.2mm and the medial is 12.7mm. These cuts begin on the superior surface and progress towards the anterior surface, with a slightly medial progression.

The severing of the ilium of [43303] and the involvement of the sacrum to examine the anatomy of the pelvis, which contains the rectum, bladder and reproductive organs, is described by Ellis. He states that 'these organs are best examined in the lateral view obtained by taking away the os innominatum of one side' (1840, 571) (Fig 183). This description is consistent with the excavated human remains recovered, as only the right ilium has been severed.

Thirty-three dissected portions, representing 16 different skeletal elements, were analysed (see Table 76). Remarkable variation in the placement of tool marks was observed, providing evidence of the practice of cadaver sharing (above). Of the seven dissected individuals with long bones, all had at least one long bone transversely sawn, and four (57.2%) had two or more long bones severed. The long bones in the leg are severed at a variety of locations with significant variation in the severing of the femur. The progression of the saw was anterior to posterior in [522] whilst [27201] was sawn from medial to lateral and [19202] from anteromedial to posterodistal. Generally the tibia was severed with a lateral to medial progression as evident in [522] and [24301].

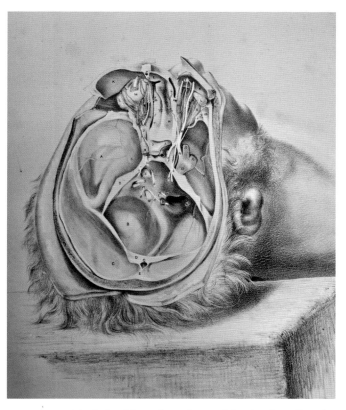

Fig 180 Base of the skull and first and second views of the orbit, from Ellis and Ford (1876, fig 4); this dissection displays the cranial nerves and the inner structures of the skull (reproduced with permission of the Thackray Museum, Leeds)

posterolateral aspect of the right ala of the sacrum, terminating on the posterior aspect and suggesting the entry was from the anterior and progressed posterodistally (Fig 182). The superior articular facets and the neural arches on the sacrum had been severed and the left pedicle removed. Several sawn surfaces could be seen on the left pedical, and a false start aligned with another on the posterolateral aspect of the right ala suggests that during the process of removing the pedicle from the sacrum with a saw, the ala was also nicked. This may indicate that the practitioner was standing on the right side of the cadaver, while sawing posteriorly at a 60° angle to remove the pedicles in order to access the spinal cord. Two parallel cut marks 3.5mm apart on the superomedial aspect of the right ala

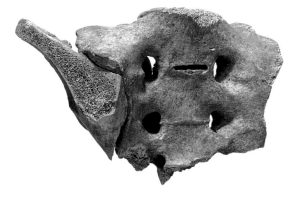

Fig 182 The sacrum and the sawn fragment of the right ilium of [43303], consistent with dissection focused on the anatomy of the pelvis (scale 1:2)

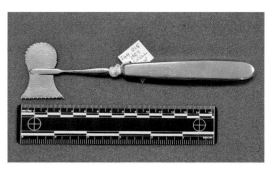
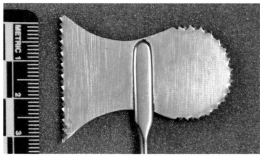

Fig 181 Cranial saw (left) and head of cranial saw (right) with 16 teeth per inch (photographed by and reproduced with permission of the Thackray Museum, Leeds)

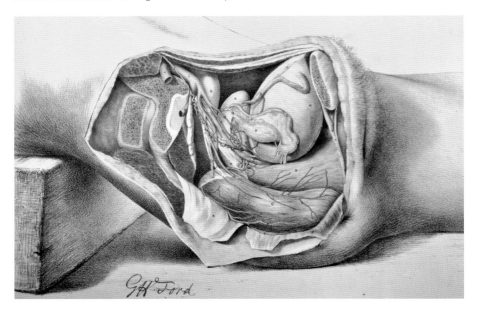

Fig 183 Plate XLI from Ellis and Ford (1876), depicting the lateral view of the viscera of the female pelvis; in order to achieve this, first the right limb was detached from the trunk, then the fat, fascia and the peritoneum were removed (reproduced with permission of the Thackray Museum, Leeds)

The elements of the upper limbs showed more consistency in an anteroposterior saw progression. Based on the symmetry and placement of the sawn locations it is likely that these elements were severed to distribute body portions from a single corpse to multiple students to learn anatomy. The symmetry of the transverse cuts on the humeri, radii and ulnae of [29401] and the similar severing of the humerus of [50804] suggest that the upper limbs were severed into three sections. The distal portion included the radius, ulna and hand, the intermediate portion included the proximal portions of the radius and ulna and the distal portion of the humerus (the elbow joint), whilst the proximal portion of the humerus remained attached to the body.

The placement of the saw marks on [522] suggest that the leg was also severed into three portions. This would allow one student to learn the anatomy of the foot and lower limb, while another student was given the intermediate portion to learn the anatomy of the knee, and a third could learn the anatomy of the hip, as well as the lower abdominal cavity (as seen in [43303]).

In most cases, the placement and variation of sawing direction used to sever the long bones is not consistent with the literature on amputation practices. The severing of the long bones of [19202] and [34301], however, could be evidence of post-mortem amputation practice on individuals that were also dissected, as referred to by Cherryson (2010, 141) and mirrored by post-mortem amputations described by Witkin (1997) at the Newcastle Infirmary and at the Royal Hospital Greenwich (Boston et al 2008). The severing at the approximate midshafts of these elements may suggest a focus on the preservation of the joints for further study. The division of the corpse provides strong evidence for anatomical instruction in a class setting, and is seen again in the skeletal elements recovered from the Craven Street anatomy school in London (Kausmally 2010).

The location of tool marks on the skeletal elements of cadavers is dependent on the structures examined by the practitioner. As all areas of the body are potentially subject to investigation, it was expected that significant variation would be found on the skeletal remains. It has also been established that in

some cases contemporary sources provide accurate descriptions of the procedures and techniques used, confirming a standard method of the procedure used to dissect cadavers in order to learn anatomy. The results indicate that during dissection, cadavers were placed in a supine position, most likely on a table that allowed the practitioner to move freely around the circumference.

Ample space was required to facilitate the sawing motions required to create the striation patterns visible on the dissected skeletal remains and this accounts for the variation in the practitioner's location while performing dissection. This, in addition to the documented evidence of cadaver sharing, indicates that more than one student would have worked on a cadaver at a time and reflects the high demand for anatomical studies in early 19th-century London, and indeed Headington's opening remarks (above, 'Cadaver sharing').

Practising surgical techniques

In the disarticulated material, 15 cranial elements contained a number of small, drilled holes. The volume of interventions indicates that this was not carried out in life but rather that the bone was being used to practise the techniques needed to create burr holes, which were drilled to relieve pressure on the brain, successfully. In the parietals and supraoccipital of an adult male from [229] five holes (three right and two left) were noted, together with scrape marks indicating defleshing (Fig 184). Twelve holes, varying in diameter from *c* 1mm to 6mm, were present in an adult left frontal from [234], whilst 30 holes with the same range of measurements were present in the supraoccipital of probable male [559] (below, 'Worked human bone', for discussion of this context). It seems probable that this represents the full range of drill bits in medical use. Burr holes and practise trephinations have also been reported on remains from Craven Street, London and Belfast (Hillson et al 1999; Cherryson 2010, 140). One adult left frontal bone showed evidence of a trephination, as previously discussed (Chapter 5.11, Fig 133).

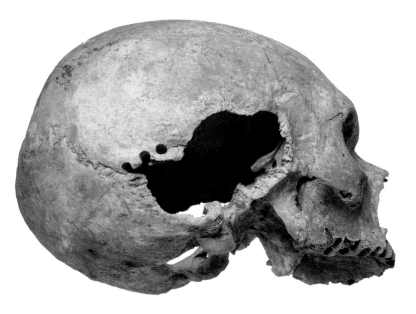

Fig 184 Burr holes and scrape marks in a disarticulated cranium from [229] (scale c 1:2)

Despite the contemporary documentary evidence and the presence of definite patterns within the portions (Fig 170), distinguishing between surgical waste, the practising of surgical techniques and anatomical dissection in disarticulated remains is extremely difficult (above, 'Osteological evidence for surgical intervention'). However, if the assemblage was predominantly composed of medical waste one might anticipate a preponderance of distal limb segments with evidence of sawing, the proximal segment having been retained by the patient who, unless the operation was both unsuccessful in outcome and they were themselves unclaimed, should not have contributed to the skeletal assemblage. An examination of the number of limb segments present in the disarticulated assemblage and the proportion in which saw marks were noted showed that the proportions of proximal and distal limb segments with evidence of sawing were remarkably similar in the upper limb, and although a slightly higher proportion of sawn distal limb

segments compared to proximal elements was present in the lower limb this was not large.

To examine this pattern further, data were collated for all disarticulated humeri and femora displaying saw cuts in the midshaft portion of the bone. Of the 26 humeral segments identified (including three sets of paired partial bones), 15 (57.7%) were proximal segments, nine were distal (34.6%), one contained an entire humerus with saw cuts and another was an ambiguous midshaft segment. This is again suggestive of a sample not predominantly derived from amputation waste. In the femur, however, 19/24 (79.2%) of such segments consisted of the proximal portion of the bone, with just one distal segment and one midshaft fragment that had been sawn at both the proximal and distal ends. Three entire bones were also noted. The presence of surgical waste within the disarticulated sample cannot therefore be completely excluded.

Worked human bone

Four disarticulated post-cranial elements also contained drilled holes not associated with articulation by means of wires or pins (below, 'Prosections and articulations'). All were adult bones from [559]. A left ulna (Fig 185) and a right fibula contained a number of drilled holes, but the most dramatic intervention was in two sections of femur. The first, a left proximal femur, had been sawn through in an anteroposterior direction beneath the lesser trochanter. The bone appeared to have been placed in a lathe, as evident from a V-shaped groove (max D 0.6mm) consistent with gripping in such a tool. At the distal end the bone had been sawn in concentric circles, probably using a circular ring saw blade that was drilled in to create a screw mechanism, a technique used in this period to create needle boxes out of animal bone (A Pipe, pers comm). The V-shaped groove suggests that this bone is the 'chuck' (the waste end piece) rather than the worked object (D Goodburn, pers comm).

In the same context as this element, though from a different individual, was a section of the proximal and midshaft of a right

Table 77 Proportion of sawn elements in the upper and lower limbs from the disarticulated assemblage associated with the early 19th-century cemetery

	Proximal	Mid	Distal
Upper limb (humerus, radius, ulna)			
Present, no marks	313	300	275
Sawn	41	53	30
Cut	1	0	0
Cut & sawn	0	0	1
Total	355	353	306
All sawn elements	41	53	31
%	11.5	15.0	10.1
Lower limb (femur, tibia, fibula)			
Present, no marks	293	268	249
Sawn	70	119	75
Cut	1	0	0
Cut & sawn	0	2	0
Total	364	389	324
All sawn elements	70	121	75
%	19.2	31.1	23.1

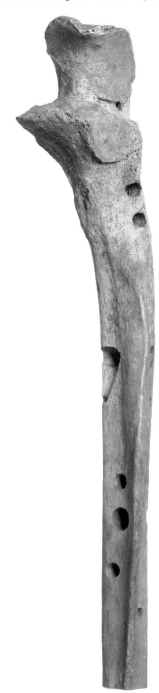

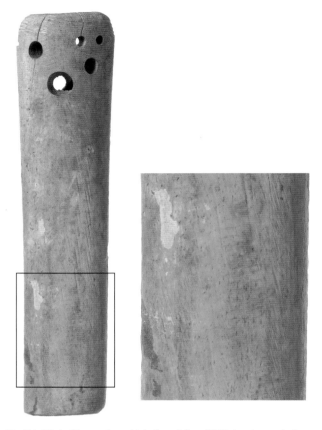

Fig 186 *Worked human bone (right femur) from [559] showing marks from being held in a vice and worked with a file (scale* c 1:1; detail 2:1)

Fig 185 *Holes drilled through the shaft of a disarticulated left ulna from [559] (scale* c 1:1)

femur, 109mm long and again sawn below the lesser trochanter. Marks indicated that it had been held in a vice and that the end of the bone had been filed down to create a smooth, rounded profile and the medullary cavity had been smoothed on the inside. Five small holes had been drilled through the proximal end of the shaft (Fig 186).

These marks clearly do not conform to common surgical techniques (amputation stumps might sometime be filed (Witkin 1997, 30) but not internally), nor do they appear to provide anatomical information. This is, instead, evidence of an attempt at the deliberate working of human remains into artefacts. The

French scholar Pierre Baume, writing in 1829, bequeathed his bones to be turned into knife handles, pin-cases and so forth, by a turner (Richardson 2001, 169), and it is tempting to think that a student reading of this might have attempted to replicate the idea using the facilities available within the hospital (Baume did not die until 1875). The surgeon James Luke is known to have ordered a lathe in 1835 (RLH, LH/A/5/21, 24). The purposes for which it was intended are unclear, but in 1841 he described a suspensory apparatus that he had invented for slinging fractures of the leg by means of a cradle and an 'elevating bedstead', and after his retirement he is known to have taken up wood carving (RCS *Plarr*, sub Luke). However, such behaviour would surely not have been considered acceptable by most of the staff and students. It is also interesting that these remains were found with an excessively drilled occipital (above, 'Practising surgical techniques'), other drilled post-cranial elements and a group of hand phalanges that had been snapped whilst the bone was wet, as if a hand had been deliberately broken or forced open during dissection. Perhaps their proximity indicates that one person was responsible for all, or that this context was a one-off clearance event? Although located within a standard row, there was only one burial in [559].

Waxes, resins and injections

The use of injected waxes started in the early 17th century and at this time the mixtures used were composed of beeswax, tallow, resin and turpentine (Tompsett 1969, 108). As early as 1760, Douglas recommended that the ducts of various glands were to be filled with mercury and wax for examination, as were the veins and arteries, the vascular system to be demonstrated through the use of both dried preparations and dissection (Douglas 1760, 199–205).

The records of the London Hospital detail the purchase in November 1829 of yellow and white wax from Mr John Cowan of Mansion House Street (RLH, LH/A/5/18, 293). Waxes may have been used for sealing bottles or jars, but they were also a vital ingredient for anatomical preparations. When the stolen body of a child was recovered from the dissecting room of St Bartholomew's in 1823 (Chapter 6), it was seen that the veins had been filled with wax (*Morning Chronicle*, 11 March 1823, issue 16814).

Shaw's 1822 anatomy manual refers to the use of dyes and injected waxes for observing the cardiovascular system. Preparations of the arteries were to be filled from the arch of the aorta and he recommended using warm solutions of glue and red lead, or tallow and turpentine varnish. The blood vessels had to be heated first by flushing them through with warm water (Shaw 1822, 20–1). He advised that a red injection was made into the ascending aorta, and the vessels kneaded to work the wax through them (ibid, 257). The right side of the heart was to be filled with blue or yellow injections (ibid, 258). As his was a practical textbook, Shaw provided two recipes for such injections. Ideally one was to use wax, resin and turpentine varnish, but as this was expensive he also recommended a cheaper mixture of 'tallow, resin, wax, venic turpentine, spirit of turpentine, colouring matter' (ibid, 415). He advised that the elderly were unsuitable subjects for injecting as the arteries were likely to be blocked. To inject the heart the sternum was bisected along its length (ibid, 256–7). The manubrium and/or sternum of 12 portions and adult [428], who had been suffering from pulmonary infections at the time of their death, had been bisected in this manner. A further example was identified in the disarticulated remains from [221].

We know that there were those at the London Hospital who had a particular interest in the heart. Dr Archibald Billing (Chapter 5.9, 'The surgeons and physicians'), worked extensively in this area during the 1820s and 1830s, trying to establish a method for rapidly diagnosing aortic aneurysm and performing both autopsy and dissection to aid his studies (Billing 1831, 236; 1833, 443; 1834, 900). This demonstrates, incidentally, that clinicians also performed such procedures.

Mercury injections were used to highlight the lymphatic system. Sir Charles Bell wrote in 1810 that the ideal subject for mercury injection should be under 25 years and 'dropsical'. A cannula was used to enter a lymph gland and then the system was filled with the liquid mercury. Mixtures of turpentine and dyes such as Prussian blue were also used (Tompsett 1969, 109).

Unusual coloration or staining of the skeletal remains was noted throughout the assemblage. A greater percentage of primary inhumations (109/173: 63%) than portions (84/463: 18.1%) were affected. Some staining resulted from contact with iron or copper objects (Table 78). The presence of such staining

Table 78 Number of contexts containing stained human remains (some contexts displayed more than one type of staining)

	No. of contexts	Iron staining		Copper-alloy staining		Other staining		Red stains	
		n	%	n	%	n	%	n	%
Primary inhumations	173	64	37.0	58	33.5	14	8.1	4	2.3
Portions	463	36	7.8	36	7.8	21	4.5	13	2.8

was difficult to interpret, for elements that were not wired or otherwise prepared (below, 'Prosections and articulations') could become stained owing to deposition in proximity to those that were, or indeed to other objects. The small fragments of iron found adhering to numerous skeletal elements probably represent the accidental inclusion of waste within the burial ground soil. The small number of coffin nails found may also have contributed.

Other colours featured in examples of staining included purple, pink, black and yellow. Endocranial pink staining was noted in two primary inhumations and has been seen in remains from a number of other post-medieval cemeteries, such as St Mary and St Michael (Henderson et al in prep). Such staining is thought to be taphonomic in origin and to relate to the colonisation of the tissue by yeasts (Molleson and Cox 1993, 13). Pink staining of the right clavicle of [208] and pink powder adhering to the hands of portion [28506] may also be taphonomic, or the remains of red pigments. Black and dark purple staining is so far of unknown origin but it is possible that this resulted from the degradation of artificially preserved tissues. Embalming was not routinely used during this period, but some practitioners recommended injection of remains with a solution of salt, nitre and alum, preservation by soaking the cadaver in a bath of the same preparation, or wrapping the remains in soaked bandages during dissection (*The Lancet*, 8 August 1835, Preservation of dead bodies for dissection, 24(623), 596–7).

Red staining was most often seen in the thorax. The vertebrae and/or ribs of seven portions and two primary inhumations (2/173: 1.2%) were affected in this way. The left side of the thoracic vertebrae and the visceral surfaces of the left ribs were the apparent focus (Fig 187). Such staining is most likely to have resulted from the employment of resin or wax to examine the aorta, as outlined above.

Perinate [476] (*c* 38 weeks *in utero*) had both green staining in the spinal column and red staining on many of the anterior and lateral surfaces of the vertebral bodies. The extensive nature of this staining suggests preparation as an anatomical specimen. Given the young age and unusual nature of the staining, it may be that this individual was purchased especially for preparation and for investigation of the circulation. The same may be true of the 32-week foetus from [574], where the cranium and mandible were extensively stained (Fig 188). This individual also displayed thick deposits of new bone on the limbs, and this underlying pathological condition – caused by an infectious

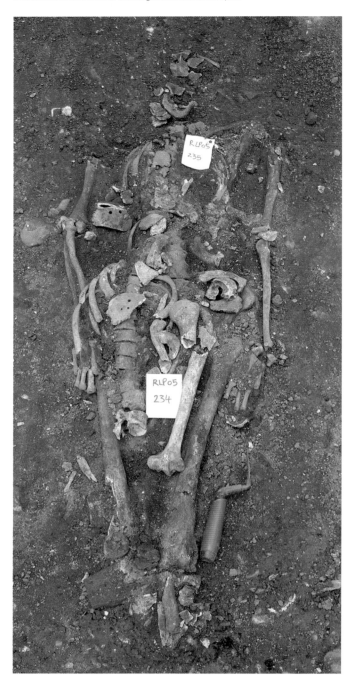

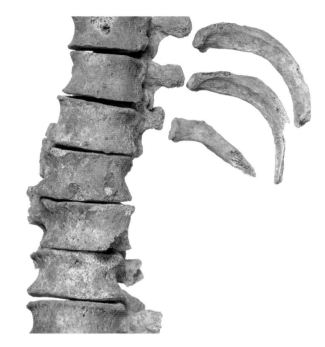

Fig 187 Staining of the ribs and vertebrae of portion [43301]: left – in situ; right – following excavation (scale c 1:2)

four sections of cranium) showed copper-alloy staining. A left frontal and left parietal from [457] were very pale in colour, with a red stain surrounding a saggittal cut that passed through both elements: 0.7% of the groups of conjoined cranial elements (4/609) were stained red (17/1770 elements: 1.0%). A sawn right ilium and ischium from [457], which articulated with a fragment of sacrum and three sections of manubrium and sternum from [263] and [484], also showed red staining. One cranium was darkly stained, the coloration affecting ten cranial elements.

Identified with the remains from seven contexts (six portions and primary inhumation [260]) were tubes of apparently calcareous material. Several were found lying

disease, nutritional deficiency or possibly infantile cortical hyperostosis, a condition whose cause remains unknown but which begins and resolves in early infancy (Lewis 2007, 144) – may have been the reason for its selection for further investigation (though it may have been purely coincidental).

Yellow powdery staining was noted on the left ilium of adult male [222]. The colour suggested that this might be a deposit of sulphur. Sulphur was medicinally used from the 17th century (Harrison et al 2009, 4). The excavators noted, however, that the ilium appeared to have been disturbed after interment and it is therefore not possible definitively to associate this material with the human remains or with the anatomy classes.

In the disarticulated material, seven cranial elements (from

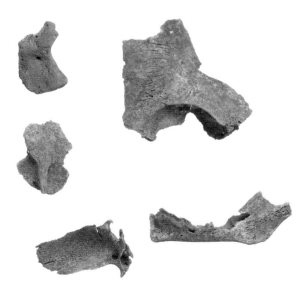

Fig 188 Red staining on the cranium of 32-week foetus [574] (scale c 1:1)

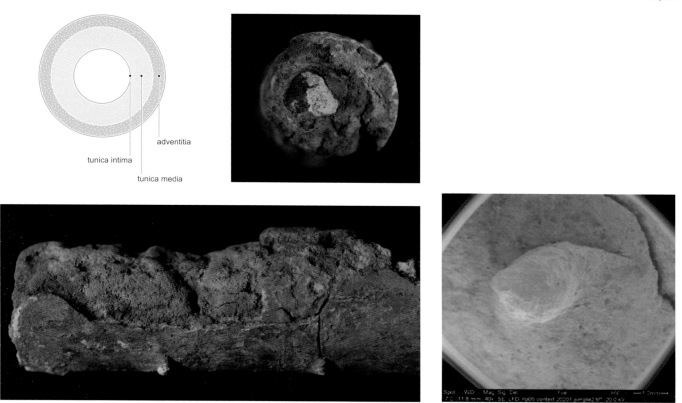

Fig 189 Aortic cast: upper left – diagramatic cross section of the aorta; upper right – detail showing the broken cross section of one of the tubes (scale c 2:1) (© A Wilson 2011); lower left – detail showing the alignment of branches on the tube surface (scale c 2:1); lower right – SEM image of one of the tubes showing side branches (approximate image width 6.7mm) (© A Wilson/University of Bradford 2011)

along the left side of the vertebral column and the dimensions (L *c* 52mm, Diam 20mm) suggested that they were casts of the major blood vessels, specifically the abdominal aorta (confirmed by K Manchester, pers comm) (Fig 189). Close examination of a sample at the University of Bradford showed that the tubes had small projections spaced regularly apart (*c* 25mm), which were *c* 5mm broad by *c* 2mm high and oriented relative to the long axis. The abdominal aorta usually has a number of branches beginning at the thoracic vertebra. Their location would tally with the branches seen on the side of these tubes. The tubes each had an outer lumen of variable thickness up to *c* 2–4mm. X-ray diffraction (XRD) for both the outer (surface) and innermost (core) regions of the tubes, using a Siemens X-ray powder diffraction (PXRD) system, identified the material as lead carbonate.

Lead degrades within the depositional environment, a common outcome being lead carbonate. Lead carbonate is white in colour and has historically been used as a pigment, but the side branches would suggest that liquid (?molten) lead was poured into the aorta to enable casting, or possibly to support the tissue during drying (Mitchell et al 2011, 7). Three examples were found within portions from grave [171], all of which had originated from group 21 (Chapter 3.4). This may suggest that the process that created such casts was introduced during the earliest years of the use of the cemetery. Only two ([16401] and [34404]) showed evidence of thoracotomy (in four instances the bones of the thorax were absent), and neither of these displayed

a bisected sternum. Most curiously, adult primary inhumation [260] had no indications of surgical intervention. Given the stacked nature of the burials it must be considered that the tubes may have originated from another individual, particularly since an intrusive, bisected sternum was found within this context.

Prosections and articulations

Five portions and a number of bones from the disarticulated samples showed evidence of wiring and articulation for presentation as prosections or teaching specimens. Two portions were from group 20 and three from group 22. Small holes, some still containing twists of copper-alloy wire, were seen in a number of ribs and vertebrae from [22901] and [23401]. They were evidently used to articulate the vertebrae together and to the ribs (the former also had iron pins inserted into the vertebral bodies); copper-alloy wires <S35> were also recovered from [234] (Fig 190).

The right foot of portion [22903] had a hole through the body of the right talus, whilst symmetrical holes had been drilled through the ilia and acetabula of a male from [20102] (Fig 191). Both would seem to be consistent with articulation of bone specimens.

One primary inhumation, probable male [504], also showed signs of post-mortem articulation. A thin iron plate (L *c* 24mm, W 13mm) protruded from the superior aspect of the body of the sternum with iron pins in each surviving costal facet. Small

<S35>

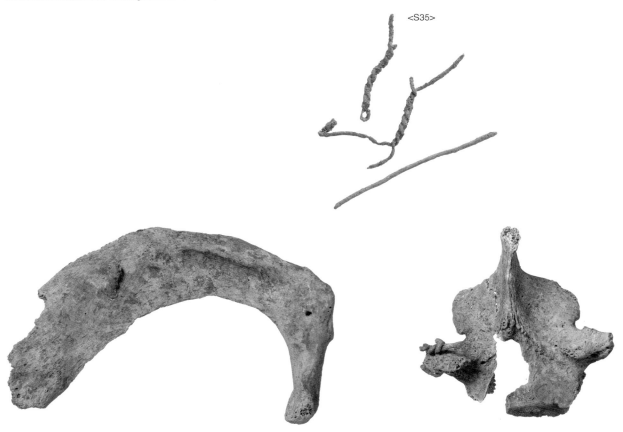

Fig 190 Copper-alloy wires <S35> from [234] and a rib and vertebra with drilled holes from portion [23401] (scale c 1:1)

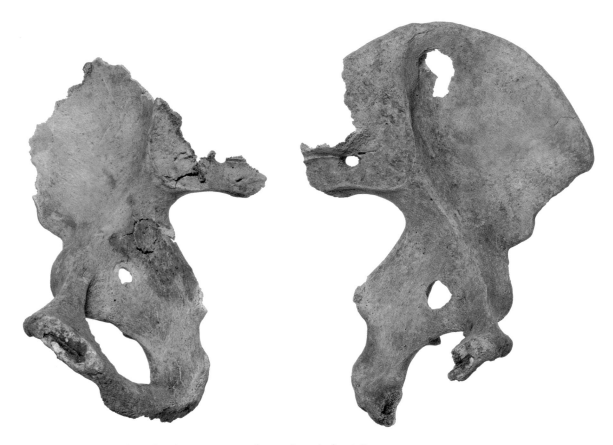

Fig 191 Drilled male os coxae from [20102], indicating preparation for articulation (scale c 1:2)

holes for copper-alloy pins (two of which remained) were present adjacent to the costal facets in the anterior and posterior surfaces of the sternum, with two further pin holes near the top of the first segment (Fig 192). This method appears to have been used to articulate ribs and sternum.

There is some possibility that a rectangular bone label (<S36>, Fig 193), with a hole for a tag and an inscribed number, found in close association with the skull of one of the individuals in the cemetery [341], might have been attached to a prosection.

From the disarticulated material within [224], eight associated ribs showed evidence of articulation using copper-alloy wires. A fragment of ilium from the same context may also originally have been wired. A similar example was seen in [431]. Two holes drilled through a manubrium from [229] and an iron pin passed through the right ilium of a probable female from [224] are also likely to relate to the articulation of dry-bone specimens. A left radius from [229] had been sawn transversely and a hole in the proximal end of the bone may once have held a copper-alloy pin that was found with this bone. A small iron fragment adhering to the lateral aspect of the distal end of the bone may also have been the remains of an inserted pin. It is of interest that [229] (and the portions from within it) accounts for a large number of the prepared specimens.

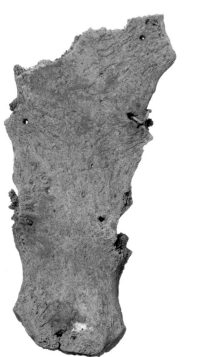
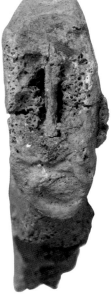

Fig 192 Articulation of the ribs and sternum of adult [504], probable male, by means of copper-alloy and iron pins (scale c 1:1; detail 2:1)

<S36>

Fig 193 Bone label <S36> (scale c 1:1)

Disarticulated first and second sacral vertebrae from [214] also showed evidence of preparation for presentation. A hole had been drilled in a medial to lateral direction through the second sacral vertebra and a rectangular copper-alloy object (8.1 × 2.8mm), with the long axis aligned coronally, was visible in the surface of the first sacral vertebra. An iron pin also protruded from the auricular surface of a female right ilium from [224]. The polished surface of several bones from the disarticulated assemblage, such as a left mandible from [457], is also highly suggestive of the longer-term retention and handling of dissected specimens. In general there were no indications of the selection of a particular specimen of interest, but a first lumbar vertebra from [341], which had been drilled for articulation, had bony changes indicative of an avulsion fracture.

Material that had previously formed part of preserved specimens, as evident from drilled holes and staining caused by copper wires, has also been found at the Old Ashmolean, Bristol Royal Infirmary and Nottingham General Hospital (Cherryson 2010, 140). This suggests that unwanted specimens may have been routinely disposed of within burial grounds, though the material at the London is significant since it had been formally buried within coffins.

Coroner's inquests and autopsy

A brief history of the inquest

Today, around 45% of deaths in England and Wales are referred to the coroner; in 2005, at the coroner's request, autopsies were carried out on 22% of all those who died (Mayor 2006). Until 1874, however, it was not compulsory to have a death medically certified (Higgs 2009, 75), and although the 19th century saw a gradual increase in the number of post-mortems associated with inquests, it was not until the early 20th century that they became routine (Burney 2000, 61). In Westminster between 1835 and 1838, just 17% of coroner's inquests included a post-mortem (ibid, 195).

Before 1860, a coroner was elected only on the basis that he was an independent freeholder, though in practice most were solicitors. They were paid a fee for each inquest held but inquests were generally called only if there was some concern that a death was suspicious or the result of accident (Burney 2000, 3). The coroner did not initiate the inquest but would receive information on a death from any one of a number of sources, including physicans and surgeons. He would then send the parish beadle to make an initial report and only after that would he decide whether an inquest was needed (in effect placing much of this power in the hands of the beadle). The inquest would involve a jury of between 12 and 24 men, drawn from the local community, who would first view the body and then hear all the evidence before deciding on a cause of death (ibid, 4). Inquests were also carried out on all prisoners who died in custody (ibid, 21). By the early 19th century, the body did not have to be present throughout the entire proceedings, but the coroner and jury had to view it together (ibid, 92). After the introduction of the Births and Deaths Registration

Act in 1836, which required the registration of all deaths, the verdict of the inquest became the registered cause of death (ibid, 62).

With no coroners' courts, inquests often took place in public houses (it was not until the 1870s that funds would be found for public mortuaries). The exception was when the death had occurred in an institution, such as a hospital, that had its own 'dead house' (Burney 2000, 80–7). This explains why the staff of the London Hospital were involved in inquests held both on and off the premises (below, 'Inquest and autopsy at the London Hospital'). A publican who refused to allow a body to be taken to their property might find that their licence had been suspended, no matter what state the remains were in; reports from Nottinghamshire indicate that the dismembered remains of those who had died in terrible accidents would be gathered up and taken to the public house for the unfortunate jury to view (Heathcote 2005, 17).

During the 18th and 19th centuries autopsy was viewed as 'an extension of clinical care' and it was not unusual for the upper classes to request a post-mortem examination (Crossland 2009, 109). Cherryson (2010, 136) noted that of a sample of 6719 post-medieval burials excavated from parish burial grounds, churches and chapels across the country, just 48 (0.7%) had been subject to autopsy. That autopsy was initially the preserve of the educated classes is reflected in the fact that the highest rates reported in an archaeological assemblage to date (1.7%) were seen in the high-status burial ground of St Marylebone, Westminster (Miles et al 2008).

Autopsy might be requested to determine cause of death for personal peace of mind or out of philanthropic motives. The will of Robert Featherby (Fotherby), written in 1750 stated 'my Body I direct and order to be opened (if I die in London) by Mr Dawkins the surgeon that now lives near Smithfield Barrs to whom for his trouble I give and bequeath Three Guineas'. If this surgeon was unable to perform the autopsy, he directed that his body be opened by one of the surgeons of St Bartholomew's Hospital, or any other surgeon whom his executors saw fit to appoint 'that the cause of my Death as much as possible may be discovered for the Benefit of Mankind' (TNA: PRO, PROB 11/776, 74). A witness to the autopsy was to swear an oath to a magistrate that the procedure had taken place and provide an affidavit to the church wardens, and it seems that the certificate was received by his family, proving the autopsy took place (TNA: PRO, C 108/250). The usefulness of autopsy as a method for studying morbid anatomy was also recognised (Cherryson 2010, 135), and would cause some controversy.

Throughout much of the period examined by this volume, the coroner for the area of Middlesex, in which the London Hospital was situated, was Mr William Baker. Like many coroners, he was a solicitor. He was also a vestry clerk (Burney 2000, 16). The Middlesex coroner's office was to prove pivotal in establishing the modern practices of the inquest, particularly regarding involvement of the medical profession.

In the autumn of 1830, upon the death of Mr Unwin, the then coroner for Middlesex, Thomas Wakley mounted an election campaign opposing William Baker. Advertisements were placed in the press and supporters' meetings convened in public houses (*Standard*, 23 August 1830, issue 1021; *Examiner*, 29 August 1830, issue 1178; *Morning Post*, 20 September 1830, issue 18650, p 1; *The Times*, 29 September 1830, issue 14344, p 3, col E). Wakley was not just campaigning for himself but for a fundamental change to the nature of the office to that of medical coroner. Some felt that they could not see why medical knowledge was essential to the deliberations over a dead body, but Wakley related that when he had arrived in London in 1815 he had found corrupt practices pervading the charitable medical institutions and stated that his exposés had saved thousands: clearly the office of coroner was for Wakley, as it stood then, also a political one. The coroner was required to consider complicated questions of anatomy and chemistry, for which he felt a medical man (rather than a lawyer) was most appropriately suited (*Morning Post*, 24 August 1830, issue 18627, p 1). Forensic medicine was in its infancy, the role of pathologist yet to be invented (the Pathological Society of London was formed in 1846 (Burney 2000, 114)), and it had not been until the 1820s that forensic medicine was taught in London. The Society of Apothecaries made the subject compulsory in 1831, and the Royal College of Physicians in 1836 (Ward 1993, 42).

Whilst some in the medical profession may have agreed, Wakley's statement that a medical coroner was necessary to ensure that 'improper' medical practices could be brought to light (*Morning Post*, 10 September 1830, issue 18642) hardly made him universally popular. Wakley had an extremely uneasy relationship with many of his colleagues, particularly Blizard, and the early years of *The Lancet* feature few reports of cases from the London Hospital for this very reason.

Wakley did not achieve his ambition until 1839 (Burney 2000, 40), but it was he who first insisted that the coroner be notified of all sudden deaths, not just those that were suspicious, an aspect of the coroner's role that had been restricted by several high court decisions in the early 19th century (ibid, 53). This 'appropriation of sudden death as an exercise in medical self-interestedness' was not at all popular with the magistrates or with the press, who noted his fondness for dissection (ibid, 54). Wakley's 'medicalisation' of the inquest was being seen merely as an excuse for gratuitous post-mortem investigation after the Anatomy Act, and a convenient way of lining the pockets of the surgeons (ibid, 56).

Inquest and autopsy at the London Hospital

The committee at the London Hospital referred to autopsy as 'that important branch of medical duty' (RLH, LH/A/5/19, 197). Not all autopsies were performed at the request of the coroner. Surgeons might undertake an autopsy to determine the cause of death of a patient from intellectual curiosity or to aid in teaching. From the end of the 18th century there appears to have been little obstacle to this, though the families of private patients were more likely to raise a complaint (Lawrence 1996, 309). At Worcester Royal Infirmary, records indicate that post-mortems took place throughout the 19th century (Western

2010, 6), whilst as early as 1750 the governors of St Bartholomew's Hospital had determined that autopsies should be performed on patients to determine cause of death. As at the London, the process was overseen by the surgeon's beadle (St Bartholomew's further stipulated that a member of staff was required to observe before the body was sewn up and placed in a coffin (Lawrence 1996, 196)). It was not just patients who might be examined – at the London in November 1822 a resolution was passed that nurses and hospital servants were not to be 'open for examination' without a relative's permission (RLH, LH/A/5/17, 169).

Physicians and surgeons from the London were frequently involved in coroner's inquests (and their associated autopsies), many of which were held at the sign of the London Hospital (eg, *The Times*, 29 September 1806, issue 6853, p 3, col C), a nearby public house that was run by a Mr Gilbert. Others were held in the hospital board room (*The Times*, 7 January 1819, issue 10564, p 3, col E) or other public houses in the vicinity. In January 1824 the house committee resolved that in future all inquests should be held in the committee room and not at a public house (RLH, LH/A/5/17, 302).

Many viewings of the bodies were held in the dead house. The necessity to do so was questioned by Blizard in September 1830, but no alternative room could be found (RLH, LH/A/5/18, 366–9). Inquests were continuing in the dead house in 1831 when William Baker wrote (RLH, LH/A/5/19, 17 November 1831, 144):

you are aware of the great difficulty I have in getting Jurymen to meet at the Hospital and although I believe it arises in some degree from there being no allowance made to them, yet I am well persuaded that it also arises from an apprehension of great danger from fever or infectious disease; this would be very much obviated by the dead bodies to be viewed by the Juries which are entirely confined to accidents being placed in a separate Depository from all other cases. At present the Juries have to pass through the general receiving room for the dead into the Depository room, and it is a matter of great complaint.

By August 1832, the fitting up of an inquest room in the corner of the waiting hall for the outpatients was nearly complete (RLH, LH/A/5/19, 296).

In one bizarre case, the viewing of the body of Catherine Moody was delayed until Hurst, the surgeon's beadle, was located with the keys. The coroner, Mr Unwin, decided meanwhile to start taking statements, and established that Moody had fallen down a set of steps whilst drunk, breaking her leg. She was taken by coach to the London Hospital for treatment. The jury was satisfied that it had been an accident and prepared again to view the body. At this point Mr Gilbert, the landlord of the public house next to the hospital in which the inquest was being held, rushed in, exclaiming 'the woman on whom you have held the inquest is still living, for I left her this moment eating stewed oysters and drinking wine [surely not part of the usual hospital diet]; the nurse who was

attending her seems to have some hopes of her recovery.' Unwin stated that he 'would never again hold an inquest on any person in the hospital, unless he previously had a letter from the beadle of that establishment, declaring the individual to be actually dead' (*The Times*, 8 October 1823, issue 11996, p 3, col D).

With forensic medicine still an emerging branch of study, a post-mortem would not always provide conclusive results. When Hannah Norton was beaten by her husband John in August 1835, she was admitted to the London Hospital with numerous lacerations and bruises, her jaw broken on both sides. Five days later in a state of delirium she died. The house surgeon, James Duncan, reported that the autopsy had been inconclusive. He felt that her constitution had been broken by years of drinking and that this made her susceptible to the punches rained on her, and he could not definitively state that the injuries had caused her death. In this case evidence was also given by a nurse, Emma Parish, as to the state in which the patient had been in the hospital (*Old Bailey Proc*, August 1835, John Norton (t18350817-1883)).

Medical witnesses were not paid until after 1836, when, with the help of Thomas Wakley, the Medical Witnesses Act was passed (Burney 2000, 108). This act required the coroner to select a medical witness, with the guidance that the medical practitioner who had most recently attended the deceased or who saw them immediately after death was to be called (Burney 2000, 109).

It seems that at the London Hospital the person who attended a patient in life was also likely to perform, or at least attend, their autopsy in death, regardless of their rank (a practice which must have left open the possibility of covering up their failures). Thus a report of 1842 indicates that a pupil, Andrew Hingston, had performed a post-mortem on a patient whom he had previously dressed, discovering that he had died of complications from a fractured skull. Hingston stated 'we' found a fracture, suggesting that he may have been in attendance on a more senior practitioner during the autopsy (*Old Bailey Proc*, June 1842, Robert Peck (t18420613-1735)).

When 16-year-old William Gage died following an organised fist fight with 15-year-old Joseph Palmer – which had lasted three quarters of an hour and during which Gage fell into a hole – John Adams, a student, performed the autopsy. After the fight, Gage started to complain of a headache, fell insensible and, after 12 hours at the London Hospital, died. Adams opened Gage after his death and examined his brain for injuries. He concluded that the quantities of blood found on the brain (probably describing a haematoma) and injuries to the internal structures were the result of the fall, rather than the pummelling Gale had taken at the hands of a far stronger boy (*Old Bailey Proc*, June 1826, Joseph Palmer, James Kendall, Joseph Spring, Samson Tasker (t18260622-30)).

Perhaps the lack of financial incentive before the passing of the Medical Witnesses Act, or simply the educational role that the hospital played, were reasons for the attendance of pupils at autopsies. As early as 1834 pupils clearly played a significant role at inquests, the coroner noting that juries often complained of the 'impertinence of the medical pupils of this hospital, and the loose and flippant manner in which they frequently give evidence', after a Mr Wells, a pupil called to give evidence at an inquest, did not know the name of the deceased and claimed that he did not have any need for notes from which to give his evidence (RLH, LH/A/26/1).

Some of the inquests held directly involved patients (RLH, LH/A/5/19, 324):

Limehouse 21st September 1832

Sir,
at the request of the Jury summoned this day to enquire into the circumstances attending the death of Elizabeth Davies who threw herself out of the window of a watercloset in the London Hospital, I beg to state to you, for the information of the House Committee that it was their unanimous opinion upon a view of the window in question that it would be desirable in the fever wards, where delirium is likely to prevail, that bars should be placed at the watercloset windows to prevent, as much as possible, the occurrence of any such calamity in future.

William Baker, Coroner.

Some of those on whom inquests were held were interred in the hospital ground. Upon completion of the inquest, the burial warrant was issued by the coroner, Mr Unwin, to permit the burial of the body. He had been issuing the warrants to the petty parish officers, who had been eventually supplying them to the hospital to allow for burial in the hospital ground but had been demanding the payment of 14s 8d from relatives. Eventually efforts from the hospital's solicitor persuaded him to deliver the warrant instead to the surgeon's beadle, who was to deliver it either to the relatives or to the house governor, if the burial was to take place in the hospital ground (RLH, LH/A/5/17, 300), although the problem persisted for a while (RLH, LH/A/17/5, 6 June 1826).

It is likely that some of those on whom autopsies were performed would have been interred in the hospital burial ground even if they had not been treated at the London Hospital, as they could have been brought to the mortuary facilities there. If such a body were unclaimed, then it is also possible that further dissection would have been performed.

Osteological evidence of autopsy

Modern autopsy procedures normally involve the performance of a craniotomy and the opening of the thoracic cavity, the former being the most commonly observed in archaeological material (Cherryson 2010, 137). There is little evidence of the standardisation of autopsy techniques until the late 19th century, however, and the areas investigated would vary depending on the presumed location of interest and sometimes on the wishes of the family of the deceased (ibid). Charles Hastings, physician at the Worcester Royal Infirmary, noted

that post-mortems were carried out between 18 and 48 hours after death and consisted of thoracotomy and/or craniotomy (Western 2010, 10).

The analysis of evidence of autopsy in archaeological skeletal remains is subject to a number of difficulties. Whilst the use of true prevalence rates (observations by element) may help to counter this, the absence of areas of the skeleton may hinder analysis of the pattern of involvement within each individual, an important factor in the interpretation of the intent behind the cutting and sawing. In cases of genuine autopsy, where the purpose was to investigate the cause of death, there may be little or no significant variation between the distribution of tool marks as the result of the interventions of a doctor or surgeon in a medical school and those from a student practising the same techniques in class. Whilst the presence of craniotomy and/or thoracic cuts alone is considered to be representative of autopsy, such cuts might also form part of dissection. In an era before refrigeration and other methods of artificially prolonging preservation, the anatomist or surgeon would have needed to proceed pragmatically. The contemporary texts recommended that the viscera were examined and removed first, to delay putrefaction for as long as possible (above, 'Tools and techniques'). It is not therefore possible to distinguish osteologically between individuals who underwent autopsy and then passed to the anatomy table, and those who went directly to the classroom.

For the purposes of statistical analysis of the primary inhumations, autopsy was considered where there was only limited investigation of the body, defined as craniotomy (circumferential sawn cuts in the horizontal plane that allowed removal of the calvarium) and internal thoracic investigation (assumed where saw cuts were observed in the ribs, sternum and/or medial clavicles) (Fig 194). Of the 55 primary inhumations with sawn elements, 48 (87.3%) included patterning characteristic of autopsy. In total, 27.7% of primary inhumations were affected, with no statistically significant difference in prevalence rate between males and females (Table 79).

Craniotomies were the most common indication of autopsy, with 79.2% (38/48) of 'autopsied' primary inhumations thus affected (Fig 195). This rose to over 95% when the maximum possible percentage was calculated (number affected plus number of absent crania, as a percentage of 'autopsied' primary inhumations). All eight females and 86.7% of males (26/30) with cuts consistent with autopsy had undergone craniotomy. The sternum was least frequently affected. The lower numbers of clavicle, rib and sternal cuts may reflect variations in the techniques for gaining entry to the thoracic cavity depending on the precise structures which were of interest (above, 'Tools and techniques'). In comparison, 11% of articulated (7/63) and 18% (53/295) of disarticulated crania recovered from Newcastle Infirmary had craniotomy cuts (Boulter et al 1998, 143). Nineteen 'autopsied' primary inhumations (19/48: 39.6%) at the London Hospital also had evidence of dissection in the form of saw cuts in areas of the body beyond the clavicles, ribs, sternum or the circumferential horizontal plane of the calvarium.

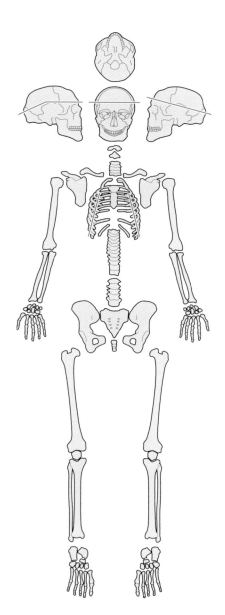

Fig 194 Diagram of 'autopsy' sawn cuts in 36–45-year-old male primary inhumation [349]

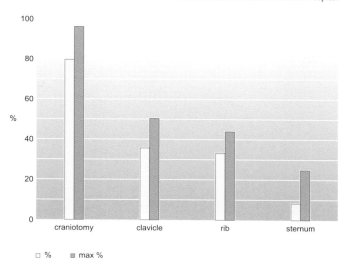

Fig 195 Percentage of primary inhumations affected with each aspect of possible autopsy (maximum percentage includes absent elements)

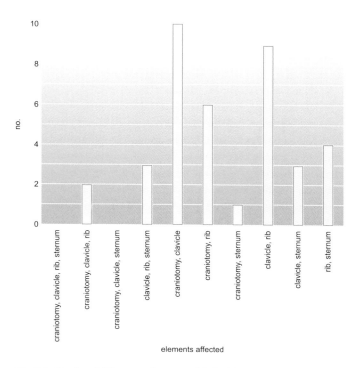

Fig 196 Number of different combinations of skeletal locations in primary inhumations affected by autopsy

Table 79 Primary inhumations with saw cuts characteristic of autopsy

	n	'Autopsied' n	%
Subadult	13	2	15.4
Female	30	8	26.7
Male	80	30	37.5
All adults	160	46	28.8
Total	173	48	27.7

The most commonly found combinations of saw cuts in the 'autopsied' primary inhumations were craniotomies and clavicles, followed by clavicles and ribs (Fig 196). Few had more than two different locations affected, but the absence of elements in some individuals impacted upon the accuracy of the graph.

Possible examples of autopsy following unsuccessful surgery were noted in female [396], where a sawn fragment of distal ulna suggested the possibility that the left hand had been amputated in life, and male [408], where the right femoral head had been removed, though the legs were partially complete.

Visual examination of the pattern of surgical intervention in the entire articulated assemblage enabled further observations of the numbers of individuals who had undergone autopsy. For the examination of patterns from the the recording diagrams, an osteological definition of autopsy was based on the presence of minimal cranial and/or thoracic intervention, with up to one other type of intervention where an archaeological parallel from a known autopsy could be established, specifically, vertical

Table 80 Location of intervention in contexts with evidence of autopsy from the articulated assemblage, by group

	No. cranium only	No. thoracic only	No. cranial & thoracic	Craniotomy only	Thoracic only	Cranial & thoracic intervention	Cranial & vertebral	Pubic cuts	Total
Group 20									
Male	0	0	10	3	0	5	0	1	9
Female	1	0	3	1	0	3	0	0	4
Other adult	0	6	0	0	6	0	0	0	6
Subadult	0	0	1	1	0	0	0	0	1
Total	1	6	14	5	6	8	0	1	20
Group 21									
Male	0	0	8	6	1	1	0	0	8
Female	1	0	1	2	0	0	0	0	2
Other adult	1	1	0	1	1	0	0	0	2
Subadult	0	0	0	0	0	0	0	0	0
Total	2	1	9	9	2	1	0	0	12
Group 22									
Male	0	2	4	2	1	1	1	1	6
Female	0	1	3	1	1	2	0	0	4
Other adult	0	0	0	0	0	0	0	0	0
Subadult	0	0	0	0	0	0	0	0	0
Total	0	3	7	3	2	3	1	0	10
Grand total	3	10	30	17	10	12	1	1	42

saw cuts removing one or several neural arches and/or the basilar cranium (with parallels at City Bunhill burial ground (Connell and Miles 2010, 48), New Bunhill burial ground (Miles 2012) – where the cuts ran from the second cervical to fifth sacral vertebra – Cross Bones burial ground, Southwark (Brickley and Miles 1999, 45) and Christ Church Spitalfields (Molleson and Cox 1993, 87)) and cuts through the pubis (seen in Perfect Dives, a male buried at Bow Baptist church (Henderson et al in prep)). The former would have been carried out to examine the spinal cord 'by the removal of the spinous processes and rings of the vertebrae along the whole length of the spine' (Stanley 1822, 360).

Examination of the recording diagrams for the entire articulated assemblage produced a surprisingly low number of contexts containing the remains of individuals who had undergone only autopsy: just 20 from group 20, 12 from group 21 and ten from group 22. The majority had both cranial and thoracic remains observable, yet the incidence of craniotomy only, with no evidence of thoracic intervention, was high, supporting the observations made in the primary inhumations (Table 80). A spatial examination of the location of those burials showing only indications of autopsy revealed no discernible pattern, with such burials spread across the cemetery (Chapter 3.4).

7.9 Burying the dissected dead

The Anatomy Act specified that the remains of each individual should be reunited following dissection in order for a 'decent burial' to take place. Valentine, the house governor, was obviously concerned that this would require changes to existing practices, and Hamilton's letter regarding the burial of remains from Lane's school suggests that this clause created some difficulties for anatomists, and that it was not always strictly observed (above, 7.6). It is only through taking a holistic approach, utilising historical records, archaeology and osteology, that the reality of an 'anatomy burial' can be revealed.

The London Hospital was not unique in its disturbance of recently buried remains in the mid 19th century (group 22; Chapter 3.4). At Newcastle Infirmary, a number of bone-filled pits found within a ravine were thought to result from the infilling of the feature to create a formal garden in 1859 (Nolan 1998, 19). An extension to the Dobson wing there was constructed in 1851–3 and included surgeons' rooms and a dead house. Construction resulted in the disturbance of a large quantity of remains (ibid, 22). Most significant was the enlargement of the hospital in 1801–3 over the existing burial ground. Estimates for the extension do not mention the impact on the burial ground but there were 'payments for extra work connected with the foundations' (ibid, 30) and at least 407 individuals were moved for this extension. Considering these remains Nolan states that 'the apparent casualness with which these remains, many belonging to the then only recently dead, were treated makes an interesting counterpoint to the popularly accepted view of mid 19th-century reverence and concern for the deceased' (ibid, 41).

Clearly this was not the case at the London, where a formal, if somewhat communal, burial appears to have been the norm prior to the Anatomy Act, perhaps as a direct result of the efforts of William Valentine. Removal of illegally anatomised

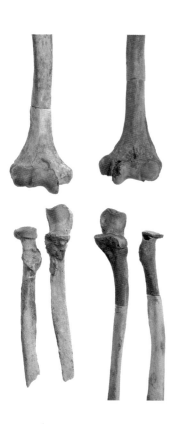
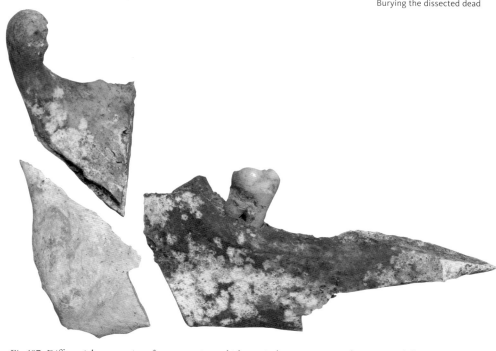

Fig 197 *Differential preservation of sawn remains, which may indicate retention or deposition in different environments or states of decomposition: left – from portion [16404] (scale c 1:4); right – disarticulated bone from context [213] (scale c 1:1)*

(ie, pre-1832) remains to a parish ground would have been somewhat risky, but dead and unclaimed patients who were not the subject of post-mortem intervention were equally separated from the parish in death. Whilst not unique in disposing of dissected remains by interring them within coffins that were arranged in rows, the London clearly showed a degree of formality in the funerary treatment of those who passed through its walls.

From the contemporary accounts of anatomy classes, it seems that body parts may have been retained above ground for some time before burial, and the archaeological evidence of prosections and possibly that of differential preservation (Fig 197) supports this. It is, however, unclear what the interval between death and burial would have been if an individual was not examined or was simply the subject of an autopsy. Given that speed was advocated in dealing with the dead, it is unlikely that the interval was great.

At Newcastle Infirmary the dead were placed on a thin layer of sawdust within a wooden coffin, which was then packed with wood shavings. Rows of graves were dug and covered by low mounds with marker sticks (Nolan 1998, 40, 72). The maximum number of individuals found within each coffin was six and the registers indicate that there were approximately 13 burials per year (A Chamberlain, pers comm).

Guthrie, writing in 1829, declared that the pretence of a decent burial should be scrapped. He claimed that as dissection was a slow process it simply was not possible to store all the separated parts for a single burial and therefore flesh was often thrown away with the rest of the rubbish (Wise 2004, 250). The archaeological evidence, however, clearly indicates that reuniting of body parts for burial regularly took place at the London Hospital. Eighteen contexts from group 20, 12 from group 21 and four from group 22 contained remains that had been sawn through or otherwise dissected but placed within the same coffin for burial. For example, the limbs of [52203] presented with multiple saw cuts portioning the body into 'standard' sections, but the remains had been reunited (Fig 198), and the head and body of male [34083] were interred together despite the neck having been severed. Preservation now prevents the evaluation of Guthrie's claim about the casual disposal methods used for soft tissue. Intrusive remains in primary inhumation [166] appeared to have been deliberately placed to make up cosmetically the deficit from the absence of the left leg. The left distal femur was sawn through and portions of femoral shaft from two other adults had been placed in the location where the lower leg should have been. In contrast, the remains recovered from the Old Anatomy School in Dublin were recorded as having been deposited in trenches and pits with no attempt to inter individuals as complete (Murphy 2011).

In order to examine the possibility that the deposition of the remains would reflect the class that was being taught at that time – in which case some contexts might contain only remains from the upper limb, others only lower limbs and so forth – the articulated remains were catalogued based on structural segment. The arm and scapula and leg and pelvis were each considered as a single unit and the number of right and left units, together with the number of skulls present in each context, was calculated, with a unit considered to be present if any portion remained, with the exception of those where only the hands, feet or a small fragment of pubis remained. Whilst this cannot provide an accurate count of the elements or individuals present, particularly since it excludes the evidence from the disarticulated assemblage (but also as this method does not prevent a segmented limb from being counted twice), it provides a broad comparison of the nature of the human remains by burial stack, sufficient to examine whether some stacks (and therefore some burial events) differed significantly from others. Perhaps surprisingly, there was little apparent variation, with almost all contexts containing articulated remains from upper and lower limbs and the head. Grave [278] contained a large number of portions (32), a high proportion of which (18) came from the lower limbs. The average number of limb zones by grave was lower in group 20 than the other two groups, but when this pattern was examined further it became clear that this was probably a result of the lower relative proportion of contexts showing evidence of dissection (in other words, segmented limbs were counted more than once in groups 21 and 22). Examination of the primary inhumations only confirmed that the head was under-represented within the

Table 81 Number of primary inhumations, by group, where a particular body zone was not represented (excluding hands/feet)

Group	No. of contexts	No upper limb	No lower limb	No head	% no upper limb	% no lower limb	% no head
20	68	14	11	33	20.6	16.2	48.5
21	55	18	10	29	32.7	18.2	52.7
22	50	2	1	20	4.0	2.0	40.0

primary burial sample (Table 81), in parallel with patterns noted in the faunal assemblage (Chapter 7.7).

Within the constraints of the project it was not possible to establish the total minimum number of individuals present in each context, but in order to examine the number of bodies placed in each coffin, four graves from groups 20 and 21 were selected for further investigation, on archaeological grounds and for their lack of truncation (Chapter 3.4; Fig 199). It should be remembered that the minimum number estimates are just that and that the graves may each have contained as many individuals as the maximum number of contexts plus disarticulated bones present.

Based on the maximum number of repeated elements grave [417] from group 20 was found to contain the remains of a minimum of six individuals (left mandible). The grave contained remains from all three categories: two primary inhumations, five portions and three contexts of disarticulated remains. All were adult and it was possible to estimate the sex of one primary inhumation and two portions, all of which were male. One portion originated from an 18–25-year-old and primary inhumation [237] was that of a 26–35-year-old. Although parts of six adults were present in the grave, most elements were repeated no more than three times, suggesting that the burial contained three largely substantial individuals and a smaller collection of additional elements. Grave [366] contained a minimum of four individuals (left distal femur and fourth lumbar vertebra). Two primary inhumations (one male, one female), seven portions (two of which were from males) and one context of disarticulated bone were recovered.

In group 21, grave [207] contained a minimum of ten individuals (left mid humerus – all bones were largely complete so no double counting has occurred) represented by four primary inhumations, 20 portions and four contexts of disarticulated bone. Grave [220] contained 30 portions and four contexts of disarticulated bone from a minimum of nine individuals (left mandible) including ten portions from males, two from females and one subadult. Most elements were repeated four times, again suggesting that there was a smaller group of largely complete individuals plus additional remains. The results show that the deeper graves of group 21 contain a larger number of individuals and suggest that an average of approximately seven burials per grave might be expected.

There does not appear to be any discernible pattern to the

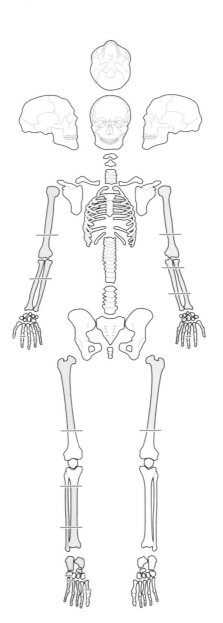

Fig 198 Context [52203] showing standardised portions reunited for burial

deposition of the human remains, other than that each coffin usually contained elements from throughout the body, as well as a demographic mix and that, whilst attempts were made to reunite dissected body parts, animal bone and 'odd' specimens were also disposed of in this way. As the three burial groups represent change over a period of time spanning the Anatomy Act (Chapter 3.4), this suggests that there was no significant change in behaviour following its implementation.

An apparent deposition pattern was noted in the faunal remains (Table 82). In group 20, the majority of the associated bone groups were recovered in association with the last (uppermost) or penultimate human burials in the grave stacks, perhaps representing the opportunistic disposal of anatomy school waste in graves that were about to be closed. In contrast,

the remains in group 21 appeared to have been deposited towards the bottom of the grave stacks. The remains from [220], for example, were associated with the first, second and third burials in that stack, whereas the three later burials had no animal remains associated with them. The burials are slightly later in date than those from group 20 and it may be that this does represent a change in behaviour after the introduction of the Anatomy Act. Group 22 burials include the possible 'odd' specimen of a hedgehog.

The reuniting of the human remains and patterns suggesting that animal bone was 'hidden' in the lowest coffins in each stack suggest that there was a degree of sensitivity in the way in which the dissected cadavers and specimens were interred or, at the very least, of sensitivity to the expectations of society.

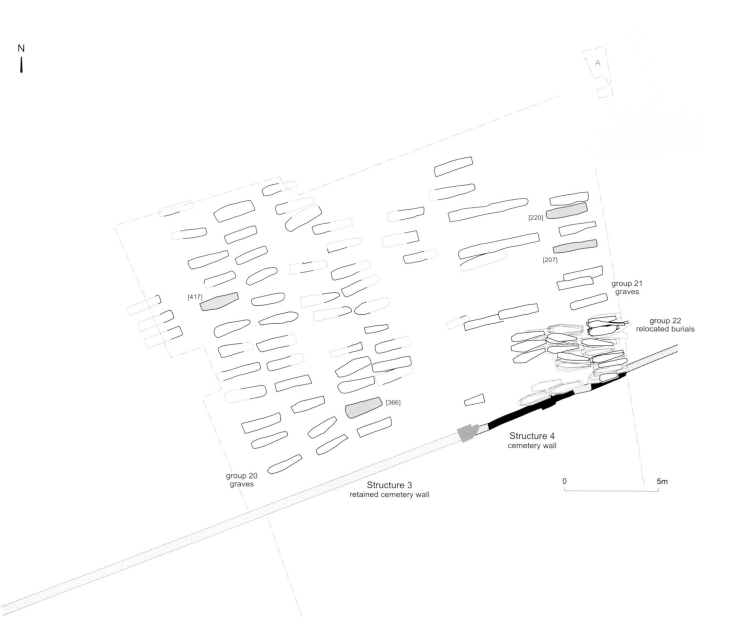

Fig 199 Location of the four graves ([417], [366], [220], [207]) examined from groups 20 and 21 (OA6, period 4) (scale 1:200); inset (top right) locates area A within the overall area of phase 1 works (see Fig 3)

Table 82 Summary of animal remains likely to originate from the hospital's anatomy school recovered from graves in groups 20, 21 and 22 (OA6, period 4)

Grave context no./subgroup	Burial	Taxon	Description
Group 20			
[331]	last of 2	primate	fibula with dissection marks
[332]	last of 3	dog	partial male adult, hind elements
		rabbit	partial, hindlimb elements
	1st of 3	rabbit	almost complete, adult, skull missing, dissection marks
[435]	last of 2	rabbit	partial skull & forelimbs, very large
[447]	last of 2	dog	complete subadult, possibly female
		rabbit	partial adult, hind elements
[464]	1st of 3	cow	dissected 1st phalanx
[470]	last of 5	dog	partial, hind foot
		dog	partial adult, hind foot (possibly associated with human neonate)
[516]	single burial	dog	partial subadult, body & hindlimb elements
[553]	last of 3	dog	complete adult, probable female, dissection marks present
[555]	4th of 5	cat	partial juvenile, body & forelimb elements
[622]	single burial	dog	partial adult, head, body & forelimbs
[803]	last of 2	dog	partial adult, head & forelimb elements
[805]	1st of 2	horse	dissected mandible (fragmented)
Group 21			
[171]	1st of 5	pig	partial infant, hind elements
[207]	3rd of 6	rabbit	partial head & front limbs, very large, juvenile
	2nd of 6	tortoise	partial Hermann's, limb bones, no carapace present
		plaice	almost complete head & vertebra
	grave fill	dog	partial infant, both hindlimbs
		dog	partial infant, head body, fore- & hindlimbs
		rabbit	complete juvenile, large rabbit
[220]	3rd of 6	dog	almost complete adult male, mandibles & some foot elements missing, pathology on hindlimb
	2nd of 6	dog	partial adult, head & body elements
		conga eel	head & first 3 vertebrae
	1st of 6	horse	partial adult, dissected head & vertebral elements
[251]	1st of 4	cow	dissection periotic bone marks
		monkey	possible mona monkey, missing head & cervical vertebrae, juvenile
[327]	grave fill	primate	2 1st metacarpals, juvenile, from different species
[458]	grave fill	cat	2 partial neonates, ribs, vertebrae & long bones
		tortoise	humerus, unknown species
Group 22			
7	2nd of 5	cow	partial neonate, head & vertebral elements
	1st of 5	dog	partial, cervical vertebra
16	last of 3	cat	partial juvenile, head & vertebral column
22	1st of 4	hedgehog	almost complete adult, feet missing
24	3rd of 4	sheep/goat	partial vertebral column

8

'Abuses, peculations and misapplications'

'Without which science must perish' (Millard 1825, title page; Agnew 1963, 176)

8.1   The case of William Millard

Of all the information recorded in the minute books, there is perhaps one story that provides us with the greatest insight into the awkward relationship the medical profession had with the practices of dissection prior to the Anatomy Act. Unlike the later cases of Burke and Hare in Edinburgh, and the 'Italian boy' murder in London, it concerned not opportunistic murderers but those who were regularly involved in the supply of 'subjects' to the London schools of anatomy. Vitally, it is a story that can now be viewed in a very different light, thanks to the archaeological evidence in support of the claims of a woman who at the time was vilified for her extreme criticism of those practising medicine in London: Mrs Ann Millard.

William Millard's arrest took place in 1823, before the burial ground (OA6; Chapter 3.4) came into use. At that time, the hospital burial ground was located immediately to the north, overlooked by Gloucester, Granby and Talbot wards in the east wing (Clark-Kennedy 1962, 232). Despite this, burials were at risk from 'resurrectionists' hoping to disinter remains that could then be sold to one of the other schools of anatomy operating in the capital. Matters reached a head in 1823. On 12 August, the house governor, William Valentine, reported to the house committee that during the previous week intruders had attempted to disinter a body buried immediately under one of the ward windows. The patients had been disturbed and had called out, frightening off the intruders, who returned the following night to try their luck again and again failed. During the same week, the dead house had been broken into and the body of a young woman stolen (according to Bransby Cooper this was the work of Vaughan (Cooper 1843, 444)). The house governor recommended to the house committee that 'a more effectual fence be placed on the surrounding walls of the burial ground and that a watchman is employed' (RLH, LH/A/17/3, 72).

The arrest

At one o'clock in the morning on Saturday 23 August 1823, William Millard and Cornelius 'Bryant' were arrested in the grounds of the London Hospital. According to the *Morning Chronicle* the hospital had set a watch on the graveyard and 'between the hours of twelve and one o'clock on Saturday morning, the inmates of the establishment were thrown into the greatest confusion and alarm' when one of the nurses spotted the two men from the window of a ward (*Morning Chronicle*, 25 August 1823, issue 16957). The minutes of the house committee state that some of the patients, together with Samuel Hicks (a hospital porter also known as 'Sam the Barber'), raised the initial alarm (RLH, LH/A/5/17, 268), and Hicks would certainly later state that a body had been interred on the Wednesday morning and that each night from Wednesday to Friday he had seen the defendant 'lurking about' (*The Times*, 12 September 1823, issue 11975, p 3, col B). In a fantastic piece of tabloid journalism, the *Morning Chronicle* claimed that 'the anxiety prevailing amongst the poor patients to secure the villains was so great, that several of them were seen, on their crutches, joining the pursuit through the sepulchres' with the servants and students. Cornelius was apparently found hiding in the privy and tried to fight his way out with a shovel, whilst Millard was caught heading over the fence (*Morning Chronicle*, 25 August 1823, issue 16957). A subsequent investigation by the solicitor Mr Lang identified those who had been most instrumental in securing the arrest of Millard and Bryant (RLH, LH/A/5/17, 268):

the Persons principally instrumental in apprehending the Prisoners are in the first place – The Patients making the discovery of their presence in the Ground and the Porter Samuel Hicks with those Patients accompanying him to the Ground and assisting in the attack, and of these Patients Sheen was the most active. The persons next in degree of merit appear to be the police officer George Ellis and Watchman Samuel Bowden who scaled the East Wall of the burial Ground upon hearing the alarm with an alacrity highly creditable to them. The watchmen John Walton and Edward Letterys Appear in the next degree prompt in rendering assistance and to the active discharge of their duty the capture of Millard is attributable. The two other police officers David Healey and Henry Paulson and the night constable James Stone were assisting only after the capture and in eliciting from Millard a declaration. Admitting his presence in the burial Ground and the purpose for which he was there the evidence of which was important in establishing the proof of his identity and intended offence.

The two men could not be arrested for stealing a body (Chapter 6.3) and, in any case, they had not got as far as disturbing a corpse. Instead they were arrested for vagrancy as they could not (or would not) give a proper account of their reasons for being in the hospital grounds at night (*The Times*, 12 September 1823, issue 11975, p 3, col B). The Vagrancy Act had been amended in 1822 and was extremely unpopular as it required that anyone challenged in the street should give 'a good account' of themselves to avoid arrest (Roberts 1988, 283).

Millard and Cornelius were perhaps unfortunate, seeing that after the recent theft of a woman's body from the dead house the governors had offered a reward of £20 to anyone who caught those responsible (RLH, LH/A/5/17, 251; *Morning Chronicle*, 25 August 1823, issue 16957; Cooper 1843, 444). Those who apprehended a vagrant were anyway rewarded with a payment of 5s (Roberts 1988, 283). The rewards paid to those instrumental in apprehending Millard and Cornelius, however, fell far short of the sum offered by the governors, with those identified in Mr Lang's report receiving the following rewards from the funds of the hospital: George Ellis £2 2s; Samuel Bowden £2 2s; John Walton £1 1s; Edward Letterys £1 1s; David Healey 10s 6d; Henry Paulson 10s 6d; Samuel Hicks £2 2s; Jeremiah Sheen £2 2s. All the men also received 'such allowance as is usual for daily pay of witnesses' (RLH, LH/A/5/17, 272).

Immediately upon their arrest an unidentified 'Member of

the Faculty' stepped forwards to post bail (*Morning Chronicle*, 25 August 1823, issue 16957). This behaviour was common in such cases: Sir Astley Cooper had paid £14 7s in bail through an intermediary to assist Vaughan in 1818, paying for his food, drink and tobacco when he was imprisoned after making a trip to Yarmouth (where Sir Astley had previously lived) to procure bodies (Cooper 1843, 396). It was the usual practice for surgeons to post bail for loyal suppliers, who, in addition to performing a vital service, posed a potential threat to their good name, should they decide to tell all to the courts. Sir Astley had reportedly 'expended hundreds of pounds for this purpose' bailing out resurrectionists and paying for the care of their wives and children (ibid, 395). Unfortunately for Millard and Bryant, the offer was rejected on the grounds that they had not been arrested for bodysnatching but under the Vagrancy Act. The two men were sentenced to be kept for three months 'at the wholesome exercise of the Tread-Wheel' in Cold Bath Fields prison (*Morning Chronicle*, 25 August 1823, issue 16957). The house committee ordered that the following placard be displayed (RLH, LH/A/5/17, 263):

London Hospital – Caution – Whereas attempts have been lately made to open the Graves in the burial Ground attached to the London Hospital with intent to steal bodies therein interred – And whereas Cornelius Bryant and William Millard have been convicted under the Vagrant Act and sentenced to be imprisoned during the space of three months and to be kept during that time to hard labour at the Tread Mill + Notice is herby given that measures have been taken to apprehend all persons who shall be found trespassing in the said burial Ground who will be prosecuted with the utmost severity of the Law. By Order of the house committee.

King of the resurrection men?

According to Bransby Cooper, Millard was originally a servant of a relation of the anatomist Mr Cline and later became superintendent of St Thomas's dissecting room, where 'a more trustworthy man for some time could scarcely exist' (Cooper 1843, 440–1). He was also superintendent of the anatomy theatre and the anatomical museum (Millard 1825, 13), in charge of preparing and caring for the anatomical specimens. Millard was of sober temperament and a great boxer, boxing at the time being a sport of fashionable gentlemen. He was reportedly fond of good food and expensive clothes (he is elsewhere described as 'of gentlemanly appearance and superior address' (*Morning Chronicle*, 25 August 1823, issue 16957), and had a lucrative sideline selling the pupils the kit and clothes they needed for classes. Cooper reported that it was the love of money that was to be Millard's downfall (1843, 440–1).

Whilst Millard was working at St Thomas's one of his duties was to receive the bodies brought in by the resurrection men for the pupils and for Mr Green and Sir Astley Cooper (Cooper 1843, 361; *The Times*, 16 May 1826, issue 12968, p 3, col C). He also negotiated the prices to be paid (*Morning Chronicle*, 25

August 1823, issue 16957). Bransby Cooper noted Millard's skill in dealing with the resurrection men, stating that his 'uncompromising courage' kept them in constant awe of him, and none of them were willing to fight him, although Millard offered to do so on occasion in order to settle disputes. Millard's wife Ann also admired her husband's skill in this regard, claiming that although he would spare 'neither pains nor expense' to help the men if they 'got into trouble' or were arrested, he was equally 'zealous and determined' to see them punished if they were guilty of any violence or outrage (Millard 1825, 14). When one of Joshua Naples's gang was arrested for a debt in August 1812, Millard paid it for him (Blake Bailey 1896, 162). Naples's diaries indicate that, at this time, St Thomas's Hospital (and therefore Millard) was a regular customer, paying £1 1s in August that year (ibid, 164).

As might be expected, Millard's relations with the resurrection men did not always run smoothly. Ann Millard recounts that when Crouch and Butler tried to raise the price for subjects to 6 guineas, the students refused to pay; whilst Crouch and Butler withheld subjects from the school the students were forced to rely on the bodies of dead patients, until eventually Millard found another supplier. On discovering this, the men broke into the dissecting room at St Thomas's, 'mangling' the bodies and threatening the students with knives (Millard 1825, 16; 'London News', Caledonian Mercury, 16 November 1816, issue 14818). Following this attack, a group of resurrection men rioted outside Millard's house in Canterbury Square, Southwark, and threatened his family, accusing Millard of employing men 'ignorant of their art' to procure subjects for the medical college. The men again demanded that their payment should be raised from 4 to 6 guineas per subject. After intervening to safeguard his family from the men, who then left the scene, Millard obtained a warrant for their arrest from the magistrates at Union Hall ('London News', Caledonian Mercury, 2 December 1816, issue 14825).

Further insight into Millard's more clandestine duties at St Thomas's is provided by a curious incident that occurred in October 1819. A man named John Williams was arrested following the discovery of two parcels containing the remains of an old woman and the head and body of an elderly man. Williams claimed that he was simply a porter who had been asked to deliver the packages to the corner of St Thomas' Street, Bermondsey, where he would be met (Williams later said that he knew the gentleman but did not wish to bring him any trouble) (The Times, 14 October 1819, issue 10750, p 3, col F). The bodies were thought to have been collected in Gillingham, Kent, though no one could definitely establish their origins. A letter to Williams in prison was intercepted, from which 'it appeared that the subjects were intended for a Mr Millan, a professional gentleman in the neighbourhood of Bermondsey' (The Times, 15 October 1819, issue 10751, p 2, col A). It is likely, given the Bermondsey address and connection to St Thomas's, that 'Millan' was in fact Millard. The coroner was so concerned that this incident had uncovered a 'very extensive system' of agents employed to forward bodies that he requested that

Williams (whom he claimed was a bodysnatcher named George Barton) should be detained for a week for questioning. The magistrate said that this was not possible as stealing a corpse was only a misdemeanour and had not been proven, so the prisoner was allowed bail (ibid).

In 1822, after many years of devoted service, Millard was dismissed (The Times, 16 May 1826, issue 12968, p 3, col C). It was alleged that he had been using money from St Thomas's Hospital to buy bodies, and then selling them on to Edinburgh at an inflated price whilst at the same time claiming there was a shortage. He was caught through a 'sting' by one of the hospital staff, who confronted him. When he claimed not to have delivered any bodies, the supplier (Murphy) stepped out and called his bluff. Murphy also accused Millard of being in league with Edward Grainger, a rival of Sir Astley Cooper, an accusation that his wife claimed was unfounded and was not investigated (Millard 1825, 21; Cooper 1843, 441–3). Ann Millard suggested that the reason her husband had fallen out of favour with the hospital authorities was actually because he refused to vote for the preferred parliamentary candidate of the hospital treasurer and perhaps also because he had been suffering some ill health, and she certainly claimed that he was told his dismissal was not because he had done anything wrong (Millard 1825, 21–3). Richardson notes that problems in the supply of the London anatomy schools caused by bodies being sent to Edinburgh, where they could reach a higher price (20 guineas in 1825), occurred during the mid 1820s (2000, 101–2).

After the disturbances of 1816 Millard's accuser, Murphy, effectively took over from Butler and Crouch the supply of subjects to St Thomas's. He was quick to seize every opportunity for making money, demanding, for example, an 'opening fee' at the start of each term for the supply of subjects to each school (Millard 1825, 17; Cooper 1843, 361–2). Cooper details a devious scheme put into practice by Murphy to dissuade one of the anatomy lecturers, who had tried to circumvent the opening fee, from acting independently. Murphy, who claimed that the money was used to bribe the watchmen and gravediggers, took the lecturer to the house of a gravedigger so that he could negotiate the fee for himself; Murphy had briefed the gravedigger to threaten the lecturer with a gun on revealing the reasons for their visit. A second outing with Murphy convinced the lecturer 'of the folly of his attempting to form alliances with sextons and grave-diggers' (Cooper 1843, 363–7).

In 1824 Mr Green, finding the price demanded by the resurrection men too heavy, stopped supplying the students of St Thomas's with subjects for dissection and told them to make their own arrangements. The students raised a sum of money and tried to negotiate with the watchmen and gravediggers of Bethnal Green burial ground. They were made to pay 'enormously' for the one or two subjects they obtained, and by the time they returned a second time the watchman had spoken to Murphy, who had briefed him to demand 10 guineas before a body was produced. In the end, Murphy and his gang took the bodies and the students were left with neither the subject nor their money (Millard 1825, 17–18).

Interrogation of Joshua Naples's diary suggests that, in the first decade of the century, the resurrectionists used the St Thomas's dissecting room for overnight storage of remains that were destined for other clients (T Kausmally, pers comm), and in 1831 John Bishop and Thomas Williams left the body of Fanny Pigburn at the hospital whilst they made arrangements to sell it to Grainger's school in Webb Street (Wise 2004, 153). If this were still the case whilst Millard was in charge then the presence of bodies that were not for hospital use could be easily explained, though perhaps the hospital administrators were unaware of this arrangement.

It might appear odd that Millard's employers would accept Murphy's testimony that Millard had been withholding bodies from the school and working in the interests of Grainger, rather than taking the word of a long-standing employee, were it not for a years-old feud. Edward Grainger, a talented pupil of Sir Astley Cooper, had been prevented from lecturing at the hospital because he did not have the funds to pay to be a dressing pupil. Instead he left the hospital and set up his own school of anatomy in 1819, infuriating Sir Astley, who was worried that Grainger's school would poach his students (Millard 1825, 19; Richardson 2001, 311). Murphy and the resurrection men exploited the rift and the price paid for subjects soared (Cooper 1843, 367). Entreated by Sir Astley, Millard built a dissecting room behind his house at Gregory Place, Southwark, at a cost of over £200, apparently as part of an attempt by Sir Astley to stem a loss of students to Grainger's school in the summer months. The room was eventually leased to Mr Morgan, an apprentice to Sir Astley, who subsequently, until he was threatened with legal action, refused to pay the rent (Millard 1825, 19–20).

Following his dismissal and encouraged by the students, who obviously had a fondness for him, Millard opened an eating house in Borough. This soon went under, losing him 'upwards of £300' (Millard 1825, 23; Cooper 1843, 443). Eventually, after promised work from Sir Astley was not forthcoming, Millard found work as superintendent with Grainger in the dissecting room at Webb Street (Millard 1825, 23–4; Power 1895a, 1390). Ann Millard later claimed that his appointment was 'received with jealousy' (The Times, 16 May 1826, issue 12968, p 3, col C).

It was only after starting work with Grainger that Millard seems to have turned to the resurrection trade himself. Perhaps Grainger was no longer willing to pay the inflated prices demanded by Murphy, and thought that Millard might be able to negotiate them down or come to the same solution as he had done with Crouch and Butler in 1816. Ann Millard states that Grainger himself went with Millard to procure subjects, suggesting that he was no longer being supplied by Murphy. Millard was warned by one of the police that Sir Astley Cooper had used his influence to direct the arrest of both men if they were caught (Millard 1825, 24). In fact, Millard had been arrested in similar circumstances only a month before his capture at the London Hospital. In July 1823 he and a Cornelius Fitzgerald were apprehended in Great Maze Pond, Southwark at five in the morning, carrying a box containing the body of a

woman tied up in a sack. They posted bail and were due to return to answer to the offence at the sessions. The body was taken to St Olave's workhouse ('Police', Morning Chronicle, 17 July 1823, issue 16924). Bransby Cooper describes a resurrectionist by the name of 'Patrick', to whom he gave a pseudonym because he was still alive when Cooper was publishing, 'and of respectable character' (Cooper 1843, 374). From Cooper's description of events it appears that Cornelius Bryant and Fitzgerald were the same person, and further it seems most likely that 'Bryant' was also a pseudonym, as the name Cornelius Fitzgerald appears in later newspaper reports.

After Millard's arrest at the London Hospital, the newspapers claimed that 'he was known amongst a certain class by the appellation of "King of the Resurrection Men"' (Morning Chronicle, 25 August 1823, issue 16957), but both Bransby Cooper and Ann Millard give this accolade to Murphy (Millard 1825, 18; Cooper 1843, 441), and this may have been hyperbole or a mistake on the part of the rabble-rousing reporters. Cornelius had been previously apprehended with Murphy in a private burial ground on Holywell Mount (Cooper 1843, 374). He was originally a sailor and then a corn porter but was persuaded into the trade by Murphy, 'whom he appeared to look up to as one of the greatest men living', when he wanted an assistant. Cooper states that Murphy and 'Patrick' always acted together, but this contradicts an earlier anecdote that he gives, when Murphy tricked an accomplice of 'Patrick' into revealing the source from which he had been acquiring subjects: he and his wife had found a lucrative supply in pretending to be relatives of those dying in workhouses in order to claim the body for burial. Cooper reports that 'Patrick' did not wish anyone to know what he did and hid his profession from his friends and the public (ibid, 440). It is not hard to imagine that two somewhat reluctant resurrectionsists, Millard and Cornelius, might feel that they had much in common and take up in business together.

Bransby Cooper claimed that, after his experience in Cold Bath Fields prison, 'Patrick' had 'entered into a business in London in which he is still engaged, and bears an excellent character for his propriety and conduct'. A Cornelius Fitzgerald, of the same age as 'Cornelius', is listed in the 1841 census living in the parish of St Mary Newington, where his occupation was given as a coffin dealer (TNA: PRO, 1841 England census, parish St Mary Newington). It does not seem too much of a leap to suggest that after the Anatomy Act he worked within the circles of undertakers and body dealers who kept the anatomy schools supplied (Hurren 2012). Time in Cold Bath Fields certainly did not put Cornelius off bodysnatching. In February 1825 he was detained for trying to obtain illegally the body of a woman who had died in St Giles' workhouse (Morning Post, 17 February 1825, issue 16899; Cooper 1843, 385) and in July that year he was involved in a disturbance at Grainger's school in Webb Street ('Police', Morning Chronicle, 28 July 1825, issue 17533; Cooper 1843, 438–40). In 1828 he evaded arrest when two accomplices were arrested after the theft of four bodies from the dead house of Newington workhouse (Morning Chronicle, 17 March 1828, issue 18254).

Then in 1832 Cornelius, 'an Irishman of reputable appearance, aged 35', was arrested in Deptford with Robert Self, 'a wooden legged man and a pensioner [an ex-serviceman] aged 35', and George Betts, 'a shabbily dressed man aged 45', for stealing the bodies of two elderly men. The group were described as having been instantly recognised by James Jeffries and Luke Kenney, two police officers who were coming off duty, as 'belonging to a desperate gang of resurrectionists, who have for this long time past been a terror to the inhabitants of Deptford, Greenwich, Camberwell, Peckham, Woolwich and the whole of the west of Kent'. The arrest came some time after the notorious case of the murders perpetrated in Edinburgh by Burke and Hare, and the rumour spread that the gang had in fact 'Burked' or murdered the men to sell for dissection. The result was that an angry mob of several thousand people besieged the police station where they were being held. The police resisted the calls of the mob to let them mete out their own justice on the 'Burkites' and an escort of 40 officers surrounded them as they were led to the magistrates in Deptford. The mob hurled bricks and missiles at the party, injuring several officers. At the magistrates' court the police 'had the utmost difficulty to prevent their prisoners being sacrificed by the indignant multitude'. The prisoners were remanded so that an attempt could be made to identify the bodies. The gang appear to have been further attacked by the crowds on their way to their re-examination by the magistrate in Greenwich. By this time the corpses had been identified by the boatswain of a prison ship, the *Justitia*, which was moored in Woolwich, who stated that they had died the night before the prisoners' arrest. Here the report takes a turn for the bizarre. The bodies having been identified, the magistrate ordered them returned to the burial ground in Plumstead. Jeffries and Kenney

were on duty the following Monday and found Hollis (Chapter 6.3) taking the same two bodies; perhaps having paid for the corpses, the gang wanted to make sure they got their money? He was taken with the others for trial at the Maidstone assizes (*The Times*, 19 April 1832, issue 14830, p 4, col C).

In Cold Bath Fields

Cold Bath Fields prison was constructed in 1794 in a swamp in north London and had a reputation for severity (Thornbury 1878) (Fig 200). By the time of Millard's sentence, the treadmill had been introduced as a punishment by hard labour (Forbes 1977, 666).

On arrival at Cold Bath Fields Millard informed Mr Webbe, the surgeon who attended the prison, that he had worked for Sir Astley Cooper for many years. On investigating this claim Webbe returned to say that Cooper denied all knowledge of Millard. Henry Green, another of the surgeons at St Thomas's Hospital, was more supportive, and visited Millard at Cold Bath Fields to intervene on his behalf, resulting in both Millard and Bryant being excused from the punishment of the treadmill (Millard 1825, 30; Cooper 1843, 444). The hospital solicitor, Mr Lang, reported to the house committee that Millard was in the infirmary and Bryant was employed picking oakum, and that neither of them had been working on the treadmill (RLH, LH/A/5/17, 273).

Cooper states that Millard found bail and then entered an appeal against his conviction once he had obtained his liberty, bringing an action against the Lambeth Street magistrate for false imprisonment (1843, 444). Ann Millard gives a slightly different story, suggesting that Edward Grainger appealed the

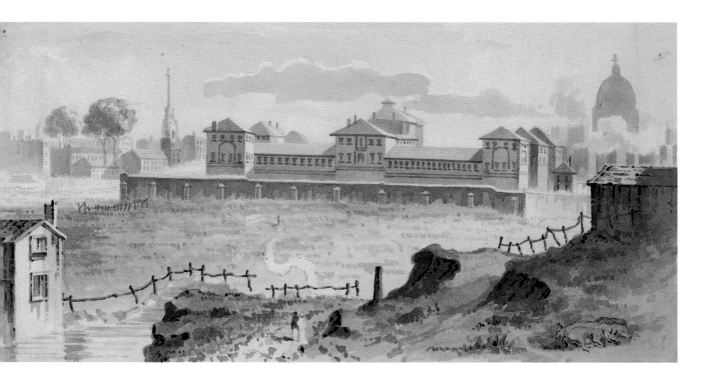

Fig 200 Cold Bath Fields prison c 1810, viewed from the north-west, with the River Fleet in the foreground and the dome of St Paul's Cathedral in the distance (far right) (Anon, pen/ink/wash: LMA, main print collection, cat no. q6074181)

decision of the magistrate on Millard's behalf whilst he was still imprisoned, thereby securing him his liberty (Millard 1825, 31). Before his appeal, Millard visited Sir William Blizard to protest at the hospital's pursuit of the case. When Blizard commented that 'we shall be very happy to accommodate any lecturer who may be in want of our assistance, but we must not have things taken away by force', Millard replied that he had always given 'value received' for any body that he had taken from the hospital. Hurst, the surgeon's beadle at the London Hospital, subsequently went to visit Millard and he was apparently reassured that the hospital did not intend to proceed with his prosecution (Millard 1825, 31–2).

On the contrary, however, the governors did wish to secure Millard's conviction and had instructed their solicitor to do so (RLH, LH/A/5/17, 268). Millard's appeal against his conviction for vagrancy took place at the sessions house in Clerkenwell on 11 September. The defence mounted by Mr Adolphus was that William Millard, as a respectable man, was able to give 'a good account of himself', and did not have to justify his reasons for being in the hospital grounds. Millard, he stated, kept a good house for which he paid 'scot and lot' and was well known in the parish. The prosecution conceded his respectability but stated that since Millard was found 'in an enclosed burial ground under circumstances pointing at an intention to commit an indictable misdemeanour' it was reasonable to ask him what he was doing there. He should account for the shovel, the sack and for having climbed a ten-foot wall. One witness stated that Millard was employed in the lecture room under Sir Astley Cooper, but 'could not say in what manner'. Millard lost his appeal and was sentenced to three months' hard labour. On hearing the verdict Mr Adolphus cried, 'it is high time to leave England'. Millard was attacked by a mob as he was led from the court, even though he was protected by the officers. The crowd pelted him with dirt and sawdust and tried to assault him (*The Times*, 12 September 1823, issue 11975, p 3, col B). He was returned to jail, refused to eat and sank further into depression (Cooper 1843, 444–5).

Past commentators, perhaps influenced by the writings of Bransby Cooper on the subject, have followed his assertion that Ann Millard's 'chief object appears to have been to vilify Sir Astley Cooper, for refusing to intercede for her husband's discharge from prison, or afterwards to settle a pension upon herself' (1843, 446), but in fact she does mention assistance that she received from Sir Astley. On the advice of a 'gentleman of high estimation in the profession', who warned her under no circumstances to mention Grainger, she made an application to him. Although at first he did not give her any money, he later asked her to return and gave her £10, and recommended that she should also call upon Mr Green, Mr Stanley and Mr Headington. Of these, Mr Green promised her £5, which she never received, Mr Stanley 'promised nothing and gave nothing', as did Blizard, but Mr Headington asked her to return the following day, whereupon she received £5 5s from Mr Luke. At this point she ran into additional problems, when a case in which Millard had acted as security for two resurrection men employed in the service of St Thomas's six years

previously was suddenly revived and a sheriff's officer took possession of their house and furniture. Mr Green eventually agreed to write to the attorneys about the case (Millard 1825, 33–5), and she and her family appear to have found accommodation with some medical students, perhaps with the assistance of Sir Astley, as she labelled one of them as the agent for his dirty work (ibid, 40).

In the meantime Millard's condition in the infirmary worsened and he asked her to appeal to Sir Astley and Mr Green for help in securing his release. Although Green was of no assistance, Sir Astley wrote to the Home Secretary, Robert Peel. The question of whether Sir Astley interceded on Millard's behalf was for many years a matter of some controversy, as a result of Bransby Cooper's assertion that Millard's 'extreme state of despondency' was partly because he had refused to do so. Believing himself to have been abandoned he was apparently heard 'to swear that he would revenge himself by inflicting some bodily harm upon him' (Cooper 1843, 445). Because of Millard's apparent threat to Sir Astley, Mr Wakefield advised him not to visit. Instead, Wakefield and Bransby Cooper visited Millard 'a week or ten days' before his death and reportedly found him 'in a state of raving madness' (ibid). This is also the point when Sir Astley relented.

In the 1960s a letter was acquired by the University of Kansas (Agnew 1963, 176) that corroborates Ann Millard's version of events:

> Sir Astley Cooper presents his best compts to Mr Peel and informs him that a person of ye name of Millard who was imprisoned for being detected in disturbing a grave at ye London Hospital lies dangerously ill in ye Cold Bath Fields Prison: Sir A C hopes that when Mr Peel considers this man's offence without which science must perish and the state of his health, he will be induced to regard him with an eye of compassion & set him at liberty.
>
> Spring Gardens
> Octr 7th 1823

She herself paraphrases it in her account of the affair (Millard 1825, 37):

> After asking a few questions, he penned a note to the Secretary of State; the purport of which was, that a man was then in confinement in the House of Correction, Cold Bath Fields, *for being found near the burial ground of the London Hospital!* That without such men science would perish; that this individual was dangerously ill, and therefore appealed to the humanity of the Secretary of State, to release him.

In addition to penning the letter to Robert Peel, Sir Astley, who appears to have been less confident than Mr Green in the abilities of Mr Webbe, wrote to a Dr Farr and requested him to attend Millard in the prison. Sir Astley was primarily guilty of procrastinating to the point at which his help could do Millard no good. On receiving the letter from Sir Astley, Peel interceded and sent an order for Millard's release, on the production of a certificate from the surgeon at Cold Bath Fields confirming his sick condition. According to Ann Millard (1825, 37), Sir Astley kept the letter for two days before giving it to her to take to the prison, by which time Millard was too sick for it to be of any use. He died of fever on 14 October 1823, aged 43 years (LMA, MA/G/CBF/417), leaving his wife and six children.

It seems clear that Millard died believing himself to have been abandoned by those he had worked for, and that his wife felt a similar animosity towards the medical establishment for their lack of assistance (below, 8.2). Despite its notoriety, Millard's arrest did not dissuade others from attempting to procure corpses from the London Hospital burial ground. In July 1829 trespassers were interrupted whilst attempting to disinter the body of an old man by the name of Hatfield by the patients shouting from the ward windows. Valentine reported to the house committee (RLH, LH/A/17/6, 2 July 1829; Fig 201) that:

> the fellows left the body in a sack partially covered, in the ground to the horror & disquiet of all who saw it. The man was 76 years of age, & being in a state of putrefaction the parts of the Body which were exposed through the broken sack, all the thighs & legs, were denuded of the skin, & of course presented a shocking sight. Having gone to see it, I directed the immediate reinterment.

8.2 Ann Millard and the fight for William Millard's reputation: an archaeological vindication?

Millard's arrest came at a time of increasing unrest amongst the providers of anatomy classes. An anatomical society, effectively a cartel, had been set up in the early 1800s to keep costs down, but for some time the hospitals had been trying to marginalise the private anatomy schools and from 1819 to 1824 Sir Astley Cooper made concerted efforts to stop the resurrectionists from selling bodies to Edward Grainger. The resurrectionists, never ones to miss an opportunity, started to increase the prices, playing the two groups off against one another (Wise 2004, 167). In 1823, Sir Astley began to discuss what could be done to break the power of the bodysnatcher, passing on the responses, most of which were soliciting covert official support of the existing – illegal – supply routes (Richardson 2001, 163), to Sir Robert Peel.

After Millard's death, his wife Ann began her campaign to clear his name. Thomas Wakley had interested himself in the case when Millard was imprisoned, and had published veiled threats against William Blizard for his conduct (*The Lancet*, 5 October 1823, Notice to correspondents, 1(1), 36):

> E. Z. May rest assured that Sir Billy Fretful shall shortly receive a pretty sharp cut from "THE LANCET", as a

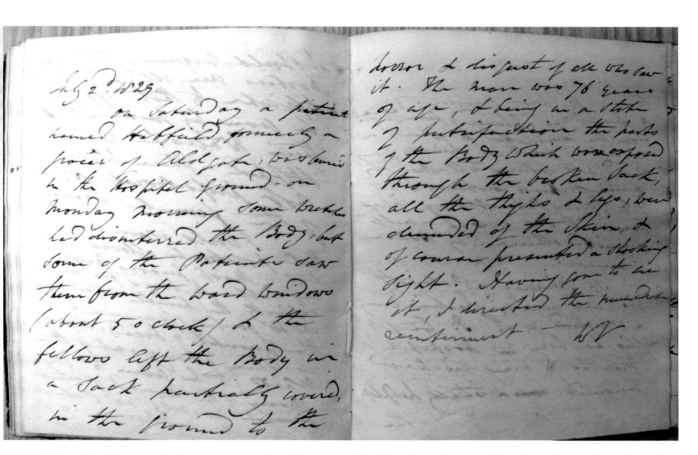

Fig 201 William Valentine's report to the house committee regarding the disinterring of a body from the London Hospital's burial ground: excerpt for 2 July 1829 from the house governor's report book (RLH, LH/A/17/6)

chastisement for his unrelenting conduct towards Mr. Millard.

Two months later he continued (*The Lancet*, 21 December 1823, Notice to correspondents, 1(12), 419):

B.Z.U. is much deceived if he imagines we have forgotten the cruel treatment of the late Wm. Millard. We shall very shortly investigate this affair most fully; and if we should succeed in getting into our possession some original letters and documents … they shall, at an early period, be presented to our professional brethren. We feel confident that the particulars of this extraordinary transaction will excite the greatest disgust and indignation.

Ann Millard believed that far from having a genuine interest in the case, Wakley had merely wanted ammunition in his own dispute with the medical establishment. As soon as he had achieved his object, he lost interest, and she turned again to Sir Astley. He suggested that she go to Sir William Blizard, who sent her back to Cooper, who in turn suggested that she apply to the house committee of the London Hospital for assistance. With the assistance of a medical student living in her house, she drew up her petition and presented it to the governors on 27 January, accompanied with a letter of introduction from Cooper (RLH, LH/A/5/17, 302–3; Millard 1825, 44–8):

Sir Astley Cooper presents his respectful Complts. To the Rev. Wm Valentine and the Gentlemen comprising the Committee of the London Hospital and begs them to hear the bearer's story.

Her petition read:

To the Governors of the London Hospital
The Petition of Ann Millard widow of Wm Millard
Showeth … That it has long been a custom to disinter the persons buried in the London Hospital Ground for the use of the Anatomical School attached to that Institution or if not required by that School for the use of any one who was willing to purchase them. That your Petrs [petitioner's] late husband Wm Millard has often fetched subjects from the above mentioned Hospital at the desire of Sir Astley Cooper and the late Mr Henry Cline in whose service W:M was for 13 years and being aware that Mr Brookes and the late Mr Grainger professors of Anatomy were during the Summer frequently supplied from the same source he as your Petitioner verily believes conceived the practice to be authorized by the Governors of the Hospital the more especially as a message or letter was always sent from some one of the Servants of the Hospital stating that there was a subject to be disposed of & at what price some of which letters are hereto subjoined.

That in pursuance of such a message received by Wm Millard he went to the burial Ground on the 23rd of August last and was there apprehended by persons lying in wait for him and

taken to Lambeth Street Police Office and was by Mr Wyatt the sitting Magistrate sentenced to 3 months imprisonment in the House of Correction Cold Bath Fields which sentence being confirmed at the next Sessions the said Wm Millard was confined in the above Prison and there being attacked by a fever frequently prevailing in the Prison, died.

That your Petitioner and her family consisting of 6 children are thereby reduced to a state of great distress.

That she believes either that the Governors of the Hopl [hospital] were ignorant of the above facts or that the prosecution against her late husband was carried on without their sanction which the latter she is the more inclined to believe as the practice of disinterment still subsists.

That your Petitioner trusts that you will take her case into your humane consideration and afford her such relief as you may deem proper.

Ann Millard – 11 Gregory Place, Southwark

The house committee called her in and asked to examine the evidence she had in her possession. This consisted of a letter from Mr Cline to Headington requesting subjects, a letter from Cobley, the anatomy assistant, to Millard offering 'a very fine subject that will be done to morrow', and an anonymous letter to Millard in which Hurst offered a 'very fine male subject … the abdomen and chest have been opened, consequently, the price will be three guineas' (Millard 1825, 24–6). The committee dismissed her claim, saying the letters were only copies and her husband had not been working for the hospital, and the minute outlining the transaction was sent to Sir Astley Cooper (RLH, LH/A/5/17, 303). Ann Millard claimed that the chairman of the house committee tried to shift responsibility for Millard's conviction on to the magistrate, although she believed that the magistrate had been strongly influenced in his decision by the governors, a suspicion apparently confirmed in the minutes of the house committee, who instructed their solicitor to pursue Millard's and Bryant's convictions (ibid, 26 August 1823, 262–3; Millard 1825, 51–2).

Valentine told Mrs Millard that when Millard and Bryant were first arrested, the hospital had enquired about Millard's character with Sir Astley Cooper, who answered that he had been discharged from St Thomas's for his dishonest practices (Millard 1825, 49–50). When Bransby Cooper learned of this accusation he called it 'a damned lie', and offered to start a subscription amongst the medical students to support Ann and her family, although she claimed that she did not receive anything, saying that 'beyond a paltry attempt at a subscription, and an offer to take one of her children as a foot-boy, nothing has been done for her'. She did, however, still have some friends in the medical profession, and acknowledged the kindness of several practitioners, including 'Mr Kent, Mr Swan, Mr College, Mr Carpue, &c &c' (ibid, 58).

Such was Ann's determination to clear her husband's name

following the treatment that she had received that she acquired a printing press, which was installed at her home in Southwark in December 1825 (SHC, QS6/14/166). She then published a pamphlet in which she made public the particulars of her husband's dealings with the medical establishment, providing detailed information on the process of acquiring subjects for dissection and identifying the staff who were involved in this, and who made money from it. Richardson (2001, 312) comments that Ann 'is usually ignored or dismissed as a vulgar hysterical woman'. Certainly Bransby Cooper felt that her petition 'was loaded with statements so evidently absurd, respecting the various metropolitan hospitals, and such violent abuse of the officers severally connected with them, that it defeated its own object, and failed to attract any attention' (1843, 446). In contrast, Richardson felt that the 'account has a ring of truth about it … The detail is so precise, and conforms so closely to other observers' comments … that I am inclined to believe her' (2001, 312). By the 1830s bodies were certainly sold on from the London Hospital to other hospitals (*The Lancet*, 21 September 1833, Vindication of the teachers of anatomy against the charge of making a profit on subjects for dissection, 20(525), 826), and there is little reason to suspect that the situation was substantially different a decade earlier.

Millard appears to have been caught up in a perfect storm between the capital's rival resurrection men and teachers of anatomy. When Edward Grainger opened his school on Webb Street, Sir Astley Cooper and other teachers of anatomy in the capital were said to be furious at the effect on the prices paid for subjects. This desire to cause problems for Grainger may perhaps explain why Sir Astley initially denied all knowledge of Millard to the surgeon at Cold Bath Fields and spoke badly of his character to the London Hospital. In spite of the warning that Ann Millard had received, not to mention her husband's position with Grainger when she went to Sir Astley, she indicates elsewhere that he knew Millard had been working with Grainger, because he had used his influence to direct that they should be arrested if caught with a body. And yet Sir Astley appears to have softened towards his old employee shortly after he was imprisoned. Perhaps Green or another persuaded him that it was in the interests of the medical profession as a whole not to turn its back on those who kept the dissecting rooms of the capital supplied.

It was the rivalries between the resurrection men that were perhaps to prove more significant. The two men were spotted, not by police officers briefed by Astley Cooper, but by patients and staff at the hospital. In a letter written to Cooper in November 1823 Joshua Brookes, who ran a private theatre of anatomy on Blenheim Street, commented on 'the very disorganised system at present pursued by the resurrection-men', who had been breaking into dead houses, targeting bodies of wealthier people and quarrelling amongst themselves, accusing their rivals and leading to the police seizing subjects from the schools (Cooper 1843, 391–3). *The Times* had reported in September that the body of a woman awaiting an inquest had been stolen from an outhouse and was later found at Brookes's house. The reporter commented that 'the resurrection-men

have lately hit upon a new mode of getting possession of prey, without the trouble and hazard of digging' (*The Times*, 27 September 1823, issue 11988, p 3, col G). Earlier in the year, the exposure of Fitzgerald and Murphy's chief source of subjects, the burial ground near Holywell Mount, had led to Murphy swearing his revenge on Vaughan, and after this discovery Cornelius and Murphy apparently also parted company. The exposure led to increased vigilance from the public and greater danger in exhuming bodies from burial grounds. Brookes's reference to resurrection men breaking into dead houses and the theft reported in *The Times* directly recall the break-in at the London Hospital the week before Millard's arrest in August. Bransby attributed the theft to Vaughan, who conveniently moved to Manchester for the autumn of 1823, and it is possible that this was the crime for which Murphy reported him when he returned to London at Christmas, and for which he served two years in Maidstone jail (Cooper 1843, 429–30). By the time of Millard's arrest, Cornelius and Millard seem to have been working together to supply the Webb Street school. Murphy, who only the previous year had been instrumental in costing Millard his job at St Thomas's, cannot have been too happy about this arrangement and the loss of this source of income. Ann Millard noted that just like Sir Astley, he could not 'bear a rival near the throne' (Millard 1825, 17).

In 1823, Sir Astley Cooper is known to have solicited the views of other anatomists on alternative potential sources of subjects for dissection during the winter season, a move that Richardson attributes to the introduction by the Royal College of Surgeons of regulations limiting qualifications to those trained in the London schools attached to hospitals, and the growing success of Grainger's Webb Street school (2001, 163, 345). It is likely, however, that Cooper acted not only because of the financial implications of the rising cost of subjects but also because the feuding between rival resurrection men was causing increasing trouble for those teaching anatomy in London during 1823, although it is unclear whether this was in turn caused in part by the higher rewards at stake or by the personalities involved. Interestingly, although he requested the opinion of his friend Joshua Brookes, of the private school on Blenheim Street, he does not appear to have asked the opinion of anyone working at the London Hospital.

Millard was at pains to point out to Sir William Blizard that he had not stolen anything from the London Hospital. Ann Millard notes that he had received a communication from Hurst about the body that he had gone to collect, and which he said he could have 'in consideration of the usual fee' (Millard 1825, 28). After the break-in by Vaughan the previous week and the reward of 20 guineas for the capture of those responsible, patients and staff were in a state of high alert. Millard and Bryant were not the culprits, but the patients were not to know that, though 'Sam the Barber' may well have done. According to Ann Millard he was keen to break the exclusive right of Hurst and Cobley to sell the bodies of patients, and he may have been tipping off Vaughan, as she notes that he was in league with 'the resurrection men' (ibid, 26). After such a public arrest the hospital had to be seen to do something, and it was unfortunate that Millard's employment with Grainger meant that he did not at first receive the recognition and character reference that he might have expected from Sir Astley Cooper. Learning that Millard had been sacked from St Thomas's for his dishonesty might well have led the London Hospital to believe that Millard and Bryant were also intent on stealing bodies from the hospital ground.

Samuel Hicks may have been more than an innocent bystander. On 4 July 1826 (RLH, LH/A/5/18, 96–7):

A complaint was made against two of the Porters of the Establishment/[?] and Hicks/ of their having been concerned with others in removing a Body from the burial ground of the Hospital/ by two persons who had been Patients in the Hospital of the names of Samuel Stones and Joseph Bentley.

Although this complaint was dismissed on the grounds that there was insufficient evidence, by 18 July the first porter had been dismissed because 'his discontented and unhappy disposition [has] been repeatedly the cause of dissention among the other servants' (RLH, LH/A/5/18, 98). Then on 28 November the minute books note that 'the committee will take the expense upon themselves of prosecuting Samuel Hicks a Porter lately dismissed as to the misdemeanour charged against him in relation to a female outpatient' (ibid, 111, 142). At the Middlesex session on St Valentine's Day 1827 Samuel was indicted at the request of the hospital governors for sexual assault (The Times, 15 February 1827, issue 13203, p 4, col B). If both porters were innocent of the initial accusations, it was certainly convenient for the hospital that they got themselves into further trouble so quickly.

Ann Millard and Wakley later fell out over the way in which he had dealt with supporting the case. Always one to court controversy, particularly if it would rile the establishment, Wakley had promised Ann that he would publish the letters and documents that she had in support of their case. When he failed to follow through with this promise she published her petition, in which she was said to have libelled Wakley, and where 'Others were assailed with charges of peculiating and misapplying public funds, and statements were made respecting the mode of procuring subjects for anatomical theatres, which, if true, it would have been better to have withheld' (The Times, 16 May 1826, issue 12968, p 3, col C). Perhaps this is the crux of the matter? Ann Millard had spoken out and it was not just the surgeons who would have preferred that she had not. If any conspiracy were present then surely it was to isolate and belittle her claims in the interest of the medical profession and, by extension, of the public?

Newspaper reports from May 1826 indicate that Wakley was suing Ann for libel in relation to her comments that he had defrauded his insurance company after a fire at his house in August 1820 and her claims that he was the person who neatly and, very publicly, decapitated the Cato Street conspirators following their execution (Thornbury 1878). The man in question was actually a resurrection man who obtained bodies for the hospitals (Morning Post, 29 September 1820, issue 15456).

Wakley reluctantly brought the case against Ann, who by this time was 'not worth 5/- in the world after payment of her just debts, save and except the wearing-apparel of herself and her six children' (The Times, 18 May 1826, issue 12970, p 3, col F). Ann and her children were seeking relief from the parish (Examiner, 21 May 1826, issue 955), though some questioned whether she was really so down at heel ('To the editor of The Morning Chronicle', Morning Chronicle, 18 May 1826, issue 17684). Wakley would rather have not prosecuted Ann at all and when the verdict was given he wrote (The Lancet, 1 July 1826, Wakley vs Millard, 5(131), 437):

The defendant … was an unfortunate person, placed in circumstances that altogether prevented the plaintiff having the slightest feeling to press for any sort of damages against her. She was the widow of a person, who, before his decease, had been employed in necessary purposes about an hospital in London, of which the least said, except in hospitals, the better. She thought she had a claim on certain persons, and she went to the plaintiff to state her case to him; he endeavoured to serve her, but she conceived that she was entitled to a great deal more.

The court asked whether they could settle the matter without a jury and both the defendant and plaintiff's counsel agreed. Wakley took the view of 'least said soonest mended' when it came to Ann's allegations regarding anatomy classes. It was bad form for a surgeon to break ranks (Richardson 2001, 50).

What happened to Ann Millard between 1826 and 1834 remains a mystery. One imagines that it must have been a difficult time, living in such reduced circumstances with a young family to support. She was vilified by many of the people who had previously been her husband's clients and Bransby Cooper's tone suggests that several people felt that William Millard had brought some of this on himself by getting ideas and airs above his proper station. In 1827 Charing Cross Hospital was founded by a former St Thomas's student, Benjamin Golding (K Chilton, pers comm), and it seems that her old connections stood Ann in good stead as she secured employment there.

On 7 April 1853 Ann Millard died of bronchitis at the Charing Cross Hospital, where she had worked as head sister for more than 19 years (The Times, 9 April 1853, issue 21398, p 9, col A) and 'where her kind care and attention to the afflicted objects of her superintendence, rendered her much respected and valued, and her loss greatly regretted' ('Births, deaths, marriages and obituaries', Daily News, 13 April 1853, issue 2151). Such was the regard in which she was held at the Charing Cross Hospital that a marble plaque was raised in her memory.

Printed and other secondary works

Agnew, L R C, 1963 Sir Astley Cooper and William Millard – a vindication, *J Hist Medicine Allied Sciences* 18, April, 176–8

Allen, M, 2008 *Cleansing the city: sanitary geographies in Victorian London*, Athens, OH

Altman, R D, 1993 Paget's disease of bone, in *The Cambridge world history of human disease* (ed K F Kiple), 911–13, Cambridge

Armitage, P, 1981 Jawbone of a South American monkey from Brooks Wharf, City of London, *London Archaeol* 4, 262–70

Armitage, P, Arnold, N, and Meddens, F, 2005 Note on the reptile remains, in Killock, D, and Meddens, F, Pottery as plunder: a 17th-century maritime site in Limehouse, London, *Post-Medieval Archaeol* 39(1), 81–2

Auden, R R, 1978 A Hunterian pupil: Sir William Blizard and the London Hospital, *Annals Roy Coll Surgeons Engl* 60, 345–9

Aufderheide, A C, and Rodríguez-Martín, C, 1998 *The Cambridge encyclopedia of human paleopathology*, Cambridge

Barnes, E, 1994 *Developmental defects of the axial skeleton in paleopathology*, Niwot, CO

Barron, C M, and Davies, M (eds), 2007 *The religious houses of London and Middlesex*, London

Bashford, L, and Sibun, L, 2007 Excavations at the Quaker burial ground, Kingston-upon-Thames, London, *Post-Medieval Archaeol* 41(1), 100–54

Bass, W M, 1987 (1971) *Human osteology: a laboratory and field manual*, 3 edn, Missouri Archaeol Soc Spec Pap 2, Columbia, MO

Battersby, W, 2008 Identification of the probable source of the lead poisoning observed in members of the Franklin expedition, *J Hakluyt Soc*, September, available online at http://www.hakluyt.com/PDF/Battersby_Franklin.pdf (last accessed 17 March 2011)

Bennett, J A, Johnston, S A, and Simcock, A V, 2000 *Solomon's house in Oxford: new finds from the first museum*, Oxford

Berry, A C, and Berry, R J, 1967 Epigenetic variation in the human cranium, *J Anat* 101(2), 81–7

Betts, I M, and Weinstein, R I, 2010 *Tin-glazed tiles in London*, London

Billing, A, 1831 London Hospital, introductory clinical lecture, *The Lancet*, 19 November, 17(429), 233–9

Billing, A, 1833 Early detection of aneurysm in the chest, *The Lancet*, 14 December, 21(537), 443

Billing, A, 1834 Diagnosis of a diminutive aneurysm of the aorta, close to the heart, *The Lancet*, 8 March, 21(549), 900

Blaine, D, 1817 *Canine pathology, or a full description of the disease of dogs: with their causes, symptoms, and mode of cure: being the whole of the author's curative practice, during 20 years extensive experience*, London

Blake Bailey, J, 1896 *The diary of a resurrectionist 1811–12, to which are added an account of the resurrection men in London and a short history of the passing of the Anatomy Act*, London

Blakely, R L, and Harrington, J M (eds), 1997 *Bones in the basement – post-mortem racism in 19th-century medical training*, Washington, DC

Boddice, R, 2011 Vivisecting major: a Victorian gentleman scientist defends animal experimentation 1876–85, *Isis* 102(2), 215–37

Bolter, D R, and Zihlman, A L, 2003 Morphometric analysis of growth and development in wild-collected vervet monkeys (*Cercopithecus aethiops*), with implications for growth patterns in Old World monkeys, apes and humans, *J Zool* 260, 99–110

Bond, G, and Gale, F, 1834 Use of plaster of Paris in the treatment of fractures, *The Lancet*, 26 July, 22(569), 616–17

Boston, C, and Webb, H, 2012 Early medical training and treatment in Oxford: a consideration of the archaeological and historical evidence, in *Anatomical dissection in Enlightenment England and beyond: autopsy, pathology and display* (ed P Mitchell), 43–68, Farnham

Boston, C, Witkin, A, Boyle, A, and Wilkinson, D R P, 2008 *'Safe moor'd in Greenwich tier': a study of the skeletons of Royal Navy sailors and marines excavated at the Royal Hospital Greenwich*, Oxford

Boulter, S, Robertson, D J, and Start, H, 1998 The Newcastle Infirmary at the Forth, Newcastle upon Tyne: Vol 2, The osteology: people, disease and surgery, unpub ARCUS (Archaeol Res Consultancy Univ Sheffield, Res Sch Archaeol) rep 290

Bowsher, J, 1998 Dreadnought Seamen's Hospital, King William Walk, London, SE10, unpub MOL rep

Braybrooke, T, 2011 Oxford University: Radcliffe Observatory Quarter, Radcliffe Infirmary site, Oxford, unpub MOL rep

Brickley, M, and Ives, R, 2008 *The bioarchaeology of metabolic bone disease*, London

Brickley, M, and Miles, A, with Stainer, H, 1999 *The Cross Bones burial ground, Redcross Way, Southwark, London: archaeological excavations (1991–8) for the London Underground Limited Jubilee Line Extension Project*, MoLAS Monogr Ser 3, London

Britton, F, 1987 *London delftware*, London

Brooks, C M, 1983 Aspects of the sugar-refining industry from the 16th to the 19th century, *Post-Medieval Archaeol* 17, 1–14

Brooks, S T, and Suchey, J M, 1990 Skeletal age determination based on the os pubis: a comparison of the Ascadi–Nemeskeri and Suchey–Brooks methods, *J Hum Evol* 5, 227–38

Brothwell, D, 1981 (1963) *Digging up bones: the excavation, treatment and study of human skeletal remains*, 3 edn, London

Buikstra, J E, and Ubelaker, D H (eds), 1994 *Standards for data collection from human skeletal remains: proceedings of a seminar at the Field Museum of Natural History*, Arkansas Archaeol Survey Res Ser 44, Indianapolis, IN

Burdett, H C, 1893 *Hospitals and asylums of the world: their origin, history, construction, administration, management, and legislation with plans of the chief medical institutions accurately drawn to a uniform scale …*, London (copy available in the Wellcome Library, London)

Burney, I A, 2000 *Bodies of evidence: medicine and the politics of the English inquest, 1830–1926*, Baltimore, MD

Caledonian Mercury 19th-century British Library newspapers, Gale databases, http://gale.cengage.co.uk/product-highlights/history/19th-century-british-library-newspapers.aspx (last accessed 10 January 2012)

Cassell's science and art of nursing: Vol 2 (n d [c 1905–10]), London

Cauch, J, 1840 *The funeral guide; or, a correct list of the burial fees, &c. of the various parish and private grounds in the metropolis, & five miles round …*, London

Chadwick, E, 1843 *Report on the sanitary condition of the labouring population of Great Britain. A supplementary report on the results of a special inquiry into the practice of interment in towns*, London

Cherryson, A, 2010 In the pursuit of knowledge: dissection, post-mortem surgery and the retention of body parts in 18th- and 19th-century Britain, in *Body parts and bodies whole: changing relations and meanings* (eds K Rebay-Salisbury, M L Stig Sørensen and J Hughes), 135–48, Oxford

Choi, H K, Aitkinson, K, Karlson, E W, Willett, W, and Curhan, G, 2004 Purine-rich foods, dairy and protein intake and the risk of gout in men, *New England J Medicine* 350(11), 1093–103

Clark-Kennedy, A E, 1962 *The London: a study in the voluntary hospital system: Vol 1, 1740–1840*, London

Clark-Kennedy, A E, 1963 *The London: a study in the voluntary hospital system: Vol 2, 1840–1948*, London

Coletta, E M, 1999 Pressure ulcers: practical considerations in prevention and treatment, in *Reichel's care of the elderly: clinical aspects of aging* (eds J J Gallo, J Busby-Whitehead, P V Rabins, R A Silliman, J B Murphy and W Reichel), 543–55, Philadelphia, PA

Connell, B, and Miles, A, 2010 *The City Bunhill burial ground, Golden Lane, London: excavations at South Islington schools, 2006*, MOLA Archaeol Stud Ser 21, London

Connell, B, and Rauxloh, P, 2007 (2003) A rapid method for recording human skeletal data, 2 edn, rev N Powers, unpub MOL rep

Cooper, A, and Travers, B, 1818 *Surgical essays: Part 1*, London

Cooper, B B, 1843 *The life of Sir Astley Cooper, Bart, interspersed with sketches from his note-books of distinguished contemporary characters, in two volumes: Vol 1*, London

Coventry, M, 2000 *Guide to herbal remedies*, London

Coysh, A W, and Henrywood, R K, 1982 *The dictionary of blue and white printed pottery 1780–1880*, Woodbridge

Coysh, A W, and Henrywood, R K, 2001 (1989) *The dictionary of blue and white printed pottery 1780–1880: Vol 2*, Woodbridge

Cox, M, and Mays, S (eds), 2000 *Human osteology: in archaeology and forensic science*, London,

Crockford 1865 *Crockford's clerical directory for 1865, being a biographical and statistical book of reference for facts relating to the clergy and the church*, 3 edn, London

Crossland, Z, 2009 Acts of estrangement: the post-mortem making of self and other, *Archaeol Dialogues* 16(1), 102–25

Cunha, D F, Frota, R B, Arruda, M S, Cunha, S F, and Teixeira, V P, 2000 Pressure sores among malnourished necropsied adults – preliminary data, *Revista do Hospital das Clinicas; Faculdade de Medicina Da Universidade de Sao Paulo* 55(3), 79–82

Daily Mail 14 April 2011 Funeral for murderer hanged in 1821 after his skeleton is found in Bristol University cupboard, http://www.dailymail.co.uk/news/article-1376395/Funeral-murderer-hanged-1821-skeleton-Bristol-University-cupboard.html (last accessed 18 May 2012)

Dandy, D J, and Edwards, D J, 1998 *Essential orthopaedics and trauma*, Edinburgh

De Groot, H, et al, n d Osteomyelitis, www.bonetumor.org/tumors-bone/osteomyelitis (last accessed 11 January 2012)

Dermott, G D, 1834 Preservation of subjects for dissection: treatment of dissection wounds, *The Lancet*, 24 May, 22(560), 319–20

Dobson, J, 1951 The 'anatomizing' of criminals, *Annals Roy Coll Surgeons Engl* 9, 112–20

Dobson, J, 1962 John Hunter's animals, *J Hist Medicine Allied Sciences* 17, 479–86

Douglas, J, 1760 *Myographiae Comparatae Specimen …*, Edinburgh

Driesch, A von den, 1976 *A guide to the measurement of animal bones from archaeological sites*, Peabody Mus Bull 1, Cambridge, MA

Elias, I, Dheer, S, Zoga, A C, Raikin, S M, and Morrison, W B, 2008 Magnetic resonance imaging findings in bipartite medial cuneiform – a potential pitfall in diagnosis of midfoot injuries: a case series, *J Med Case Reports* 2, 272 (also available online, www.ncbi.nlm.nih.gov/pmc/articles/PMC2542399, last accessed 11 January 2012)

Ellis, G V, 1840 *Demonstrations of anatomy; being a guide to the dissection of the human body*, London

Ellis, G V, and Ford, G H, 1876 *Illustrations of dissections: in a series of original colored plates the size of life, representing the dissection of the human body*, New York

Ellis, J, 1986 *LHMC 1785–1985. The story of the London Hospital Medical College, England's first medical school*, London

Emery, P A, and Wooldridge, K, 2011 *St Pancras burial ground: excavations for St Pancras International, the London terminus of High Speed 1, 2002–3*, Gifford Monogr Ser, London

Evans, J, and Blandy, J 1992 Richard Clement Headington 1774–1831, *London Hospital Gazette* 19, 32–4

The Examiner 19th-century British Library newspapers, Gale databases, http://gale.cengage.co.uk/product-highlights/history/19th-century-british-library-newspapers.aspx (last accessed 10 January 2012)

Faden, M A, Krakow, D, Ezgu, F, Rimoin, D L, and Lachman, R S, 2009 The Erlenmeyer flask bone deformity in the skeletal dysplasias, *American J Medical Genetics – Part A*, 149A, 1334–45

Finnegan, M, 1978 Non-metric variation of the infracranial skeleton, *J Anat* 125, 23–37

Forbes, T R, 1977 A mortality record for Coldbath Fields prison, London, in 1795–1829, *Bull New York Acad Medicine* 53(7), 666–70

Fothergill, B, Thomas, R, and Morris, J, in prep Avian tibial dyschondroplasia in 19th-century turkey (*Meleagris gallopavo* L 1758) remains from the Royal London Hospital, *Int J Paleopathol*

Galloway, A (ed), 1999 *Broken bones: anthropological analysis of blunt force trauma*, Springfield, IL

Gascoyne 1703 A map of the hamlet of Mile-End old-town in the parish of Stepney alias Stebunheath, reproduced in Ravenhill, W, and Johnson, D J, 1995 *Joel Gascoyne's engraved maps of Stepney 1702–4*, London Topogr Soc Publ 150 in assoc Guildhall Library, London

The Gentleman's Magazine March 1836, Obituaries, ns 5, 330

Glencross, B, and Stuart-Macadam, P, 2001 Radiographic clues to fractures of distal humerus in archaeological remains, *Int J*

Osteoarchaeol 11, 298–310

Godden, G A, 2003 (1964) *Encyclopaedia of British pottery and porcelain marks*, 2 edn, London

Gordon, J A, 1833 *An introductory lecture to a course of lectures on clinical medicine, delivered in the theatre of the London Hospital, Saturday, January 31, 1829*, 2 edn, London

Grant, A, 1982 The use of toothwear as a guide to the age of domestic ungulates, in Wilson et al, 91–108

Grant, R E, 1841 *Outlines of comparative anatomy*, London

Greenwood, C, and Greenwood, J, 1827 'Map of London from an actual survey', reproduced in Margary, H, 1982, *'Map of London from an actual survey' by C and J Greenwood, 1827*, Margary in assoc Guildhall Library, Kent, available online at http://www.bl.uk/onlinegallery/onlineex/crace/m/ 007000 000000006u00225000.html (last accessed 21 May 2012)

Guerrini, A, 2004 Anatomists and entrepreneurs in early 18th-century London, *J Hist Medicine Allied Sciences* 59, 219–39

Gustafson, G, and Koch, G, 1974 Age estimation up to 16 years of age based on dental development, *Odontologisk Revy* 25, 297–306

Hackett, C J, 1975 An introduction to diagnostic criteria of syphilis, treponarid and yaws (treponematoses) in dry bones, and some implications, *Virchows Archiv A, Pathological Anatomy and Histology* 368, 229–41

Hamilton-Dyer, S, 2003 Animal bone, in Hull, 16–19

Hamilton-Dyer, S, 2009 Animal bones, in Drury, P, with Simpson, R, *Hill Hall: a singular house devised by a Tudor intellectual*, 45–51, London

Hammon, A J, 1998 Appendix F: animal bones found in association with human remains from Newcastle Infirmary: cutmark evidence, in Boulter et al

Hancock, J, 1830 Observations: on the vapour bath, *The Lancet*, 29 May, 14(352), 334–5

Hardy, T, 1994 *The collected poems of Thomas Hardy* (ed M Irwin), Ware

Harrison, J, Kulkarni, K, Baguneid, M, and Prendergast, B, 2009 *Oxford handbook of key clinical evidence*, Oxford

Hart, L, Wood, M, and Hart, B, 2008 *Why dissection?: animal use in education*, Oxford

Hartwig, R H, and Louis, D S, 1979 Multiple carpometacarpal dislocations: a review of four cases, *J Bone Joint Surgery (American)* 61, 906–8

Heathcote, B V, 2005 *Viewing the lifeless body: a coroner and his inquests held in Nottinghamshire public houses during the 19th century, 1828–66*, Nottingham

Henderson, D, Collard, M, and Johnston, D A, 1996 Archaeological evidence for 18th-century medical practice in the Old Town of Edinburgh: excavations at 13 Infirmary Street and Surgeons' Square, *Proc Soc Antiq Scotl* 126, 929–41

Henderson, M, Miles, A, and Walker, D, with Connell, B, and Wroe-Brown, R, in prep *'He being dead yet speaketh': excavations at three post-medieval burial grounds in Tower Hamlets, East London, 2004–8*, MOLA Monogr Ser 64, London

Hempel, S, 2006 *The medical detective. John Snow, cholera and the mystery of the Broad Street pump*, London

Higgs, M, 2009 *Life in the Victorian hospital*, Stroud

Hillson, S, 1996 *Dental anthropology*, Cambridge

Hillson, S, Waldron, T, Owen-Smith, B, and Martin, L, 1999 Benjamin Franklin, William Hewson and the Craven Street bones, *Archaeol Int* 2, 14–17

Holmes, Mrs B [I M Holmes], 1896 *The London burial grounds: notes on their history from the earliest times to the present day*, London

Home, E, 1806 Observations on the camel's stomach respecting the water it contains and the reservoirs, in which that fluid is inclosed: with an account of some peculiarities in the urine, *Philos Trans Roy Soc London* 96, 357–84

Horne, J, 1989 *English tin-glazed tiles*, London

Horwood, R, 1813 Plan of the cities of London and Westminster, the borough of Southwark, 3 edn (compiled 1792–9), reproduced in Margary, H, 1985 *The A–Z of Regency London*, Margary in assoc Guildhall Library, Kent

Howard, J, 1791 *An account of the principal lazarettos in Europe*, 2 edn, London

Hughes, B, 1992 'Infant Orphan Asylum Hall' crockery from Eagle Pond, Snaresbrook, *London Archaeol* 6(14), 382–7

Huijg, A, 1978 *De bijbel op tegels*, Boxtel

Hull, G, 2003 The excavation and analysis of an 18th-century deposit of anatomical remains and chemical apparatus from the rear of the first Ashmolean Museum (now The Museum of the History of Science), Broad Street, Oxford, *Post-Medieval Archaeol* 37(1), 1–28

Hull Packet 19th-century British Library newspapers, Gale databases, http://gale.cengage.co.uk/product-highlights/history/19th-century-british-library-newspapers.aspx (last accessed 10 January 2012)

Hunnius, T E von, Roberts, C A, Boylston, A, and Saunders, S R, 2006 Histological identification of syphilis in pre-Columbian England, *American J Phys Anthropol* 129, 559–66

Hunter, J, 1861 *Essays and observations on natural history, anatomy, physiology, psychology and geology*, London

Huntsman, R G, Bruin, M, and Holttum, D, 2002 Twixt candle and lamp: the contribution of Elizabeth Fry and the Institution of Nursing Sisters to nursing reform, *Medical Hist* 46, 351–80

Hurren, E T, 2012 *Dying for Victorian medicine: English anatomy and its trade in the dead poor, c 1834–1929*, Basingstoke

Iscan, M Y, Loth, S R, and Wright, R K, 1984 Age estimation from the rib by phase analysis: white males, *J Forensic Sci* 29, 1094–104

Iscan, M Y, Loth, S R, and Wright, R K, 1985 Age estimation from the rib by phase analysis: white females, *J Forensic Sci* 30, 853–63

Iserson, K V, and Moskop, J C, 2007 Triage in medicine: Part I, Concept, history, and types, *Annals Emergency Medicine* 49(3), 275–81

Jackson, W A, 2005 *The Victorian chemist and druggist*, Aylesbury

Jeffries, N, 2011 Medieval and post-medieval pottery (c 1050–1900), in Braybrooke

Jones, H, 1991 Preliminary report of archaeological excavations at New London Bridge House, London Bridge Street, SE1, unpub MOL rep

Jukes, E, 1831 *On indigestion and costiveness … illustrated by coloured engravings*, 2 edn, London

Kalof, L, 2007 *Looking at animals in human history*, London

Kaufman, M H, and Wakelin, S J, 2004 Amputation through the hip joint during the pre-anaesthetic era, *Clinical Anat* 17, 36–44

Kausmally, T, 2010 William Hewson and the Craven Street anatomy school, *American J Phys Anthropol* 141(50), 140

Keynes, G (ed), 1928 *The anatomical exercises of Dr William Harvey. De motu cordis 1628: De circulatione sanguinis 1649: the first English text of 1653 newly edited*, London

Kingsford, C L (ed), 1971 (1908) *A survey of London by John Stow, reprinted from the text of 1603* (2 vols), repr with additions, Oxford

Knüsel, C, 2000 Bone adaptation and its relationship to physical activity in the past, in Cox and Mays, 381–402

Kohn, G C (ed), 2008 (1995) *Encyclopedia of plague and pestilence: from ancient times to the present*, 3 edn, New York

The Lancet The Lancet.com, http://www.thelancet.com/journals/lancet/issue/current?tab=past

Lane, J, 2001 *A social history of medicine: health, healing and disease in England 1750–1950*, London

Langdon-Davies, J, 1952 *Westminster Hospital: two centuries of voluntary service 1719–1948*, London

Lansbury, C, 1985 *The old brown dog: women, workers and vivisection in Edwardian England*, Madison, WI

Lapidus, P W, 1940 'Dorsal bunion': its mechanics and operative correction, *J Bone Joint Surgery (American)* 22, 627–37

Lawrence, S, 1996 *Charitable knowledge: hospital pupils and practitioners in 18th-century London*, New York

Levine, M, 1982 The use of crown height measurements and eruption–wear sequences to age horse teeth, in Wilson et al, 223–50

Lewis, M E, 2004 Endocranial lesions in non-adult skeletons: understanding their aetiology, *Int J Osteoarchaeol* 14, 82–97

Lewis, M E, 2007 *The bioarchaeology of children*, Cambridge

Lovell, N C, 1997 Trauma analysis in palaeopathology, *Yearbook Phys Anthropol* 40, 139–70

Lovejoy, C, Meindl, R, Pryzbeck, T, and Mensforth, R, 1985 Chronological metamorphosis of the auricular surface of the ilium: a new method for the determination of age at death, *American J Phys Anthropol* 68, 47–56

Lucas, G, 2002 Disposability and dispossession in the 20th century, *J Material Culture* 7(1), 5–22

Lysons, D, 1811 (1795) *The environs of London*, 2 edn, extra-illustrated in 10 vols, London

Maat, G J R, and Mastwijk, R W, 2000 Avulsion injuries of vertebral endplates, *Int J Osteoarchaeol* 10, 142–52

Maclise, J, 1846 Remarks on fractures of the thigh-bone and the apparatus used for their treatment, *The Lancet*, 17 January, 47(1168), 67–9

McRae, R, 2003 *Pocketbook of orthopaedics and fractures*, Edinburgh

Maresh, M M, 1970 Measurements from roentgenograms, in *Human growth and development* (ed R W McCammon), 157–200, Springfield, IL

Martinez, A E, Li, S M, Ganz, R, Beck, M, 2006 Os acetabuli in femoro-acetabular impingement: stress fracture or unfused secondary ossification centre of the acetabular rim?, *Hip Int* 16(4), 281–6 (also published online, www.ncbi.nlm.nih.gov/pubmed/19219806, last accessed 10 January 2012)

Matos, V, and Santos, A L, 2006 On the trail of pulmonary tuberculosis based on rib lesions: results from the human identified skeletal collection from the Museu Bocage (Lisbon, Portugal), *American J Phys Anthropol* 130, 190–200

Mayor, S, 2006 One in four autopsy reports in UK is substandard, report finds, *Brit Med J* 333(7573), 824 (published online 19 October 2006, http://www.bmj.com/content/333/7573/824.3, last accessed 20 March 2012 [doi: 10.1136/bmj.333.7573.824-b])

Mays, S A, 2005 Paleopathological study of hallux valgus, *American J Phys Anthropol* 126, 139–49

Mays, S A, Brickley, M, and Ives, R, 2006 Skeletal manifestations of rickets in infants and young children in an historic population from England, *American J Phys Anthropol* 129, 362–74

Medical Times and Gazette Obituaries, 11 April to 26 September 1846, vol 14, 135–6

Miles, A, with Connell, B, 2012 *New Bunhill Fields burial ground, Southwark: excavations at Globe Academy, 2008*, MOLA Archaeol Stud Ser 24, London

Miles, A, and Powers, N, 2006 Bishop Challoner Catholic collegiate school, Lukin Street, London, E1, London borough of Tower Hamlets: a post-excavation assessment and updated project design, unpub MOL rep

Miles, A, Powers, N, and Wroe-Brown, R, with Walker, D, 2008 S*t Marylebone church and burial ground in the 18th to 19th centuries: excavations at St Marylebone school, 1992 and 2004–6*, MoLAS Monogr Ser 46, London

Millard, A, 1825 *An account of the circumstances attending the imprisonment and death of the late William Millard: … with particulars of … abuses, peculations, and misapplications of the funds … and the barter and sale of the patients' dead bodies for the purposes of dissection …*, London

Mitchell, P D, Boston, C, Chamberlain, A, Chaplin, S, Chauhan, V, Evans, J, Fowler, L, Powers, N, Walker, D, Webb, H, and Witkin, A, 2011 The study of anatomy in England from 1700 to the early 20th century, *J Anat* 219(2), 91–9

Molleson, T, and Cox, M, with Waldron, A H, and Whittaker, D K, 1993 *The Spitalfields project: 2, The anthropology: the middling sort*, CBA Res Rep 86, York

Moorrees, C F A, Fanning, E A, and Hunt, E E Jr, 1963a Formation and resorption of three deciduous teeth in children, *American J Phys Anthropol* 21, 205–13

Moorrees, C F A, Fanning, E A, and Hunt, E E Jr, 1963b Age variation of formation stages for ten permanent teeth, *J Dental Res* 42(6), 1490–1502

Morning Chronicle 19th-century British Library newspapers, Gale databases, http://gale.cengage.co.uk/product-highlights/history/19th-century-british-library-newspapers.aspx (last accessed 10 January 2012)

Morning Post 19th-century British Library newspapers, Gale databases, http://gale.cengage.co.uk/product-highlights/history/19th-century-british-library-newspapers.aspx (last accessed 10 January 2012)

Morris, J, 2011 *Investigating animal burials: ritual, mundane and beyond*, BAR Brit Ser 535, Oxford

Morrison, K, 1999 *The workhouse: a study of poor-law buildings in England*, Swindon

Munk's Roll 2 Munk, W, 1861 *Roll of the Royal College of Physicians of London: Vol 2 (1701–1800)*, London

Munk's Roll 3 Munk, W, 1878 *Roll of the Royal College of Physicians of London: Vol 3 (1801–25)*, London

Munk's Roll 4 Brown, G H, 1955 *Lives of the Fellows of the Royal College of Physicians of London: Vol 4 (1826–1925)*, London

Murphy, C, 2011 What can an osteological investigation reveal about medical education in 18th-century Dublin?, *Archaeol Ireland* 25(3), 30–4

Neale, G, 2005 *Miller's encyclopaedia of British transfer-printed pottery patterns 1790–1930*, London

Nightingale, F, 1863 *Notes on hospitals*, 3 edn, London

Nolan, J, 1998 The International Centre for Life, The Newcastle Infirmary at the Forth, Newcastle upon Tyne: Vol 1, The archaeology and history, unpub Northern Counties Archaeological Services rep

Old Bailey Proc Old Bailey proceedings online, www.oldbaileyonline.org, version 6.0 (last accessed 17 April 2011)

O'Regan, H, Turner, A, and Sabin, R, 2006 Medieval big cat remains from the royal menagerie at the Tower of London, *Int J Osteoarchaeol* 16, 385–94

Ortner, D J, 2003 *Identification of pathological conditions in human skeletal remains*, London

Oswald, A, 1975 *Clay pipes for the archaeologist*, BAR Brit Ser 14, Oxford

Pearce, J, Birchenough, A, Bull, R, and Davis, S, in prep Industrial development and suburban growth in London during the 17th and 18th centuries, *London Middlesex Archaeol Soc*

Pemberton, N, and Worboys, M, 2007 *Mad dogs and Englishmen: rabies in Britain, 1830–2000*, Basingstoke

Phillips, W, 1855 *The wild tribes of London*, London

Pipe, A, 1992 A note on exotic animals from medieval and post-medieval London, *Anthropozoologica* 16, 189–91

Pluis, J, 1997 The Dutch tile: designs and names, Leiden

Porter, R, 1997 *The greatest benefit to mankind: a medical history of humanity from antiquity to the present*, London

Power, D, 1895a The medical institutions of London: the rise and fall of the private medical schools in London, *Brit Med J*, 22 June 1895, 1388–91

Power, D, 1895b The medical institutions of London: the rise and fall of the private medical schools in London, *Brit Med J*, 29 June 1895, 1451–53

Powers, N (ed), 2008 *Human osteology method statement*, available online at http://www.museumoflondon.org.uk/NR/rdonlyres/2D513AFA-EB45-43C2-AEAC-30B256245FD6/0/MicrosoftWordOsteologyMethodStatementMarch2008.pdf

Radley, W C, 1835 On the treatment of fractures without the aid of splints, *The Lancet*, 31 October, 25(635), 168–72

Ralston, W, 1879 Notes at a London hospital, *The Graphic*, 27 December 1879, 20 [not paged]

RCS Plarr The Royal College of Surgeons of England, *Plarr's lives of the Fellows online*, http://livesonline.rcseng.ac.uk/home.htm (last accessed 6 January 2012)

Regan, M H, Case, D T, and Brundige, J C, 1999 Articular surface defects in the third metatarsal and third cuneiform: nonosseous tarsal coalition, *American J Phys Anthropol* 109, 53–65

Resnick, D, 2002 *Diagnosis of bone and joint disorders*, Philadelphia, PA

Richardson, R, 2001 (1988) *Death, dissection and the destitute*, 2 edn with new afterword, London

Rielly, K, 2011 The leather-production industry in Bermondsey: the archaeological evidence, in *Leather tanneries: the archaeological evidence* (eds R Thomson and Q Mould), 157–86, Oxford

Rivett, G, 1986 *The development of the London hospital system, 1823–1982*, London

Rixson, D, 2000 *The history of meat trading*, Nottingham

Roberts, C A, 2007 A bioarchaeological study of maxillary sinusitis, *American J Phys Anthropol* 133, 792–807

Roberts, C A, and Buikstra, J E, 2003 *The bioarchaeology of tuberculosis: a global view on a re-emerging disease*, Gainesville, FL

Roberts, C A, and Connell, B, 2004 Guidance on recording palaeopathology, in *Guidelines to the standards for recording human remains* (eds M Brickley and J McKinley), Inst Fld Archaeol Pap 7, 34–9, Southampton and Reading

Roberts, C A, and Cox, M, 2003 *Health and disease in Britain*, Stroud

Roberts, C A, and Manchester, K, 2005 *The archaeology of disease*, 3 edn, New York

Roberts, M J D, 1988 Public and private in early 19th-century London: the Vagrant Act of 1822 and its enforcement, *Social Hist* 13(3), 273–94

Rocque, J, 1746 'A Plan of the Cities of London Westminster and Southwark with contiguous buildings from an actual survey' by John Rocque, reproduced in Margary, H, 1971 *'A Plan of the Cities of London Westminster and Southwark' by John Rocque, 1746*, Margary in assoc Guildhall Library, Kent

Rogers, J, 2000 The palaeopathology of joint disease, in Cox and Mays, 163–82

Rogers, J, and Waldron, T, 1995 *A field guide to joint disease in archaeology*, Chichester

Rousham, E K, and Humphrey, L T, 2002 The dynamics of child survival, in *Human population dynamics: cross-disciplinary perspectives* (eds H Macbeth and P Collinson), Biosocial Society Symposium Series 14, 124–40, Cambridge

Ryan, M (ed), 1832 *The London Medical and Surgical Journal; exhibiting a view of the improvements and discoveries in the various branches of medical science* 2(32), 165–8, London

Santos, A L, and Roberts, C A, 2001 A picture of tuberculosis in young Portuguese people in the early 20th century: a multidisciplinary study of the skeletal and historical evidence, *American J Phys Anthropol* 115, 38–49

Savigny, J H, *c* 1798 *A collection of engravings, representing the most modern and approved instruments used in the practice of surgery, with appropriate explanation*, London

Sawyer, R T, 1981 Why we need to save the medicinal leech, *Oryx* 16, 165–8

Schaap, E, with Chambers, L H, Hendrix, M L, and Pierpoline, J, 1984 *Dutch tiles in the Philadelphia Museum of Art*, Philadelphia, PA

Scheuer, J L, and Black, S, 2000 *Developmental juvenile osteology*, San Diego, CA

Scheuer, J L, Musgrave, J H, and Evans, S P, 1980 The estimation of late foetal and perinatal age from limb-bone length by linear and logarithmic regression, *Annals Hum Biol* 7, 257–65

Schumacher, S A, n d, Stiff big toe joint, www.footdoc.ca/www.FootDoc.ca/Website%20Stiff%20Big%20Toe%20Joint.htm (last accessed 11 January 2012)

Schwarz, L D, 1985 The standard of living in the long run: London, 1700–1860, *Econ Hist Rev* ns 38(1), 24–41

Scripps, W A, 1837 *The literary gazette and journal of the belles lettres, arts, sciences, &c*, London

Serjeantson, D, 1989 Animal remains and the tanning trade, in *Diets and crafts in towns* (eds D Serjeantson and T Waldron), BAR Brit Ser 199, 129–46, Oxford

Shaw, C, 1832 Recollections of service, *Caledonian Mercury*, 10 September 1832, issue 17337

Shaw, J, 1822 *A manual of anatomy containing rules for displaying the structure of the body ... being an outline of the demonstrations delivered ... in the school of Great Windmill Street*, 2 edn, London

Shelley, M, 2004 (1818), *Frankenstein*, London

Smith, J, 1816 *Explanation or key to the various manufactories of Sheffield with engravings of each article*, repr 1975 with new introduction and appendices (ed J S Kebabian), Early American Industries Association, South Burlington, VT

South, J F, 1970 (1884) *Memorials*, repr edn, London

The Standard 19th-century British Library newspapers, Gale databases, http://gale.cengage.co.uk/product-highlights/history/19th-century-british-library-newspapers.aspx (last accessed 10 January 2012)

Stanley, E, 1822 *A manual of practical anatomy, for the use of students engaged in dissections*, London

Stow, J, 1592 *The annales of England, faithfully collected out of the most autenticall authors, records and other monuments of antiquitie, from the first inhabitation until this present yeere 1592*, London

Summers, L, 2003 Yes they did wear them: working-class women and corsetry in the 19th century, *Costume* 36, 65–74

Sykes, N, and Symmons, R, 2007 Sexing cattle horncores: problems and progress, *Int J Osteoarchaeol* 17, 514–23

The Times The Times Digital Archive 1785–2006, Gale databases, http://gale.cengage.co.uk/times.aspx (last accessed 7 January 2012)

Thomas, J L, Blitch, E L, Chaney, D M, Dinucci, K A, Eickmeier, K, Rubin, L G, Stapp, M D, and Vanore, J V, 2009 Diagnosis and treatment of forefoot disorders: Section 2, Central metatarsalgia, *J Foot Ankle Surgery* 48(2), 239–50

Thomas, R, 2010 Translocated Testudinidae: the earliest archaeological evidence for land tortoise in Britain, *Post-*

Medieval Archaeol 44, 165–71

Thompson, A, Grew, F, and Schofield, J, 1984 Excavations at Aldgate 1974, *Post-Medieval Archaeol* 18, 1–148

Thornbury, W, 1878 Coldbath Fields and Spa Fields, in *Old and New London: Vol 2*, 298–306, http://www.britishhistory.ac.uk/report.aspx?compid=45101, last accessed 4 April 2011

Tompsett, D H, 1969 Anatomical injections, *Annals Roy Coll Surgeons Engl* 45, 108–14

Trotter, M, 1970 Estimation of stature from intact long limb bones, in *Personal identification in mass disasters* (ed T Stewart), 71–83, Washington, DC

Tyrrell, A, 2000 Skeletal non-metric traits and the assessment of inter- and intra-population diversity: past problems and future potential, in Cox and Mays, 289–306

Valentin, F, and d'Errico, F, 1995 Skeletal evidence of operations on cadavers from Sens (Yonne, France) at the end of the 15th century, *American J Phys Anthropol* 98(3), 375–90

Vuolteenaho, J, Wood, L, and Powers, N, 2008 Royal London Hospital, Whitechapel Road, London, E1 1BB: a post-excavation assessment and updated project design, unpub MOL rep

Walker, D, 2008 Assessment of human remains recovered from St Bartholomew's Hospital, London EC1, unpub MOL rep, HUM/REP/03/08

Walker, D, and Henderson, M, 2010 Smoking and health in London's East End in the first half of the 19th century, *Post-Medieval Archaeol* 44(1), 209–22

Walker, P L, Bathurst, R R, Richman, R, Gjerdrum, T, and Andrushko, V A, 2009 The causes of porotic hyperostosis and cribra orbitalia: a reappraisal of the iron-deficiency-anemia hypothesis, *American J Phys Anthropol* 139, 109–25

Walters, A N, 1997 Conversation pieces: science and politeness in 18th-century England, *Hist Sci* 35, 121–54

Ward, J, 1993 Origins and development of forensic medicine and forensic science in England 1823–1946, unpub PhD thesis, Open University (British Thesis Service DX175924)

Washburn, S L, 1943 The sequence of epiphyseal union in Old World monkeys, *American J Anat* 72, 339–60

Weiss, J, 1831 *Catalogue of surgical instruments*, London

West, B A, 1980 The sawn human bone, *Barts J* (spring issue), 24–6

Western, A G, 2010 Osteological analysis of human remains from the Worcester Royal Infirmary, Castle Street, Worcester. A report for Worcestershire Historic Environment and Archaeology Service, unpub Ossafreelance rep OA1030

Weston, D A, 2008 Investigating the specificity of periosteal reactions in pathology museum specimens, *American J Phys Anthropol* 137, 48–59

Wheeler, M, 1956 *Still digging: interleaves from an antiquary's notebook*, London

Wheeless, C R, 2011 Accessory navicular, www.wheelessonline.com/ortho/accessory_navicular (last accessed 11 January 2012)

Whitaker, I S, Raob, J, Izadi, D, and Butler, P E, 2004 Historical article: Hirudo medicinalis: ancient origins of, and trends in the use of medicinal leeches throughout history, *Brit J Oral Maxillofacial Surgery* 42, 133–7

Williams, T, and Price, H, 2005 *Uncle Jack: the best-selling true story of John Williams – Jack the Ripper*, London

Wilson, B, Grigson, C, and Payne, S (eds), 1982 Ageing and sexing animal bones from archaeological sites, BAR Brit Ser 109, Oxford

Wise, S, 2004 *The Italian boy: murder and grave-robbery in 1830s London*, London

Witkin, A, 1997 The cutting edge: aspects of amputations in the late 18th and early 19th century, unpub PhD thesis, Univ Sheffield

Witkin, A, 1998 Appendix, in Boulter et al

Wood, J W, Milner, G R, Harpending, H C, and Weiss, K M, 1992 The osteological paradox, problems of inferring prehistoric health from skeletal samples, *Current Anthropol* 33(4), 343–70

Yeomans, L, 2006 A zooarchaeological and historical study of the animal product based industries operating in London during the post-medieval period, unpub PhD thesis, Inst Archaeol, Univ Coll London (British Thesis Service DXN099220)

INDEX

Compiled by Margaret Binns

Page numbers in **bold** indicate illustrations, maps and plans
All street names and locations are in London unless specified otherwise
County names within parentheses refer to historic counties